1150 C

Other Saunders References

Dorland's Illustrated Medical Dictionary

Dorland's Pocket Medical Dictionary

Miller—Keane: Encyclopedia and Dictionary of Medicine and Nursing

Cole: The Doctor's Shorthand

Sloane: The Medical Word Book—A Spelling and Vocabulary Guide
    to Medical Transcription

THE LANGUAGE OF MEDICINE

A worktext explaining medical terms

DAVI–ELLEN CHABNER, B.A., M.A.T.

Adjunct Professor, Montgomery College
Takoma Park, Maryland

W. B. SAUNDERS COMPANY • Philadelphia • London • Toronto

W. B. Saunders Company: West Washington Square
Philadelphia, PA 19105

1 St. Anne's Road
Eastbourne, East Sussex BN21 3UN, England

1 Goldthorne Avenue
Toronto, Ontario M8Z 5T9, Canada

This book is printed on recycled paper.

The Language of Medicine   ISBN 0-7216-2480-4

Last digit is the print number: 9   8   7   6   5

For Bruce, Brandon, and Elizabeth (Noonie)

Three special people who, with love and patience, balance the passion for work in my life.

PREFACE

This worktext of medical terminology is an outgrowth of my experiences in teaching semester courses in the medical language to those preparing for and serving in the allied health professions in the Washington, D.C., area. My students desperately needed a workbook — a text which would present the material in a simple and logical fashion and also a book in which they could practice word analysis by filling in answers and working through exercises. The worktext before you is the product of constant revision and change dictated by the needs and critical evaluations of my students over the past four years. Their comments, questions, and suggestions are continually reflected in these pages.

This book is designed both for classroom use and for independent study by allied health personnel and premedical students. My students have included medical assistants and medical secretaries, nurses, laboratory technologists, radiologic technologists, dental assistants and hygienists, hospital personnel, medical-technical writers, computer analysts, and high school and college students embarking on medical careers.

There are two basic assumptions underlying the design of the worktext. One is that medical terminology can be taught as a *language*, emphasizing logical and rational understanding of word parts rather than rote memorization of terms. Another assumption is that the learning of the medical language must be organized according to body systems and should include an elementary but fundamental understanding of the anatomy, physiology, and disease processes of each body system. Several important learning aids are included in this worktext, such as simple anatomical diagrams and concise explanations of the physiological or pathological implications of most medical terms.

The general plan of the book is as follows: The first five chapters constitute the foundation of the book, and introduce the overall approach to understanding the medical language. These chapters cover basic suffixes, prefixes, and combining forms, as well as terms involving the human body as a whole. Each of the next thirteen chapters (6 through 18) explores a body system and the medical terms which describe the anatomy, physiology, and disease processes of that system. Chapters 19 through 24 deal with specialized areas of medicine — cancer medicine, radiology and nuclear medicine, and pharmacology.

In my personal experience teaching medical terminology, I have found it difficult to cover all the systems included in this worktext in a one-semester course. Hence, in such a course it may be advisable to emphasize certain chapters and omit others, depending on the particular interests and needs of the students; for example, the radiologic technologist will spend more time on the chapters related to her or his field, perhaps at the expense of the skin and the endocrine system. Nonetheless, this text covers all the major areas of medical terminology and provides a resource for the student's further independent study should the need arise.

The review sheets after each chapter have proved invaluable for preparing the student for frequent and necessary quizzes and for emphasizing the most important terms in each worksheet. Frequent oral drills using these review sheets are recommended. I have also found that use and familiarity with a medical dictionary is crucial in the study of this new language; thus, I urge purchase of a pocket-size edition for all my students.

Above all, I hope each student using this book comes away with the feeling that learning and understanding the medical language may be hard work but is truly rewarding and fun. I hope that this worktext stirs interest in continuing a self-education in the medical language by giving the student the essential language tools to travel onward. The allied health professional need not be merely a word technician but rather may understand the proper use and meaning of medical terms.

DAVI-ELLEN CHABNER

ACKNOWLEDGMENTS

In many ways, this book has been a collaborative effort. Kathleen Moore, a friend and former medical terminology student, has helped in almost all aspects of the book. She tirelessly and meticulously typed and retyped the manuscript in all its various phases. Her fine attention to detail and sense of design are evident in the many charts and flow diagrams throughout the text, while her penchant for thoroughness and accuracy is reflected in the completeness of the book's glossary and index. I owe her much thanks.

Throughout the time that I was writing this book, I continued to teach medical terminology classes at Montgomery College and the National Institutes of Health. I want to express gratitude to Catherine F. Scott, Chairperson, Secretarial Studies Department, Montgomery College, Takoma Park, Maryland, for her personal friendship and staunch enthusiasm for the methods and materials that I was developing while teaching during the past four years. I am also indebted to Jenean McKay, Employee Development Specialist, and Dr. Margaret Dunn, Educational Services Officer, at NIH, for organizing my first terminology classes and providing assistance and encouragement all along the way.

My husband, Dr. Bruce A. Chabner, an oncologist and cancer researcher, patiently read the text, chapter by chapter, and I am grateful for his helpful criticisms and comments which were both scientific and stylistic in content.

I wish to express particular appreciation to Elizabeth J. Taylor, Associate Medical Editor, W. B. Saunders Company, for her careful editing and guiding hand in coordinating all aspects of the publication.

Finally, I must acknowledge the invaluable contributions of my students, past and present. Their comments, criticisms, questions, and supportive statements have become an integral part of the composition of this book. I offer this worktext with the hope that it may help, inspire, and fire the imaginations of countless future students of the medical language.

D-E.C.

CONTENTS

CHAPTER 1

BASIC WORD STRUCTURE

In this chapter you will:

Become familiar with basic objectives to keep in mind as you study the medical language;

Learn to divide medical words into their component parts;

Learn basic combining forms, prefixes, and suffixes of the medical language; and

Use these combining forms, prefixes, and suffixes to build medical words.

This chapter is divided into the following sections:

I. Objectives in Studying the Medical Language

II. Basic Word Structure

III. Combining Forms, Suffixes, and Prefixes

IV. Exercises

I. OBJECTIVES IN STUDYING THE MEDICAL LANGUAGE

There are three major objectives to keep in mind as you study medical terminology.

1. To Analyze Words Structurally

Your goal is to learn the **tools** of word analysis which will make the understanding of complex terminology easier. For example, we will learn to divide words into basic elements such as **roots, suffixes, prefixes, combining vowels,** and **combining forms.** With this knowledge of word construction and the meanings of the specific word elements, even the longest and most complicated terms can be handled and understood.

You may or may not already know the meanings of the following terms, but this is how we will learn to analyze them structurally:

GASTROENTEROLOGY

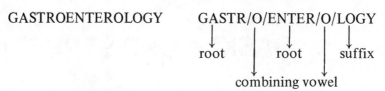

The root **gastr** means **stomach**
The root **enter** means **intestines**
The suffix **-logy** means **process of study**
The combining vowel o links root to root and root to suffix

The entire word (always reading the meaning of terms starting from the suffix **back** to the first part of the word) means then: **the process of study of the stomach and intestines**.

ELECTROCARDIOGRAM

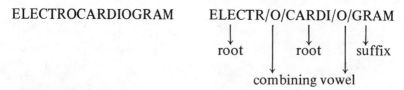

The root **electr** means **electricity**
The root **cardi** means **heart**
The suffix **-gram** means **record**

The entire word means: **the record of the electricity of the heart**.
Try another:

ONCOGENIC

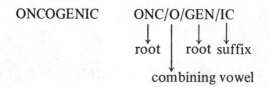

The root **onc** means **tumor**
The root **gen** means **producing**
The suffix **-ic** means **pertaining to**

The entire word means: **pertaining to tumor producing**.
Note that the combining vowel (o), usually placed between the root and suffix, is dropped in this word because the suffix (ic) begins with a vowel. However, combining vowels are usually **retained** between two roots in a word even if the second root begins with a vowel. For example:

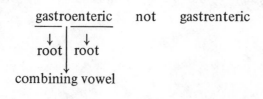

To summarize: Three important rules to remember as you study the medical language are:

(a) Read the meaning of medical terms from the suffix back to the first part of the word.

(b) Drop the combining vowel (usually o) before a suffix beginning with a vowel: gastric **not** gastroic.

(c) Retain the combining vowel between two roots in a word.

2. To Correlate an Understanding of Word Elements with the Basic Anatomy, Physiology, and Disease Processes of the Human Body

This text will continually emphasize not only the division of terms into structural elements but also the relationship of the medical words to the functioning of the body, in both health and disease.

For example, the term **hemat/o/logy** means the study of the blood. This term, however, will mean more to you as you learn the many different components of blood, how they function in the body, and the various disease conditions associated with blood. This text is structured so that the terms presented have relevance to the anatomy, physiology, and disease processes of the body. Memorization of terms, while essential to retention of the language, should not become the primary objective of your study.

3. To Be Continually Aware of Spelling and Pronunciation Problems

Spelling is especially critical in the medical language because many words are pronounced alike but spelled differently and have entirely different meanings. For example:

ileum is a part of the small intestine

and

ilium is a part of the pelvic, or hip, bone

It should be obvious as well that a misspelled word may give the wrong meaning to a diagnosis. For example:

hepat/oma: tumor of the liver

hemat/oma: blood tumor

Words spelled correctly but incorrectly **pronounced** may be easily misunderstood. For example:

urethra (u-rē′thrah)   is the urinary tract tube leading from the urinary bladder to the external surface

ureter (u-re′ter)   is one of two tubes leading from the kidney to the urinary bladder

Figure 1–1 illustrates the difference between the urethra and ureters.

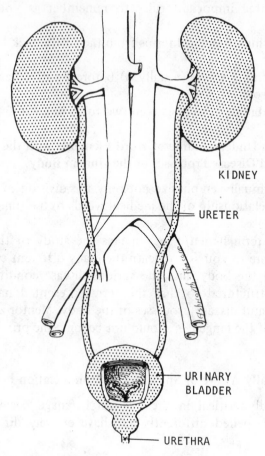

KIDNEY

URETER

URINARY
BLADDER

URETHRA

Figure 1–1 Urinary system.

II. BASIC WORD STRUCTURE

Studying medical words is very similar to learning a new language. The words at first sound strange and complicated although they may stand for commonly known English terms. The words **gastralgia**, meaning "stomach ache," and **ophthalmologist**, meaning "eye doctor," are examples.

The medical language is fascinatingly logical in that each term, complex or simple, can be broken down into its basic component parts and then understood.

These basic component parts of medical words are:

1. **Word root:** foundation of the word

gastr/ic
↓
root
(stomach)

2. **Suffix**: word ending

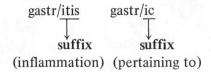

gastr/itis   gastr/ic

suffix   suffix
(inflammation) (pertaining to)

3. **Prefix**: word beginning

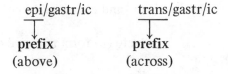

epi/gastr/ic   trans/gastr/ic

prefix   prefix
(above)   (across)

4. **Combining vowel**: a vowel (usually o) linking the root to the suffix or to another root

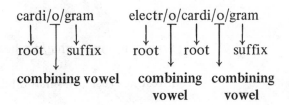

cardi/o/gram   electr/o/cardi/o/gram

root │ suffix   root │ root │ suffix

combining vowel   combining combining
                      vowel   vowel

5. **Combining form**: the combination of a word root with the combining vowel

cardi/o/gram

combining form

III. COMBINING FORMS, SUFFIXES, AND PREFIXES

In previous examples you have been introduced to the combining forms gastr/o (stomach) and cardi/o (heart). In the following lists, there are new combining forms, suffixes, and prefixes. Read them, say them aloud, and then proceed with the exercises which test your understanding.

If you wish to check your pronunciation of these word parts, consult the glossary at the end of the book.

Combining Forms

aden/o	gland
arthr/o	joint
bi/o	life

carcin/o	cancerous
cardi/o	heart
cephal/o	head
cerebr/o	brain, or cerebrum (the largest part of the brain)
cis/o	to cut (used primarily in words like incision—to cut into—and excision—to cut out, remove)
crin/o	secrete (to form and give off)
cyt/o	cell
derm/o, dermat/o	skin
electr/o	electricity
encephal/o	brain (en = in, cephal/o = head)
enter/o	intestines (usually small intestines)
erythr/o	red
gastr/o	stomach
gen/o	producing, beginning
gnos/o	knowledge
gynec/o	woman, female
hem/o, hemat/o	blood
leuk/o	white
nephr/o	kidney
neur/o	nerve
onc/o	mass, tumor
ophthalm/o	eye
oste/o	bone
path/o	disease

physi/o	nature
psych/o	mind
radi/o	rays (usually x-rays)
rhin/o	nose
scop/o	examination (usually visual)
secti/o	to cut (used primarily in words like section—cutting into—and resection—cut back, or out)
thromb/o	clot
tom/o	to cut
ur/o	urine or urinary tract

Suffixes

Suffixes may be short and simple (ic, al, gram) or long and complex, being composed of a root and a final suffix. For example:

-algia (alg = pain, ia = condition)

-logy (log = study, y = process)

-tomy (tom = cut, y = process)

-ac	pertaining to
-al	pertaining to
-algia	pain
-cyte	cell
-ectomy	to cut out, excision, resection, surgical removal
-emia	blood condition
-gram	record
-ia	condition, process

-ic	pertaining to
-ist	one who specializes in
-itis	inflammation
-logy	process of study
-oma	tumor
-opsy	to view
-osis	condition, usually abnormal (when used with blood cell terms, it means an increase in cell numbers)
-scope	instrument to visually examine
-tome	instrument to cut
-tomy	process of cutting, to section, make an incision
-y	process, condition

Prefixes

a, an	no, not, without
auto	self
ana	up
dia	complete, through
endo	within
epi	above
ex	out
exo	outside, outer
hyper	above, excessive
hypo	deficient, below, under
re	back

retro	behind
peri	surrounding
pro	before
trans	across

IV. EXERCISES

After you have completed the exercises below, a good way to review the terms in this chapter is to cover the terms on one side of the page and write their meanings, and then repeat the process, covering the other side of the page.

A. Complete the following:

1. Word beginnings are called ___prefix___.

2. Word endings are called ___suffix___.

3. The foundation of a word is called the ___root___.

4. A letter linking a suffix and a root or two roots in a word is called the ___combining vowel___.

5. The combination of a root and a combining vowel is known as the ___combining form___.

B. Using slashes (/), divide the following terms into component parts; write the word root; and give the meaning of the entire medical term:

	Root	Meaning
1. adenoma	_____	_____
2. cerebral	_____	_____
3. pathogenic	_____	_____
4. hypogastric	_____	_____
5. leukocytic	_____	_____
6. rhinitis	_____	_____
7. arthrotomy	_____	_____

C. *Using slashes, divide the following terms into component parts; identify the combining forms; and give the meaning of the entire term:*

	Combining Form	Meaning
1. carcinogenic	_____	_____
2. electroencephalogram	_____	_____
3. osteotome	_____	_____
4. erythrocytosis	_____	_____
5. nephrologist	_____	_____
6. encephalopathy	_____	_____

D. *Find the suffixes in the following words and give the meaning of the entire term:*

	Suffix	Meaning
1. leukemia	_____	_____
2. gastrectomy	_____	_____
3. hematoma	_____	_____
4. nephritis	_____	_____
5. gastroscope	_____	_____
6. dermatosis	_____	_____

E. *Identify the prefixes in the following terms and give the meaning of the entire term:*

	Prefix	Meaning
1. anatomy	_____	_____
2. pericarditis	_____	_____
3. retrogastric	_____	_____
4. hypodermic	_____	_____

	Prefix	*Meaning*
5. hyperemia	_____	_____
6. endocrine	_____	_____
7. diagnosis	_____	_____
8. prognosis	_____	_____

F. *The following are some of the fields of medicine with which you should be familiar. First use vertical slashes to divide up the words into root, combining vowel, and suffix; and then give the meaning of the term:*

1. Urology _____

2. Gynecology _____

3. Hematology _____

4. Oncology _____

5. Nephrology _____

6. Cardiology _____

7. Neurology _____

8. Dermatology _____

9. Radiology _____

10. Ophthalmology _____

11. Gastroenterology _____

12. Endocrinology _____

G. *Give the meaning of the following combining forms:*

1. aden/o _____   4. arthr/o _____

2. leuk/o _____   5. cerebr/o _____

3. cephal/o _____   6. cyt/o _____

7. oste/o _____   14. rhin/o _____

8. dermat/o _____   15. nephr/o _____

9. erythr/o _____   16. carcin/o _____

10. encephal/o _____   17. gnos/o _____

11. bi/o _____   18. onc/o _____

12. physi/o _____   19. tom/o _____

13. path/o _____   20. gynec/o _____

H. *Fill in the suffixes for the following English terms:*

1. Inflammation _____

2. Resection, or surgical removal _____

3. Section _____

4. Condition (usually abnormal) _____

5. Process of study _____

6. Instrument to examine visually _____

7. Instrument to cut _____

8. Pertaining to producing _____

9. Pertaining to _____ _____ _____

10. Blood condition _____

11. Tumor _____

12. Pain _____

13. Record _____

14. Cell _____

15. To view _____

I. *Give the prefixes for the following English terms:*

1. Surrounding _____   8. Deficient _____

2. Across _____   9. Self _____

3. Complete, through _____   10. Up _____

4. Above _____   11. Behind _____

5. Before _____   12. Outside, outer _____

6. Within _____   13. Back _____

7. Excessive _____   14. Out _____

15. No, not, without _____

J. *Build medical terms:* (These may seem hard, but don't give up!)

1. Blood tumor _____

2. Inflammation of a gland _____

3. Record of the electricity of the heart _____

4. Abnormal condition of clotting cells (increase in numbers) _____

_____

5. Pertaining to across the stomach _____

6. Process of study of the skin _____

7. Pain in the head _____

8. White blood (abnormally high white blood count) _____

9. Instrument to cut bone _____

10. Removal of the stomach _____

11. Instrument to visually examine the eye _____

12. Cancerous tumor _____

13. To view life _____

14. Inflammation of bones and joints _____

15. One who specializes in the study of tumors _____

16. Pertaining to producing disease _____

17. Incision of the stomach _____

ANSWERS

A. 1. Prefixes
   2. Suffixes
   3. Word root
   4. Combining vowel
   5. Combining form

B. 1. aden/oma – tumor of a **gland.**
   2. cerebr/al – pertaining to the **brain,** or **cerebrum.**
   3. path/o/gen/ic – pertaining to **disease producing.**
   4. hypo/gastr/ic – pertaining to under the **stomach.**
   5. leuk/o/cyt/ic – pertaining to **white** (blood) **cells.**
   6. rhin/itis – inflammation of the **nose.**
   7. arthr/o/tomy – incision of a **joint.**

C. 1. carcin/o/gen/ic – pertaining to producing **cancer.**
   2. electr/o/encephal/o/gram – record of the **electricity** in the **brain.**
   3. oste/o/tome – instrument to cut **bone.**
   4. erythr/o/cyt/osis – abnormal condition (elevation in number) of **red** (blood) **cells.**
   5. nephr/o/logist – one who specializes in the study of the **kidney.**
   6. encephal/o/pathy – disease condition of the **brain.**

D. 1. leuk/emia – **blood condition** of excessive numbers of white blood cells.

      There will be instances of terms which defy simple definitions by structural analysis. In those cases, as with the term "leukemia," you will have to understand not only how the word is constructed but also a more complete meaning of the term. Your dictionary should help with those terms.

   2. gastr/ectomy – **removal** of the stomach.
   3. hemat/oma – **tumor** of blood; collection or swelling of blood.
   4. nephr/itis – **inflammation** of the kidney.
   5. gastr/o/scope – **instrument to examine** the stomach.
   6. dermat/osis – **abnormal condition** of the skin.

E. 1. ana/tomy – process of cutting **up.**
   2. peri/cardi/tis – inflammation **surrounding** the heart.

      Note that one i is dropped when -itis is preceded by a root ending in a vowel.

   3. retro/gastr/ic – pertaining to **behind** the stomach.

4. hypo/derm/ic – pertaining to **under** the skin.
5. hyper/emia – blood condition – **increased** flow to a region.
6. endo/crine – secretion **within**.

> *Glands are classified as to their method of secretion. Some glands are endocrine, meaning they produce hormones which enter the bloodstream directly and thus influence organs and other glands all over the body; examples are the pituitary, adrenal, and thyroid glands. Other glands are exocrine, meaning they produce chemicals which leave the gland via ducts and travel to cavities which lead to the outside of the body; examples of exocrine glands are tear, digestive, and sweat glands.*

7. dia/gnosis – **complete** knowledge.

> *A diagnosis is made on the basis of extensive knowledge about the patient – family history, laboratory tests, x-rays, urinalysis, physical examination.*

8. pro/gnosis – **before** knowledge.

> *A prognosis is made by a doctor after a diagnosis about the nature of the patient's illness. It is a prediction (knowledge before) about the outlook of the disease.*

F.
1. Study of urinary system.
2. Study of the female.
3. Study of blood.
4. Study of tumors.
5. Study of the kidney.
6. Study of the heart.
7. Study of nerves.
8. Study of the skin.
9. Study of x-rays.
10. Study of the eye.
11. Study of stomach and intestines.
12. Study of the glands of internal secretion.

G.
1. gland
2. white
3. head
4. joint
5. brain
6. cell
7. bone
8. skin
9. red
10. brain
11. life
12. nature
13. disease
14. nose
15. kidney
16. cancer
17. knowledge
18. tumor
19. to cut
20. female

H.
1. -itis
2. -ectomy
3. -tomy
4. -osis
5. -logy
6. -scope
7. -tome
8. -genic
9. -al, -ac, -ic
10. -emia
11. -oma
12. -algia
13. -gram
14. -cyte
15. -opsy (an autopsy is a viewing of a dead body and its organs with one's own eyes)

I.
1. peri
2. trans
3. dia
4. epi
5. pro
6. endo
7. hyper
8. hypo
9. auto
10. ana
11. retro
12. exo
13. re
14. ex
15. a, an

J.
1. Hematoma.

> *A hematoma is not a tumor in the usual sense. It is a collection of blood outside a blood vessel but confined within a space or cavity; "black and blue" marks are hematomas.*

2. Adenitis.

3. Electrocardiogram.
4. Thrombocytosis.
5. Transgastric.
6. Dermatology.
7. Cephalalgia (may be shortened to cephalgia).
8. Leukemia.
9. Osteotome.
10. Gastrectomy.
11. Ophthalmoscope.
12. Carcinoma.
13. Biopsy (excision of living tissue for microscopic examination).
14. Osteoarthritis.

> There is no overall rule designating which root goes first in a term that has two roots. Sometimes it is what sounds best; sometimes, as in the digestive system terminology, the roots are placed according to anatomic position in the system. For example, the stomach (gastr/o) always precedes the intestines (enter/o); therefore, **gastroenterology**, not enterogastrology.

15. Oncologist.
16. Pathogenic.
17. Gastrotomy.

> When building medical terms, use the combining form **tom/o**. Don't forget, however, that a **gastrotomy** is the same as a **gastric section** or **incision**; similarly, a **gastrectomy** is the same as a **gastric resection** or **excision**.

REVIEW SHEET 1

This review sheet and the others following each chapter are complete lists of the word elements and important terms contained in that chapter. The review sheets are designed to pull together the terminology and to reinforce your learning by giving you the opportunity to write out the words and test yourself. Check the answers you are unsure of with the information in the chapter or with the glossary at the end of the book.

Combining Forms

aden/o	_____	encephal/o	_____
arthr/o	_____	enter/o	_____
bi/o	_____	erythr/o	_____
carcin/o	_____	gastr/o	_____
cardi/o	_____	gen/o	_____
cephal/o	_____	gnos/o	_____
cerebr/o	_____	gynec/o	_____
cis/o	_____	hem/o	_____
crin/o	_____	hemat/o	_____
cyt/o	_____	hepat/o	_____
derm/o	_____	leuk/o	_____
dermat/o	_____	psych/o	_____
nephr/o	_____	radi/o	_____
neur/o	_____	rhin/o	_____
onc/o	_____	scop/o	_____
ophthalm/o	_____	secti/o	_____
electr/o	_____	oste/o	_____

path/o _____   thromb/o _____

physi/o _____   tom/o _____

ur/o _____

Suffixes

-ac _____   -ist _____

-al _____   -itis _____

-algia _____   -logy _____

-cyte _____   -oma _____

-ectomy _____   -opsy _____

-emia _____   -osis _____

-gram _____   -scope _____

-ia _____   -tome _____

-ic _____   -tomy _____

-y _____

Prefixes

a, an _____   hyper _____

ana _____   hypo _____

dia _____   peri _____

endo _____   pro _____

epi _____   re _____

ex _____   retro _____

exo _____   trans _____

CHAPTER 2

ANALYSIS OF A MEDICAL PAPER

In this chapter you will:

Gain practice in reading and understanding the medical language in context;

Acquire knowledge of the anatomy and physiology of the lymphatic system in the body; and

Learn new combining forms, prefixes, and suffixes, and use them in building and giving the meaning of medical terms.

This chapter is divided into the following sections:

I. INTRODUCTION: BACKGROUND INFORMATION

The clinical medical paper included in this chapter describes the course of an illness called **lymphosarcoma**. The term lymph/o/sarc/oma is analyzed in the following manner:

-oma = **tumor**. A tumor is a new growth, or **neoplasm**. (**Neo** is a prefix meaning new, and **-plasm** is a suffix meaning formation or growth.)

lymph/o = **lymph**. Lymph is a clear fluid which is formed in all body tissues. Lymph flows from tissue spaces into small channels called lymph vessels which then lead through filters called lymph nodes (glands) and into special veins in the neck and chest where the lymph enters the bloodstream (Figure 2–1). Major sites of lymph node concentration are the axillary (armpit), cervical (neck), and inguinal (groin) regions of the body.

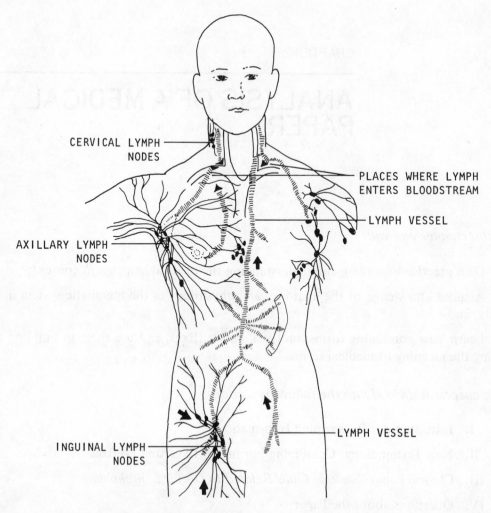

CERVICAL LYMPH NODES

PLACES WHERE LYMPH ENTERS BLOODSTREAM

LYMPH VESSEL

AXILLARY LYMPH NODES

INGUINAL LYMPH NODES

LYMPH VESSEL

Figure 2-1 Lymph seeps out of tiny blood vessels, bathes the tissue spaces, and enters tiny branches of lymph vessels. It then flows through the lymph nodes into the bloodstream. Most of the lymph enters the bloodstream through veins in the left and right upper chest regions of the body.

sarc/o   = **flesh**. The root **sarc** indicates that this is a special type of tumor, a "flesh tumor." This means that the tumor, or new growth, was derived or originated from connective tissue, such as lymph, fat, muscle, and blood.

A lymphosarcoma, then, is a flesh tumor of the lymph nodes. Most sarcomas, as well as carcinomas, are **malignant** tumors. Malignant (mal = bad) means that the tumor grows rapidly and may eventually display **metastasis** (meta = change, beyond; stasis = stopping, control). Metastasis means that the tumor spreads from its primary location to secondary sites around the body. Hence, the tumor is literally "beyond control." A **benign** (bene = good) tumor is slow growing and does not metastasize. Benign tumors are limited in extent and often are surrounded by a capsule. An example of a benign tumor is a thyroid adenoma.

II. NEW TERMINOLOGY

Some of the terms are familiar; others are totally new. Read them over and refer back to them as you explore the medical paper which follows.

Combining Forms

abdomin/o	abdomen
aden/o	gland
angi/o	vessel
axill/o	armpit
cervic/o	neck
cutane/o	skin
	Used to describe the organ; derm/o and dermat/o are used to build words about skin conditions.
hepat/o	liver
inguin/o	groin
lapar/o	abdominal wall, abdomen
later/o	side
lymph/o	lymph (clear fluid which bathes tissue spaces)
peritone/o	peritoneum (membrane surrounding the organs in the abdominal cavity)
phag/o	eat, swallow
pyel/o	renal pelvis (central section of the kidney where urine is collected)
ren/o	kidney
	Used in words describing the organ; nephr/o is used to build most words about kidney conditions.
sarc/o	flesh
thromb/o	clot
tom/o	to cut

ureter/o	ureters (tubes carrying urine from kidneys to bladder)
ven/o	vein

Suffixes

-crit	to separate
-gram	record
-lysis	to break down, destroy, separate out
-megaly	enlargement
-osis	abnormal condition (in blood cells, an increase in number)
-ous	pertaining to
-pathy	disease process
-plasia	condition expressing growth, formation
-plasm	growth, formation
-penia	decreased number (of blood cells)
-stasis	control, stop
-tomy	incision, to cut into

Prefixes

bi	two
endo	within
eso	inward
inter	between
intra	within
meta	beyond, near, change
neo	new
pan	all

per   through

post   after

re   back

retro   behind

Additional Terms

bilirubin
SGOT $\Big\}$ indicators of liver function.
alkaline phosphatase

chlorambucil $\Big\}$ drugs used to treat malignant tumors.
prednisone

diaphoresis   sweating.

fulminant   severe and sudden with great rapidity.

IVP   intravenous pyelogram, a record of the renal pelvis made by taking x-ray pictures of the kidney (renal pelvis) after dye is injected into a vein.

lysed   broke.

malaise   vague feeling of bodily discomfort.

neutrophils
eosinophils $\Big\}$ types of white blood cells (leukocytes).
monocytes
bands

occult   hidden; hard to find.

rigors   chills.

tomogram   a method of taking x-ray pictures so that "cuts" or "slices" of regions of the body are obtained by special processing of the x-ray machine.

III. CLINICAL PAPER: *SHAKING CHILLS RELATED TO OCCULT LYMPHOMA*

Use the list of terms given above and your medical dictionary as you read this medical paper (Figure 2–2). Then answer the questions which follow.

Reprinted from MEDICAL ANNALS OF THE DISTRICT OF COLUMBIA
Vol. 38, No. 1, January, 1969
Printed in U.S.A.

Shaking Chills Related to Occult Lymphoma

Report of a Case

BRUCE A. CHABNER, M.D.,* JOHN EASTON, M.D.,† AND VINCENT T. DeVITA, M.D.‡

SHAKING CHILLS have long been considered one of the most reliable signs of infection and can be a helpful clue in evaluating unexplained fever. In the case to be discussed the patient's course and autopsy findings indicate that lymphosarcoma may also be the cause of extreme rigors in association with spiking fevers, thus mimicking the clinical picture of occult infection.

Report of Case

A 63-year-old retired Negro engineer entered the Clinical Center on July 7, 1967 because of chills and fever (NIH No. 07-11-16). In 1963 a prostatic mass was resected and found to be a poorly differentiated lymphosarcoma. The patient was well thereafter until December 1966, when he was found to have massive retroperitoneal adenopathy, scalp nodules, and partial bilateral ureteral obstruction. Intravenous Cytoxan® led to apparent complete remission except for persistence of several small scalp nodules. Maintenance therapy consisting of prednisone and chlorambucil was continued for 6 months.

In late June of 1967 the patient began to have marked fatigue and malaise followed several days later by daily episodes of intense rigors, spiking fevers, and profuse diaphoresis. On admission his temperature was 40°C. Positive physical findings included only several 2 cm. scalp nodules which were unchanged since previous evaluations.

The hematocrit was 36.5 per cent, and the white blood cell count was 4,200 per cu. mm. with 63 per cent neutrophils, 14 per cent bands, 2 per cent lymphocytes, 1 per cent eosinophil, and 19 per cent monocytes. Urinalysis revealed 11 to 20 red blood cells and white blood cells per high-power field. All blood chemistries were normal, including liver and renal function tests and uric acid.

Twelve blood cultures, plus urine, sputum, and spinal-fluid cultures and smears were negative. A toxoplasma hemagglutination titer was negative, as were fungal and PPD skin tests. A chest X-ray film and IVP tomograms were normal. Abdominal and pelvic lymph nodes, as demonstrated by residual lymphangiogram dye, were of normal size.

During the first 4 weeks of hospitalization the patient experienced daily shaking chills, usually at 11:00 a.m., lasting 15 to 30 minutes, succeeded by a spiking fever to 39–40°C and several hours later profuse diaphoresis as the fever lysed. In the absence of demonstrable tumor and because of the presence of severe chills, occult infection was suspected, but routine diagnostic measures, including bone-marrow and percutaneous liver biopsies, yielded negative results. Two weeks of cephalothin (Keflin®) and kanamycin (Kantrex®) failed to affect the patient's course. Laparotomy for diagnostic purposes was strongly considered but was ultimately rejected when pancytopenia (white blood cells 1,500 per cu. mm., hemoglobin 8 Gm. per 100 c.c., platelet count 19,000 per cu. mm.) developed in the third hospital week. Bone-marrow biopsy showed hypoplasia of all cellular elements, and chlorambucil was discontinued. The fever and chills continued unabated.

During the fifth hospital week hepatomegaly and rapidly progressive hepatic failure became evident. SGOT rose to 310 units, alkaline phosphatase to 29 King-Armstrong units, and bilirubin to 23.1 mg. per 100 c.c. direct and 31.2 mg. per 100 c.c. total. A second liver scan now showed generally diminished uptake with several large filling defects. Hepatorenal failure supervened, and the patient expired on the forty-second hospital day.

Postmortem examination (A67-208) revealed massive lymphosarcomatous infiltration of the liver (figure 1), which weighed 1,760 Gm. A moderate degree of infiltration of the spleen (weight 350 Gm.) and bone marrow was present. Lymph nodes, though normal in size, also demonstrated a moderate degree of tumor invasion. Focal infiltrates were found in the skin, kidneys, lungs, esophagus, endocardium, and pericardium.

Other findings included a chronic penetrating ulcer in the first portion of the duodenum, cholemic nephrosis, and 4 gallstones, 1 mm. in size. There was no evidence of an acute or chronic septic process which might explain the patient's clinical symptoms. Cultures of the heart's blood taken several hours after death yielded 3 organisms (group D streptococcus, diphtheroids, and *Corynebacterium acnes*), all thought to represent contaminants or terminal sepsis.

*Clinical Associate, Laboratory of Chemical Pharmacology, National Cancer Institute, National Institutes of Health.

†Pathologist, Pathologic Anatomy, Clinical Center, National Institutes of Health.

‡Senior Investigator, Medicine Branch, National Cancer Institute, National Institutes of Health, Bethesda, Md. 20014. (Reprint requests to Dr. DeVita.)

Figure 2–2

SHAKING CHILLS RELATED TO OCCULT LYMPHOMA—CHABNER ET AL   *January, 1969*

Discussion

Several previous studies[1,2] have dealt with the difficult problem of differentiating between infection and tumor as the cause of fever in patients with cancer. Few observations, aside from positive bacteriologic evidence and a response to antibiotics, can identify the source of fever. However, according to Fenster and Klatskin,[3] shaking chills may be a "noteworthy" sign pointing toward infection. In reviewing the case histories of 81 pa-

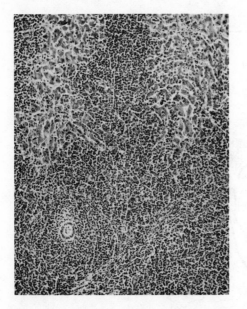

FIG. 1. Section of liver showing massive lymphosarcoma infiltrates in the portal-tract tissues and hepatic lobules. The hepatic cells adjacent to the tumor are degenerated and necrotic, and in other sections of the liver there were even larger areas of hepatocellular necrosis.

tients with hepatic metastases due to a variety of tumors these authors found 19 cases in which fever appeared to be secondary to malignancy. In none of these cases were chills present.

In the case under discussion the uncommon association of shaking chills with malignancy is documented. Frank chills have been observed in at least 1 previous case of rapidly growing lymphoma. The patients described by Aledort et al[4] developed sudden renal failure along with spiking fever and chills, and at autopsy massive renal invasion by lymphosarcoma without evidence of infection was found. Rare and less well documented reports of the occurrence of chills in association with renal,[5] stomach,[6] and bowel[6] carcinomas are also to be found in the older literature.

We conclude that, although uncommon, malignant lymphoma and probably other forms of cancer should be considered in the differential diagnosis of a patient having rigors and fever. Aggressive diagnostic measures, including early laparotomy, should be undertaken in the hope that a treatable infection or tumor will be found.

The mechanism by which the tumor led to chills in this patient is obscure. Although extensive hepatocellular necrosis was found at autopsy, tissue necrosis does not appear to have been a factor, since severe rigors were present at a time when liver chemistries, biopsy, and scan were all normal. The extreme rapidity of tumor growth is indicated by the progression to hepatic failure 3 weeks after these negative liver studies.

Death due to massive hepatic invasion and parenchymal necrosis as in this patient has been reported in 1 previous case of malignant lymphoma. In 1934 the Viennese physician, Carl Sternberg,[7] described a 32-year-old man who died of hepatic failure after a fulminant 7-week illness.

Summary

A case has been presented of a 63-year-old man in apparent remission from lymphosarcoma who had shaking chills and fever and who died of fulminant hepatic failure. At autopsy massive hepatic invasion by lymphosarcoma was found; no source of infection was uncovered that might explain the patient's presenting complaints. It is concluded that shaking chills may occur secondary to lymphoma and that an infectious etiology cannot be assumed in evaluating a patient with these complaints.

References

1. BOGGS, D. R., AND FREI, E., III: Clinical studies of fever and infection in cancer. Cancer, 1960, 13, 1240.
2. BROWDER, A. A., HUFF, J. W., AND PETERSDORF, R. G.: Significance of fever in neoplastic disease. Ann. Intern. Med., 1961, 55, 932.
3. FENSTER, L. F., AND KLATSKIN, G.: Manifestations of metastatic tumors of the liver: a study of 81 patients subjected to needle biopsy. Amer. J. Med., 1961, 31, 238.
4. ALEDORT, L. M., HODGES, M., AND BROWN, J. A.: Irreversible renal failure due to malignant lymphoma. Ann. Intern. Med., 1966, 65, 117.
5. ISRAEL, J.: Ueber Fieber bei malignen Nieren-und Nebennierengeschwülsten. Deutsche med. Wchnschr., Leipz. u. Berl., 1911, 37, 57.
6. FINLAYSON, J.: On the occurrence of pyrexia, shiverings, and pyaemia in cases of malignant disease. Lancet, 1888, 2, 710.
7. STERNBERG, C.: Über Lymphosarkomatose der Leber. Wien. med. Wchnschr., 1934, 84, 417.

Figure 2–2 *(Continued)*

IV. QUESTIONS ABOUT THE PAPER

1. (a) On admission the patient had "retroperitoneal adenopathy." The peritoneum is a membrane which surrounds the organs in the abdominal cavity (Figure 2–3). What are some of the organs in the abdominal

cavity? _____

_____

(b) What is the location of a retroperitoneal organ? _____

_____

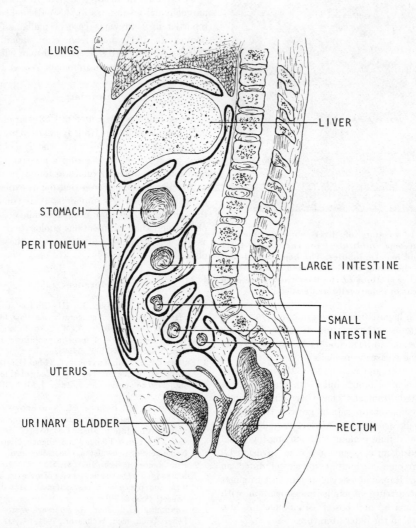

Figure 2–3 Peritoneum. This thin, moist membrane surrounds the walls and internal organs (liver, intestines, stomach) of the abdominal cavity.

    (c) What does adenopathy mean? _____

_____

2. What does "bilateral ureteral obstruction" mean? _____

_____

3. By what route was Cytoxan given? _____

4. What is the hematocrit? _____

_____

_____

5. What is a lymphocyte? _____

6. Where were 11 to 20 erythrocytes found? (See paragraph 3 under Report of

Case.) _____

7. What is an IVP tomogram? _____

_____

_____

8. What recording (x-ray) showed the condition of the patient's abdominal and

pelvic lymph nodes? _____

9. Why was a laparotomy not performed in the third hospital week?

_____

10. Platelet counts tell the number of thrombocytes. What are thrombocytes?

_____

11. (a) How was hypoplasia of all cellular elements detected? _____

_____

    (b) What is hypoplasia? _____

12. In the fifth hospital week, what happened to the patient's liver?

_____

13. What was the cause of the patient's death? _____

_____

14. On autopsy, tumor was found in various organs. Where is the:

(a) esophagus _____

(b) endocardium _____

(c) pericardium _____

15. In the summary of the case, the authors mention "fulminant hepatic failure."

What does that mean? _____

_____

16. What is the authors' conclusion about the case? _____

_____

_____

V. EXERCISES

A. *Build medical words:*

1. Blood vessel tumor _____

2. Inflammation of the liver _____

3. Incision of abdominal wall _____

4. Lack of red blood cells _____

5. Process of visually examining the peritoneum _____

6. Inflammation of the renal pelvis _____

7. Abnormal conditions of white cells (too many) _____

8. Platelet _____

9. Heart enlargement _____

10. Excessive formation _____

B. *Give the meaning of the following medical terms:*

1. percutaneous _____

2. esophagotomy _____

3. phagocyte _____

4. lymphosarcoma _____

5. resection _____

6. ureterectomy _____

7. hematocrit _____

8. osteolysis _____

9. intravenous _____

10. bilateral _____

C. *Give the answers called for:*

1. What are the medical terms for three regions of the body where there are large collections of lymph nodes?

   _____

   _____

   _____

2. What are **metastases**? _____

   _____

   _____

3. What is the difference between a **benign** and a **malignant** tumor?

   _____

   _____

   _____

4. What is a **neoplasm**? _____

5. What is an **IVP tomogram**? _____

_____

_____

_____

ANSWERS

Answers to medical paper

1. (a) Stomach, intestines, liver, gallbladder, pancreas, spleen.
   (b) Behind the peritoneum. The kidneys are organs which are retroperitoneal.
   (c) Disease of glands. The glands which are diseased are the lymph glands.
2. Both ureters were obstructed by the tumor (bilateral means two sides).
3. Cytoxan was given intravenously (within a vein).
4. Hematocrit means blood separation. The hematocrit is the percentage of red blood cells within the total blood volume. The hematocrit is obtained by spinning blood very quickly in a machine (centrifuge) so that the red cells become separated from the rest of the blood.
5. A lymph cell (type of white blood cell).
6. In urinalysis (separating out urine to investigate its contents).
7. Intravenous pyelogram. A tomogram is a "slice" view of the organ taken by focusing the x-ray camera at the organ at different levels. Dye is first injected into veins and pictures are taken of the renal pelvis.
8. Lymphangiogram (x-rays of lymph vessels after dye is injected into lymphatic system).
9. Pancytopenia developed (decrease in number of all blood cells).
10. Clotting cells (a platelet is a thrombocyte).
11. (a) Bone marrow biopsy (microscopic examination of bone interior where blood cells are formed).
    (b) Decrease in formation, growth (hypo = deficient, -plasia = formation).
12. It became enlarged (hepatomegaly) and began to fail to function (hepatic failure).
13. Hepatorenal failure (lack of functioning of the **liver** and **kidneys**).
14. (a) Tube leading from the throat to the stomach (eso = inward, phag/o = swallowing).
    (b) Inner membrane within the heart.
    (c) Outer membrane surrounding the heart.
15. Sharp, rapid, sudden lack of functioning of the liver.
16. Shaking chills may not always be associated with infection but may be secondary to (occur with) a lymphosarcoma.

Answers to exercises

A.
1. hemangioma
2. hepatitis
3. laparotomy (abdominal section)
4. erythrocytopenia
5. peritoneoscopy
6. pyelitis
7. leukocytosis
8. thrombocyte (clotting cell)
9. cardiomegaly
10. hyperplasia

B.
1. Through the skin.
2. Incision into the esophagus.
3. Cell that eats other cells.
4. Tumor (flesh) of lymph (a malignant tumor).
5. To cut out, remove.
6. Excision of a ureter.
7. Separation of blood (percentage of red blood cells).
8. Destruction of bone.
9. Pertaining to within a vein.
10. Pertaining to two (both) sides.

C. 1. Axillary (armpit); cervical (neck); inguinal (groin).
  2. Metastases (singular: metastasis) means the spreading of malignant tumors away from their primary (first) location to distant (secondary) sites all over the body.
  3. Benign tumors are limited in growth, are encapsulated, and do not metastasize.
     Malignant tumors are rapid and unlimited in their growth, are not encapsulated, and they metastasize.
  4. New growth; tumor.
  5. IVP means intravenous pyelogram. This is an x-ray record (-gram) of the renal pelvis (pyel/o). It is taken by first injecting contrast dye into a vein (intravenous) and then taking x-ray pictures of the kidney region. Tomograms are a series of special x-ray pictures showing different depths or levels of a structure by blurring detail in the images of structures not in the specific plane to be viewed.

REVIEW SHEET 2

Combining Forms

abdomin/o	_____	lymph/o	_____
aden/o	_____	peritone/o	_____
angi/o	_____	phag/o	_____
axill/o	_____	pyel/o	_____
cervic/o	_____	ren/o	_____
cutane/o	_____	sarc/o	_____
hemat/o	_____	thromb/o	_____
hepat/o	_____	tom/o	_____
inguin/o	_____	ureter/o	_____
lapar/o	_____	ven/o	_____
later/o	_____		

Suffixes

-crit	_____	-megaly	_____
-gram	_____	-osis	_____
-lysis	_____	-ous	_____
-pathy	_____	-penia	_____
-plasia	_____	-stasis	_____
-plasm	_____	-tomy	_____

Prefixes

bi	_____	pan	_____
endo	_____	per	_____
eso	_____	peri	_____
inter	_____	post	_____
intra	_____	re	_____
meta	_____	retro	_____
neo	_____		

CHAPTER 3

TERMS PERTAINING TO THE BODY AS A WHOLE

In this chapter you will:

Learn terms which apply to the structural organization of the body;

Identify the body cavities and recognize the organs contained within those cavities;

Locate and identify the anatomical and clinical divisions of the abdomen;

Locate and learn the names of the anatomical divisions of the back;

Become acquainted with terms which describe positions, directions, and planes of the body; and

Learn new word elements and use them to build and understand the meaning of medical terms.

This chapter is divided into the following sections:

I. Structural Organization of the Body

II. Body Cavities

III. Anatomical Divisions of the Abdomen

IV. Clinical Divisions of the Abdomen

V. Anatomical Divisions of the Back (Spinal Column)

VI. Positional and Directional Terms

VII. Planes of the Body

VIII. Combining Forms and Prefixes

IX. Exercises

I. STRUCTURAL ORGANIZATION OF THE BODY

The Cell

The cell is the fundamental unit of every living thing (animal or plant). Cells are everywhere in the human body — every tissue, every organ, is made up of these individual units.

Similarity in Cells. All cells are similar in that they contain a gelatinous substance composed of water, protein, sugar, acids, fats, and various minerals. This substance is called **protoplasm**. All parts of a cell are described below and pictured schematically in Figure 3–1 as they might look when photographed with an electron microscope. Label the structures on Figure 3–1 as you learn how they function as part of the activity in the cell:

(1) *Cell membrane.* This structure surrounds and protects the internal environment of the cell, determining what passes in and out of the cell.

(2) *Nucleus.* The nucleus is the controlling structure of the cell. It controls the way a cell reproduces, and contains genetic material which determines the functioning and structure of the cell. All the material within the nucleus is called **nucleoplasm** or **karyoplasm** (kary/o = nucleus).

(3) *Chromosomes.* These are 23 pairs of thin strands of genetic material (DNA) located within the nucleus of a cell. These 23 pairs of chromosomes contain regions

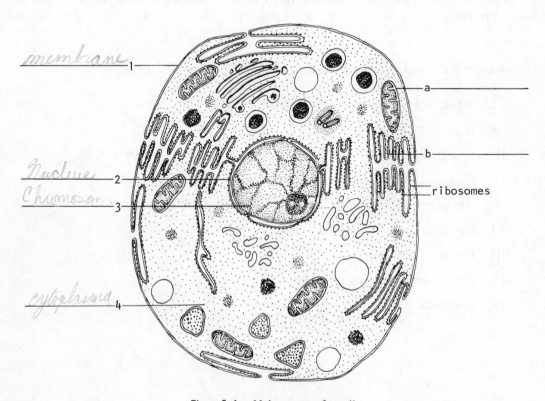

membrane 1

Nucleus 2

Chromosom 3

cytoplasm 4

a

b

ribosomes

Figure 3–1   Major parts of a cell.

known as **genes** which determine our hereditary makeup. The DNA within chromosomes regulates the activities of each cell by guiding the formation of another substance, called RNA, which can leave the cell nucleus, enter the cytoplasm, and direct the activities of the cell.

Chromosomes can be studied and classified as to size, arrangement, and number. This classification is called a **karyotype**. Karyotyping of chromosomes is useful in determining whether chromosomes are normal in number and structure.

(4) *Cytoplasm.* Cytoplasm is the protoplasmic material outside the nucleus. It carries on the work of the cell (in a muscle cell, it does the contracting; in a nerve cell, it transmits impulses). The cytoplasm contains:

(a) *Mitochondria*—small bodies which carry on the production of energy in the cell by burning food in the presence of oxygen. This process is called **catabolism** (cata = down; bol = to cast or throw). During catabolism complex structures are broken down into simpler substances and energy is released.

(b) *Endoplasmic reticulum*—a series of canals within the cell. Some canals contain small bodies called **ribosomes** which help make substances (proteins) for the cell. This synthesizing (building-up) process is called **anabolism** (ana = up; bol = to cast). Together the processes of catabolism and anabolism constitute the total **metabolism** of the cell.

Difference in Cells. Cells are different, or specialized, throughout the body to carry out their individual functions. For instance, a muscle cell is long and slender and contains fibers which aid it in contracting and relaxing; an epithelial, or skin, cell may be square and flat to provide protection; a nerve cell may be quite long and have various fibrous extensions which aid it in its job of carrying impulses; a fat cell contains large, empty spaces for fat storage. These are only a few of the many types of cells in the body. Study the different types of cells pictured in Figure 3–2 and label the **nerve** cell, **epithelial** cell, **fat** cell, and **muscle** cell.

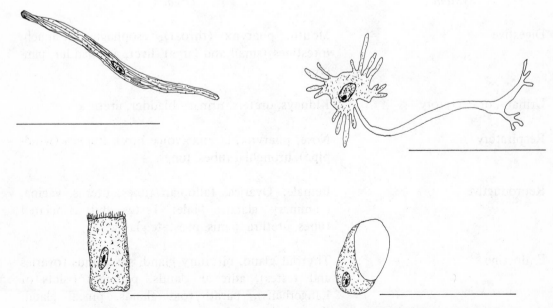

Figure 3-2   Types of cells. Label muscle cell, nerve cell, epithelial cell, and fat cell.

Tissues

A tissue is a group of similar cells working together to do a specific job. A histologist is one who specializes in the study of tissues. Some types of tissues are:

Epithelial Tissue. Epithelial tissue is located in glands, skin, the digestive tract, and the urinary tract. It is necessary for protection, lining tubes, and secretion.

Muscle Tissue. Voluntary muscle is found in arms and legs and parts of the body where movement is voluntary, while involuntary muscle is found in the heart and digestive system, as well as other places where movement is not under conscious control.

Connective Tissue. This can be fat (also called adipose tissue), cartilage (elastic, fibrous tissues attached to bones), bone, or blood.

Nerve Tissue. Nerve tissue conducts impulses all over the body.

Organs

These are structures composed of several kinds of tissue. For example, an organ like the stomach is composed of muscle tissue, nerve tissue, and glandular epithelial tissue. The medical term for internal organs is **viscera** (singular: **viscus**).

Systems

These are groups of organs working together to perform complex functions. For example, the mouth, esophagus, stomach, and small and large intestines are organs which compose the digestive system.

Examine the list of the nine body systems below and become familiar with some of the organs within each system:

System	*Organs*
Digestive	Mouth, pharynx (throat), esophagus, stomach, intestines (small and large), liver, gallbladder, pancreas.
Urinary, or excretory	Kidneys, ureters, urinary bladder, urethra.
Respiratory	Nose, pharynx, larynx (voice box), trachea (windpipe), bronchial tubes, lungs.
Reproductive	Female: Ovaries, fallopian tubes, uterus, vagina, mammary glands. Male: Testes and associated tubes, urethra, penis, prostate gland.
Endocrine	Thyroid gland, pituitary gland, sex glands (ovaries and testes), adrenal glands, pancreas (islets of Langerhans), parathyroid glands, pineal gland, thymus gland.

Nervous	Brain, spinal cord, nerves, and collections of nerves.
Cardiovascular	Heart, blood vessels (arteries, veins, and capillaries), lymphatic vessels and nodes, spleen, thymus gland.
Muscular	Muscles.
Skeletal	Bones and joints.

II. BODY CAVITIES

A body cavity is a space within the body which contains internal organs (viscera). Label Figure 3–3 as you learn the names of the body cavities. Some of the important viscera contained within those cavities are listed as well.

Cavity	*Organs*
(1) Cranial	Brain

(2) Thoracic   Lungs, heart, esophagus, trachea, thymus gland, aorta (large artery).

The thoracic cavity can be divided into two smaller cavities:
(a) The **pleural cavities**—the areas surrounding the lungs. Each pleural cavity is lined with a double-folded membrane called **pleura**; visceral pleura is closest to the lungs, and parietal pleura is closest to the outer wall of the cavity.
(b) The **mediastinum** — the area between the lungs. It contains the heart, aorta, trachea, esophagus, and thymus gland.
(Study Figure 3–4, which reviews the divisions of the thoracic cavity.)

(3) Abdominal   Stomach, large and small intestines, spleen, liver, gallbladder, pancreas.

The peritoneum is the double-folded membrane surrounding the abdominal cavity. The layer of peritoneum closest to the outer wall of the cavity is the parietal peritoneum; the layer closest to the internal organs is the visceral peritoneum.

(4) Pelvic   Urinary bladder, urethra, ureters; uterus and vagina in the female.

(5) Spinal   Nerves of the spinal cord.

The cranial and spinal cavities are considered **dorsal** body cavities because of their location on the back portion of the body. The thoracic, abdominal, and pelvic cavities are considered **ventral** body cavities because they are on the front, or belly side, of the body.

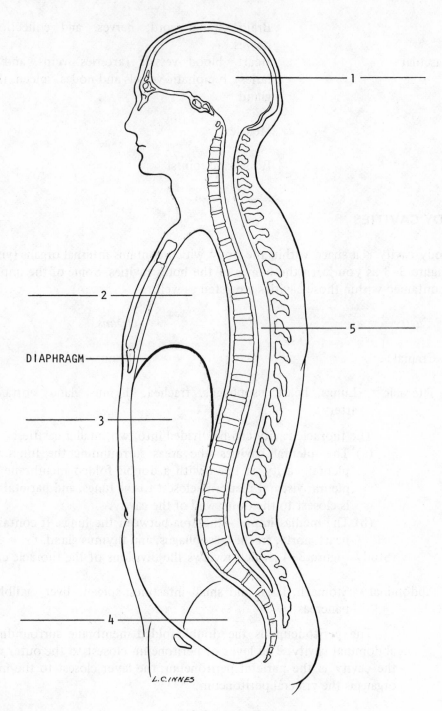

DIAPHRAGM

L.C.INNES

Figure 3–3   Body cavities.

The thoracic and abdominal cavities are separated by a muscular partition called the **diaphragm**. The abdominal and pelvic cavities are not separated by a partition and together they are frequently called the abdominopelvic cavity.

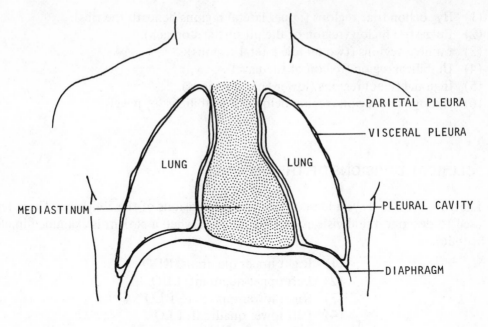

Figure 3–4   Divisions of the thoracic cavity.

III. ANATOMICAL DIVISIONS OF THE ABDOMEN

Label Figure 3–5 as you learn the anatomical divisions of the abdomen. These divisions are used in anatomy texts to describe the regions in which organs and structures are found.

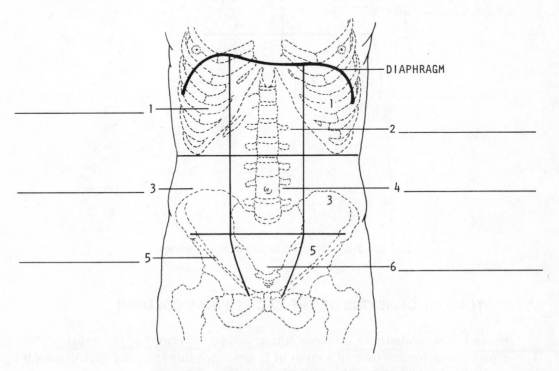

Figure 3–5   Anatomical divisions of the abdomen.

(1) Hypochondriac regions (upper lateral regions beneath the ribs).
(2) Epigastric region (region of the pit of the stomach).
(3) Lumbar regions (two middle lateral regions).
(4) Umbilical region (region of the navel).
(5) Inguinal (iliac) regions (lower lateral regions).
(6) Hypogastric region (region below the umbilicus, or navel).

IV. CLINICAL DIVISIONS OF THE ABDOMEN

Label Figure 3–6 as you identify the clinical divisions of the abdomen. These terms are used to describe the divisions of the abdomen when a patient is examined in clinic (at bedside).

(1) Right upper quadrant, RUQ
(2) Left upper quadrant, LUQ
(3) Right lower quadrant, RLQ
(4) Left lower quadrant, LLQ

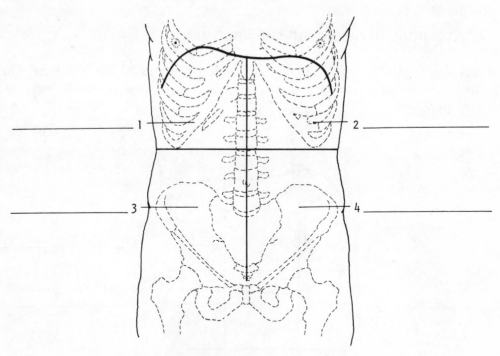

Figure 3–6 Clinical divisions of the abdomen.

V. ANATOMICAL DIVISIONS OF THE BACK (SPINAL COLUMN)

The back is separated into divisions corresponding to regions of the spinal column. The spinal column is composed of a series of bones extending from the neck downward to the tailbone. Each bone is called a **vertebra** (plural: vertebrae).

Label the divisions of the back on Figure 3–7 as you study the following:

Division of the Back	Abbreviation	Location
(1) Cervical	C	first 7 vertebrae.
(2) Thoracic	T or D (D = dorsal)	8th to 19th vertebrae.
(3) Lumbar	L	20th to 24th vertebrae.
(4) Sacral	S	25th–29th bones, which are fused to form the sacral bone, or sacrum.
(5) Coccyx		tailbone.

An important distinction should be made between the spinal column (the vertebrae) and the spinal cord (nerves running through the column). The former is bone, or osseous tissue, while the latter is composed of nerve tissue.

The spaces between the vertebrae (intervertebral spaces) are identified according to the two vertebrae between which they lie; e.g., L5-S1 lies between the 5th lumbar and the 1st sacral vertebrae.

VI. POSITIONAL AND DIRECTIONAL TERMS

Afferent	conducting **toward** a structure. Example: Veins are called afferent vessels since they take blood toward the heart.
Efferent	conducting **away from** a structure. Example: Arteries are efferent blood vessels since they take blood away from the heart.
Anterior (ventral)	**in front** of the body. Example: The abdomen is located anterior to the spinal cord. Ventral and anterior mean the same position in the human.
Posterior (dorsal)	**back** of the body. Example: The posterior lobes of the brain are in the back of the head and are called the occipital lobes. Dorsal means the same position as posterior.
Central	pertaining to the **center**. Example: The heart is located in the central portion of the thoracic cavity; it lies between the lungs in the mediastinum.

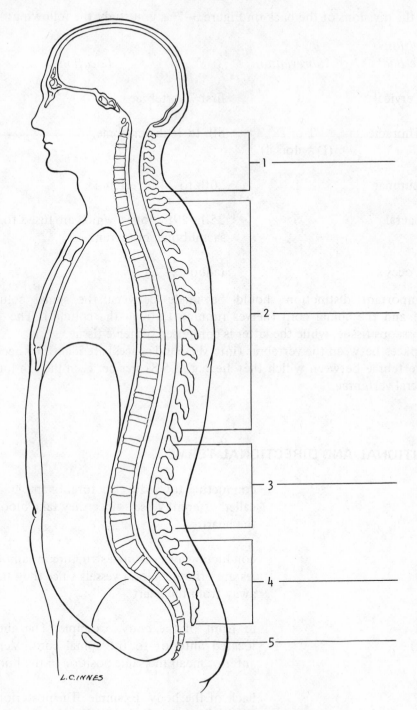

Figure 3–7   Anatomical divisions of the back (spinal column).

| Deep | away from the surface. Example: The lesion penetrated deep into the abdomen, away from the surface of the body. |
| Superficial | near the surface. Example: The wound was a superficial one, just penetrating the skin. |

| Distal | away from the beginning of a structure; away from the center. Example: At its distal end, the thigh bone (femur) joins with the knee cap (patella). |

Proximal — pertaining to the beginning of a structure. Example: The proximal end of the femur joins with the pelvic (hip) bone.

Inferior (caudal) — away from the head; situated below another structure. Example: The feet are the caudal parts of the human body.

Superior (cephalic) — pertaining to the head; situated above another structure. Example: In a cephalic presentation of the fetus, the head comes through the birth canal first.

Lateral — pertaining to the side. Example: The little toes are lateral to the big toes.

Medial — pertaining to the middle. Example: In the anatomical position, the fifth finger lies medial to the other fingers.

VII. PLANES OF THE BODY

A plane is an imaginary flat surface. Label Figure 3–8 as you study the terms for the planes of the body:

(1) Frontal (coronal) — vertical plane which divides the body or structure into anterior and posterior portions.

○ longitudinal

(2) Sagittal — lengthwise vertical plane which divides the body or structure into right and left portions. The midsagittal plane divides the body into right and left halves.

(3) Transverse — plane running across the body parallel to the ground (horizontal). It divides the body or structure into upper and lower portions.

VIII. COMBINING FORMS AND PREFIXES

| abdomin/o | abdomen | abdominal | _____ |
| adip/o | fat | adipose | _____ |

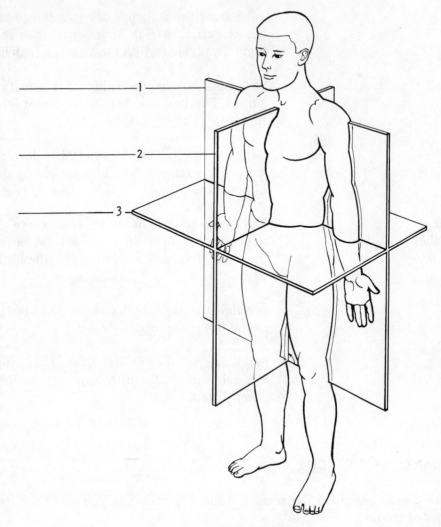

Figure 3–8   Planes of the body.

anter/o	front	anterior _____
bol/o	cast, throw	catabolism _____
caud/o	tail, lower part of the body	caudal _____
cervic/o	neck	cervical _____
chondr/o	cartilage *(type of connective tissue)*	chondroma _____
chrom/o	color	chromosomes _____

coccyg/o	coccyx (tailbone)	coccygeal _____
crani/o	skull	craniotomy _____
dist/o	far	distal _____
dors/o	back portion of the body	dorsal _____
hist/o	tissue	histology _____
ili/o	ilium *(part of the pelvic bone)*	iliac _____
inguin/o	groin	inguinal _____
kary/o	nucleus	karyoplasm _____
later/o	side	lateral _____
lumb/o	lower back	lumbosacral _____
medi/o	middle	medial _____
my/o	muscle	myoma _____
pelv/o pelv/i	hip, pelvic cavity	pelvic _____
poster/o	back	posterior _____
prot/o	first	protoplasm _____
proxim/o	near	proximal _____
sacr/o	sacrum *(lower portion of the backbone)*	sacral _____
spin/o	spine	spinal _____
spondyl/o	vertebrae *(series of bones which surround the spinal cord)*	spondylitis _____ *Use spondyl/o when building medical words about condition or diseases of the vertebrae.*
thel/o	nipple	epithelium _____

thorac/o	chest	thoracic _____
ventr/o	belly side of the body	ventral _____
vertebr/o	vertebrae, backbones	vertebral _____
viscer/o	internal organs	visceral _____
ana	up	anabolism _____
cata	down	catabolism _____
epi	above	epigastric _____
inter	between	intervertebral _____
meta	change, beyond	metabolism _____

IX. EXERCISES

A. Build medical words:

1. Process of study of tissues _____

2. Pertaining to the skull _____

3. Incision into the chest _____

4. Pertaining to the lower back _____

5. Pertaining to under the stomach _____

6. Pertaining to the neck _____

7. Pertaining to below the cartilage _____

8. Abnormal condition of vertebrae _____

9. Pertaining to internal organs _____

10. Pertaining to the side _____

11. Pertaining to the middle _____

12. Process of food breakdown to produce energy ("casting down")

_____

13. Tumor of muscle _____

14. Inflammation of skin _____

B. *Give the answers called for:*

1. Where is the mediastinum? _____

_____

What organs are contained within the mediastinum? _____

_____

2. What does sacroiliac mean? _____

_____

3. Where are the inguinal regions of the abdomen? _____

_____

4. Give the meanings of: cephal/o _____

encephal/o _____

crani/o _____

cerebr/o _____

cervic/o _____

5. What is adipose tissue? _____

6. What is epithelial tissue? _____

_____

7. What is the endoplasmic reticulum? _____

_____

8. Describe the location and function of chromosomes. _____

_____

_____

C. Give the **opposites** of the following terms:

1. deep _____   4. ventral _____

2. afferent _____   5. posterior _____

3. proximal _____   6. caudal _____

D. Identify the following planes:

1. Which plane divides the body into anterior and posterior portions?

_____

2. Which plane divides the body into upper and lower portions?

_____

3. Which plane divides the body into left and right halves?

_____

E. Fill in the blanks:

1. The bones of the spinal column are called _____

2. One of these bones is called a _____

3. The combining forms for this structure are _____

_____

4. What does L5-S1 mean? _____

_____

ANSWERS

A. 1. histology
2. cranial
3. thoracotomy
4. lumbar
5. subgastric, hypogastric
6. cervical
7. hypochondriac

8. spondylosis
9. visceral
10. lateral
11. medial
12. catabolism
13. myoma
14. dermatitis

B. 1. Between the pleural cavities within the thoracic cavity.
The heart, esophagus, trachea, thymus gland, and aorta are some of the organs within the mediastinum.
2. Pertaining to the sacrum (lower back region) and ilium (part of the pelvic bone).
3. Lower lateral regions, near the ilium of the pelvic bone.
4. cephal/o = head   cerebr/o = brain
encephal/o = brain   cervic/o = neck
crani/o = skull
5. Fat tissue; a kind of connective tissue.
6. Literally means "upon a nipple" – refers to all the outer skin tissue of the body and the inner linings of membranous tubes within the body.
7. Structures in the cytoplasm of the cell which build up proteins; they carry on anabolism.
8. Chromosomes are located in the nucleus of a cell. They contain DNA (deoxyribonucleic acid) which is the hereditary material of the cell.

C. 1. superficial
2. efferent
3. distal

4. dorsal
5. anterior
6. cephalic

D. 1. frontal
2. transverse
3. midsagittal

E. 1. Vertebrae.
2. Vertebra.
3. Spondyl/o or vertebr/o.
4. Refers to the region between the 5th lumbar vertebra and the 1st sacral vertebra.

REVIEW SHEET 3

Combining Forms

Give the meaning: *Give the combining form:*

abdomin/o _____   _____ groin

adip/o _____   _____ nucleus

anter/o _____   _____ side

bol/o _____   _____ lower back

caud/o _____   _____ muscle

cervic/o _____   _____ hip bone

coccyg/o _____   _____ first

crani/o _____   _____ sacrum

dist/o _____   _____ flesh

dors/o _____   _____ vertebra (2)

hist/o _____   _____ chest

ili/o _____   _____ internal organs

ventr/o _____

Suffixes

-tomy _____   -logy _____

-ectomy _____   -oma _____

-osis _____   -itis _____

Prefixes

ana _____   hypo _____

cata _____   meta _____

inter _____   epi _____

Name the anatomical divisions of the abdomen:

Lower lateral regions _____

Upper lateral regions _____

Upper middle region (pit of the stomach) _____

Navel region _____

Middle lateral regions _____

Region below the navel or umbilicus _____

Name the anatomical divisions of the spinal (vertebral) column:

Neck region _____   Region of the sacrum _____

Chest region _____   Tailbone region _____

Lower back region _____

Name the planes of the body:

Vertical plane which divides the body into anterior and posterior portions

_____

Horizontal plane dividing the body into upper and lower portions

_____

Vertical plane dividing the body into right and left portions

_____

Name the positional and directional terms:

Pertaining to the head (above another structure) _____

Away from the beginning of a structure _____

Conducting toward _____

Conducting away from _____

In front of the body _____

Away from the head (below another structure) _____

Pertaining to the beginning of a structure _____

Away from the surface _____

Back of the body _____

Pertaining to the side _____

Near the surface _____

Pertaining to the center _____

Pertaining to the middle or midline _____

From the following list of terms, pick the one which fits the definition best:

ribosomes	pleural cavity	anabolism
mediastinum	endoplasmic reticulum	metabolism
mitochondria	chromosomes	
diaphragm	catabolism	

_____ Structures in the cytoplasm of the cell which produce energy by chemically burning food in the presence of oxygen.

_____ Contains the hereditary material (DNA) of the cell.

_____ Building-up, or synthesizing, process in the cell.

_____ Contains the heart and other structures between the lungs in the thoracic cavity.

_____ Breaking-down, or destruction, process in the cell.

_____ Structures in cytoplasm of cell which are the site of protein synthesis.

_____ Surrounds the lungs in the thoracic cavity.

_____ Network of canals in cell.

_____ Total of building-up and breaking-down processes in cell.

_____ Muscular wall dividing the abdominal and thoracic cavities.

CHAPTER 4

SUFFIXES

In this chapter you will:

Learn new suffixes and review those presented in previous chapters;

Gain practice in word analysis by using these suffixes with combining forms to build and understand terms; and

Learn the names and functions of the different types of blood cells in the body.

The chapter is divided into the following sections:

I.   Introduction

II.   Combining Forms

III.   Suffixes and Terminology

IV.   Appendices

V.   Exercises

I. INTRODUCTION

This chapter has three purposes. The first is to teach many of the most common suffixes in the medical language. As you work through the entire book, the suffixes mastered in this chapter will appear often. An additional group of basic suffixes is presented in Chapter 7.

The second purpose is to teach new combining forms and use them to make words with suffixes. Your analysis of the terminology in Section III of this chapter will increase your medical language vocabulary.

The third purpose is to expand your understanding of terminology beyond basic word analysis. The appendices in Section IV give explanations of many terms listed. In particular, emphasis is placed on learning the names and functions of different types of blood cells. These terms are basic to the vocabulary of a person working in the paramedical field.

II. COMBINING FORMS

Read this list and underline those combining forms which are unfamiliar.

abdomin/o	— abdomen
acr/o	— extremities, top, extreme point
acu/o	— sharp
arteri/o	— artery
arthr/o	— joint
bi/o	— life
carcin/o	— cancer
cephal/o	— head
chir/o	— hand
chondr/o	— cartilage
chron/o	— time
col/o	— colon, large intestine
dactyl/o	— fingers or toes
encephal/o	— brain
eosin/o	— rosy, dawn-colored
gon/o	— seed
granul/o	— granules
hepat/o	— liver
hydr/o	— water
isch/o	— to hold back
lapar/o	— abdomen, abdominal wall
laryng/o	— larynx (voice box)

lith/o	— stone, calculus
maxill/o	— upper jaw
morph/o	— shape, form
muc/o	— mucus
myel/o	— bone marrow, spinal cord
	(context of usage indicates which meaning is intended)
necr/o	— death (of cells or whole body)
ophthalm/o	— eye
oste/o	— bone
ot/o	— ear
peritone/o	— peritoneum
phag/o	— to eat, swallow
phil/o	— like, love, attraction to
phob/o	— fear
plas/o	— development, formation
pneum/o	— lungs
radi/o	— rays
rect/o	— rectum
staphyl/o	— clusters, grapes
strept/o	— twisted chains
thorac/o	— chest
thromb/o	— clot
tonsill/o	— tonsils
trache/o	— trachea (windpipe)
ven/o	— vein

III. SUFFIXES AND TERMINOLOGY

Noun Suffixes. The following is a list of the most common noun suffixes. A medical term is given to illustrate the use of the suffix. The basic rule for building a medical word is that the combining vowel, such as **o**, is used to connect the root to the suffix, with the exception that the combining vowel is **not** used before suffixes which begin with a vowel. For example: gastr/itis, **not** gastr/o/itis

Suffix	Meaning	Terminology	Meaning
-algia	pain	arthralgia _____	
		otalgia _____	
		neuralgia _____	
-cele	hernia[1]	rectocele _____	
-centesis	surgical puncture to remove a fluid	thoracocentesis _____ (thoracentesis)	
		abdominocentesis _____	
-coccus (plural: -cocci[3])	berry-shaped	streptococcus[2] _____	
		staphylococcus[2] _____	
-cyte	cell	erythrocyte[4] _____	
		leukocyte _____	
		thrombocyte _____	
-ectomy	removal, excision	laryngectomy[5] _____	
-emia	blood condition	anemia[6] _____	
		ischemia[7] _____	
-genesis	condition of producing, forming	carcinogenesis _____	
		oncogenesis _____	

---

[1] See Appendix A
[2] See Appendix B
[3] See Appendix C
[4] See Appendix D
[5] See Appendix E
[6] See Appendix F
[7] See Appendix G

-gram	record	electroencephalogram _____
-graph	instrument for recording	electroencephalograph _____
-graphy	process of recording	electroencephalography _____
-itis	inflammation	nephritis _____
-lysis	breakdown, destruction	hemolysis _____
-malacia	softening	osteomalacia _____
		chondromalacia _____
-megaly	enlargement	acromegaly[8] _____
-odynia	pain	gastrodynia _____
-ology	study of	ophthalmology _____
-oma	tumor	hepatoma _____
-opsy	to view	autopsy _____
		biopsy _____
-osis	condition, usually abnormal	necrosis _____
		hydronephrosis _____
		erythrocytosis[9] _____
-ostomy	to make a new opening	colostomy _____
-otomy	incision, to cut into	laparotomy _____
-pathy	disease	cardiopathy _____
-penia	deficiency	erythropenia _____
		leukopenia _____

[8] See Appendix H
[9] See Appendix I

-pexy	fixation, put in place	nephropexy _____
-phobia	fear	hydrophobia _____
		acrophobia _____
-plasia	development, formation	chondroplasia _____
-plasty	surgical repair	thoracoplasty _____
-poiesis	formation	hemopoiesis _____
-ptosis[10]	drooping, sagging, prolapse	visceroptosis _____
-sclerosis	hardening	arteriosclerosis _____
-scope	instrument for examination	endoscope _____
-stasis	stopping, controlling	metastasis _____
-therapy	treatment	hydrotherapy _____
-tome	instrument to cut	osteotome _____
-trophy	nourishment, development	hypertrophy _____
		atrophy _____

The following are shorter noun suffixes which are usually attached to roots in words:

-ia	condition	leukemia _____
-y	condition, process	nephropathy _____
-ole	little, small	arteriole _____
-ule	little, small	venule _____
-or	one who	chiropractor[11] _____

---

[10] See Appendix J
[11] See Appendix K

-er   one who   radiograph<u>er</u> _____

-ist   one who   nephrolog<u>ist</u> _____
                     specializes in

Adjective Suffixes. The following are adjective suffixes:

Suffix	Meaning	Terminology	Meaning
-ic	pertaining to	dactyl<u>ic</u> _____
		osteogen<u>ic</u> _____
		chron<u>ic</u> _____

What does acute mean? _____

-tic	pertaining to	plas<u>tic</u> _____
-al	pertaining to	periton<u>eal</u> _____
-ac	pertaining to	cardi<u>ac</u> _____
-ar	pertaining to	gland<u>ular</u> _____
-ary	pertaining to	submaxill<u>ary</u>[12] _____
-ous	pertaining to	muc<u>ous</u> _____

What is mucus?[13] _____

-oid	resembling	lith<u>oid</u>[14] _____
		epiderm<u>oid</u> _____

IV. APPENDICES

Appendix A

A hernia may be a bulging forth, or protrusion, of an organ or the muscular wall of an organ through the cavity which normally contains it. Some examples of hernias are a hiatus hernia (stomach protrudes upward into the mediastinum through the esophageal opening in the diaphragm) and an inguinal hernia (part of the intestine

---

[12] See Appendix L
[13] See Appendix M
[14] See Appendix N

protrudes downward into the groin region and commonly into the scrotal sac in the male). A rectocele is a hernial protrusion of part of the rectum into the vagina.

Appendix B

Streptococci are berry-shaped bacteria which grow in twisted chains. There are two groups of streptococci—hemolytic and viridans. **Hemolytic streptococci** (called hemolytic because the bacteria cause hemolysis, or breakdown of blood, in the growth medium) are responsible for such conditions as "strep" throat, tonsillitis, rheumatic fever, and certain kidney ailments. **Streptococci viridans** (viridans means green, and these bacteria produce a green color on the growth medium) are less virulent (poisonous) than the hemolytic form and cause infections in teeth, in the sinuses (cavities) of nose and face, and sometimes in the valves of the heart, where they cause bacterial endocarditis.

Staphylococci are bacteria which grow in small clusters, like grapes. Staphylococci lesions may be external (skin abscesses, boils, styes) or internal (abscesses in bone and kidney). (An abscess is a collection of pus, white blood cells, and protein, which are present at the site of infection.) Figure 4—1 illustrates the pattern of growth of streptococci and staphylococci.

Other bacteria which are coccal in shape include **pneumococci** (pneum/o = lungs), which are the most common cause of bacterial pneumonia in adults, and **gonococci** (gon/o = seed), which infest the reproductive organs.

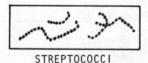
STREPTOCOCCI

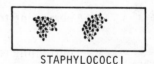
STAPHYLOCOCCI

Figure 4–1   Types of coccal bacteria.

Appendix C

Words ending in -us commonly form their plural by dropping the -us and adding -i. Thus, nucleus becomes nuclei and coccus becomes cocci (kok-sī). A guide to formation of plurals is found at the end of the book.

Appendix D

Study Figure 4–2 as you read the following to note the differences between the three different types of cells in the blood.

1. **Erythrocytes** (red blood cells). These cells are made in the bone marrow (soft tissue in the center of some bones in the body) and are important in that they transport oxygen (O_2) from the lungs through the bloodstream to the cells all over the body. The oxygen is then used up by body cells in the process of converting food to energy (catabolism). **Hemoglobin**, containing iron (globin = protein), is an important

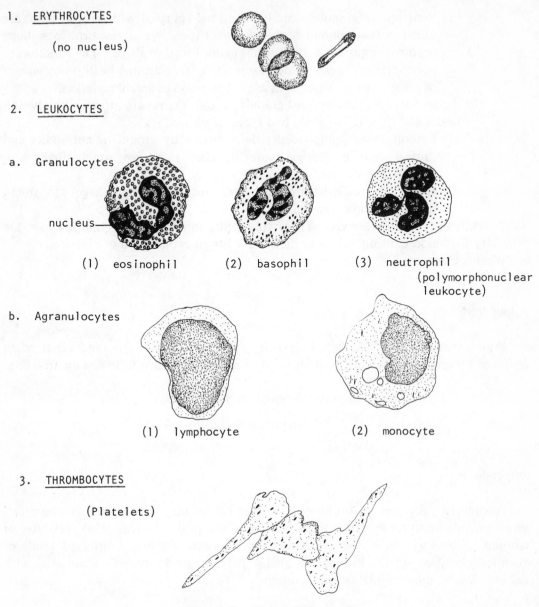

1. ERYTHROCYTES

   (no nucleus)

2. LEUKOCYTES

   a. Granulocytes

   nucleus—

   (1) eosinophil   (2) basophil   (3) neutrophil
                                            (polymorphonuclear
                                            leukocyte)

   b. Agranulocytes

   (1) lymphocyte   (2) monocyte

3. THROMBOCYTES

   (Platelets)

Figure 4–2   Types of blood cells.

protein in erythrocytes which helps to carry the oxygen as it travels through the bloodstream. Erythrocytes also carry away carbon dioxide (CO_2), a waste product of catabolism of food in cells, from the body cells to the lungs where it is expelled in the process of breathing.

   2. **Leukocytes** (white blood cells). There are several types of leukocytes:

   (a) **Granulocytes** (cells with granules in their cytoplasm) are formed in bone marrow. There are three types of granulocytes:

   (1) **Eosinophils** (granules stain red with acid stain) are thought to be active and elevated in allergic conditions such as asthma.

   (2) **Basophils** (granules stain blue with basic stain). The function of baso-phils in the body is unclear.

(3) **Neutrophils** (granules stain blue and red [purple] with neutral stain) are called **polymorphonuclear leukocytes** (poly = many; morph/o = shape or form) because the nucleus has many forms or shapes. The function of polymorphonuclears is defense of the body against bacteria by means of phagocytosis. These cells are called **polys** as an abbreviation.

(b) **Agranulocytes** (cells without granules in cytoplasm) are produced by lymph nodes and spleen. There are two types of agranulocytes:

(1) **Lymphocytes** (lymph cells) fight disease by producing antibodies and thus destroying foreign material. They may also attach directly to foreign material and destroy it.

(2) **Monocytes** (cells with a very large nucleus) ingest (phagocytose) and destroy foreign material.

3. **Platelets** or **thrombocytes**. These tiny cells, formed in the bone marrow, are necessary for blood clotting. See your dictionary for an explanation of platelets.

What is hemostasis?

Appendix E

Pronunciation clue: The letters **g** and **c** are soft (as in genes and cent) when followed by an **i** or **e**, and are hard (as in good and could) when followed by an **o** or **a**.

For example: laryngitis   (lar-in-jĭ′-tis)

laryngocele (lar-ing′-gō-sēl)

Appendix F

Anemia literally means "no blood." In medical language and usage, anemia refers to a medical condition in which there is a **reduction** in the number of erythrocytes or amount of hemoglobin in the circulating blood. There are many different kinds of anemias, classified on the basis of the many different problems which can arise with red blood cells, their circulation, and content.

Appendix G

Tissue that becomes **ischemic** loses its normal flow of blood and thus becomes devoid of oxygen. The ischemia can be caused by mechanical injury to a blood vessel, by blood clots lodging in a blood vessel, or by the gradual closing off (occlusion) of a vessel due to arteriosclerosis (hardening of the arteries).

Appendix H

Acromegaly is an example of an endocrine disorder. The **pituitary gland** in the brain produces an excessive amount of growth hormone after the completion of puberty. Hence, a person with acromegaly is of normal height, because the long bones have stopped growth after puberty, but has an abnormally large growth of bones and tissue in the hands, feet, and face. An excessive amount of growth hormone before completion of puberty produces excessive growth of long bones (giantism) as well as acromegaly.

Appendix I

When **-osis** is used as a suffix with blood cells, it means an abnormal condition in which there is a slight increase in number of circulating blood cells. When **-emia** is used as a suffix with blood cells (-cyte is usually dropped, as in leukemia), the condition is an abnormally high or excessive increase in number of blood cells. For example, erythrocytosis means an elevation of red blood cells, but erythremia is an excessively high increase of red blood cells.

Appendix J

The suffix **-ptosis** is pronounced tō′sis. The rule is that when two consonants begin a word, the first is silent. If the two consonants are found in the middle of a word, both are pronounced. For example, visceroptosis (vis-er-op-tō′-sis).

Appendix K

A **chiropractor** is a nonmedical person who manipulates the bones of the vertebral column to relieve pressure on nerves.

Appendix L

Submaxillary means under the upper jaw (maxilla) and actually refers to the lower jaw bone.

Appendix M

Mucus is a sticky secretion produced by mucous membranes and glands. It contains a protein called mucin, water, salts, and other substances. Mucosa is another term for a mucous membrane.

Appendix N

The combining form **lith/o** refers to a **stone**, or **calculus**, within the body. Stones are usually composed of mineral salts.

V. EXERCISES

A. Construct medical words:

1. Instrument to visually examine the larynx _____

2. Pain in the fingers _____

3. Enlargement of the liver _____

4. Surgical repair of nerves _____

5. Incision of the chest _____

6. Deficiency of white blood cells _____

7. Softening of the brain _____

8. One who specializes in the study of the eye _____

9. New opening of the kidney _____

10. Fear of water _____

11. Formation of red blood cells _____

12. Formation of bone _____

13. Condition of hardening of arteries _____

14. Prolapse of the kidney _____

15. Fixation of the internal organs _____

16. Removal of tonsils _____

17. Resembling a stone _____

B. Give the meaning of the following medical terms:

1. mucus _____

2. otitis _____

3. staphylococci _____

4. arthropathy _____

5. ischemic _____

6. laryngectomy _____

7. peritoneal _____

8. hypertrophy _____

9. otalgia _____

10. cardiomegaly _____

11. eosinophil _____

_____

12. hydrocele _____

13. myeloid _____

14. thrombocytopenia _____

15. electroencephalography _____

16. mucosa _____

17. tracheostomy _____

C. *Test your knowledge by giving the meaning of the following **noun** suffixes:*

1. -gram _____	10. -emia _____
2. -plasty _____	11. -coccus _____
3. -osis _____	12. -trophy _____
4. -itis _____	13. -otomy _____
5. -genic _____	14. -ectomy _____
6. -graphy _____	15. -ostomy _____
7. -oma _____	16. -megaly _____
8. -graph _____	17. -malacia _____
9. -tome _____	18. -odynia _____

19. -poiesis _____   23. -stasis _____

20. -centesis _____   24. -therapy _____

21. -opsy _____   25. -ptosis _____

22. -pexy _____   26. -lysis _____

D. *Provide answers to the following questions:*

1. What is aplastic anemia? _____

   _____

2. What is granulocytopenia? _____

3. Which blood cells are phagocytic? What is phagocytosis? _____

   _____

   _____

4. What are polys? _____

   _____

ANSWERS

A. 1. laryngoscope
   2. dactylalgia, dactylodynia
   3. hepatomegaly
   4. neuroplasty
   5. thoracotomy
   6. leukocytopenia (leukopenia)
   7. encephalomalacia
   8. ophthalmologist
   9. nephrostomy
   10. hydrophobia
   11. erythropoiesis (-poiesis is commonly used to refer to all blood formation)
   12. osteogenesis, osteoplasia
   13. arteriosclerosis
   14. nephroptosis
   15. visceropexy
   16. tonsillectomy
   17. lithoid

B. 1. Sticky secretion from a mucous membrane or gland.
   2. Inflammation of the ear.
   3. Berry-shaped bacteria arranged in clusters.
   4. Condition of disease in joints.

5. Pertaining to holding back blood from a tissue. In a heart attack, blood is held back from heart muscle.
6. Excision of the voice box, or larynx.
7. Pertaining to the peritoneum.
8. Excessive development of an organ. Weight lifters often have hypertrophy of chest muscles.
9. Pain in the ear.
10. Enlargement of the heart.
11. A white blood cell whose granules stain red with the addition of acid stain.
12. Hernia of water — usually in the scrotal sac.
13. Resembling bone marrow or spinal cord.
14. Lack of clotting cells.
15. Process of recording the electricity of the brain.
16. Mucous membrane.
17. New opening into the windpipe (trachea).

C.
1. record
2. surgical repair
3. abnormal condition
4. inflammation
5. pertaining to producing
6. process of recording
7. tumor
8. instrument to record
9. instrument to cut
10. blood condition
11. berry-shaped (bacteria)
12. development, nourishment
13. process of cutting
14. process of removing
15. to cut a new opening
16. enlargement
17. softening
18. pain
19. formation, usually of blood or bone marrow
20. surgical puncture to remove a fluid
21. to view
22. to fix, put in place
23. to stop, control
24. treatment
25. prolapse, drooping
26. breakdown, destruction

D.
1. Aplastic anemia is a form of anemia in which there is a lack of formation (a = no, not; plastic = pertaining to development) of all blood cell elements (leukocytes, erythrocytes, and thrombocytes) in the bone marrow.
2. Lack of granulocytes (eosinophils, basophils, neutrophils).
3. Neutrophils and monocytes. Phagocytosis is the process of eating or killing other cells by engulfing them.
4. Polys are polymorphonuclear leukocytes or neutrophils. These white blood cells have nuclei which are of many shapes (multi-lobed).

REVIEW SHEET 4

Noun Suffixes

-algia	_____	-malacia	_____
-cele	_____	-megaly	_____
-centesis	_____	-odynia	_____
-coccus	_____	-ole	_____
-cyte	_____	-ology	_____
-ectomy	_____	-oma	_____
-emia	_____	-opsy	_____
-er	_____	-or	_____
-genesis	_____	-osis	_____
-gram	_____	-ostomy	_____
-graph	_____	-otomy	_____
-graphy	_____	-pathy	_____
-ia	_____	-penia	_____
-ist	_____	-pexy	_____
-itis	_____	-phobia	_____
-lysis	_____	-plasia	_____
-plasty	_____	-therapy	_____
-poiesis	_____	-tome	_____
-ptosis	_____	-trophy	_____
-sclerosis	_____	-ule	_____
-scope	_____	-y	_____
-stasis	_____		

Adjective Suffixes

-ic _____   -ary _____

-al _____   -ous _____

-tic _____   -oid _____

-ar _____   -ac _____

Combining Forms

Give the combining form:

joint _____   red _____

cancer _____   liver _____

head _____   muscle _____

brain _____   spinal cord or
bone marrow _____

kidney _____

nerve _____   windpipe _____

tumor _____   chest _____

eye _____   neck _____

ear _____   clot _____

nose _____   tonsil _____

peritoneum _____   death _____

Give the meaning:

chondr/o _____   col/o _____

oste/o _____   bi/o _____

acr/o _____   lith/o _____

acu/o _____   lapar/o _____

chir/o _____   dactyl/o _____

muc/o _____   eosin/o _____

laryng/o _____   hydr/o _____

arteri/o _____   gon/o _____

chron/o _____   isch/o _____

maxill/o _____   granul/o _____

phil/o _____   strept/o _____

phob/o _____   staphyl/o _____

rect/o _____   abdomin/o _____

radi/o _____   viscer/o _____

pneum/o _____   morph/o _____

leuk/o _____   ven/o _____

Prefixes

a, an _____   hyper _____

auto _____   meta _____

hypo _____   sub _____

CHAPTER 5

PREFIXES

In this chapter you will:

Learn basic prefixes used in the medical language;

Analyze medical terms which combine prefixes and other word elements; and

Learn about the Rh condition as an example of an antibody-antigen reaction.

The chapter is divided into the following sections:

I. INTRODUCTION

This chapter on prefixes, like the preceding chapter on suffixes, is designed to give you practice in word analysis and provide a foundation for the study of the terminology of body systems which directly follows.

The list of combining forms, suffixes, and their meanings in Section II will help you analyze the terminology in the rest of the chapter. The appendices are included to give more complete understanding of the terms and to explain the words with reference to the anatomy, physiology, and diseases of the body.

II. COMBINING FORMS AND SUFFIXES

amni/o — amnion, sac in which the embryo develops

bol/o — to throw or cast off

cib/o	–	meals
cis/o	–	to cut
cost/o	–	rib
duct/o	–	to lead, carry
furc/o	–	forking, branching
gloss/o	–	tongue
glyc/o	–	sugar
gnos/o	–	knowledge
morph/o	–	shape, form
mort/o	–	death
nat/i	–	birth
nect/o	–	to bind, tie, connect
norm/o	–	rule, order
ox/o	–	oxygen
pne/o	–	breathing, breath
secti/o	–	to cut
seps/o	–	infection
somn/o	–	sleep
son/o	–	sound
the/o	–	to put, place
thel/o	–	nipple
thyr/o	–	shield
top/o	–	place, position, location
tox/o	–	poison

ven/o — vein

-blast — embryonic, immature

-crine — to separate, secrete

-cyesis — pregnancy

-drome — to run

-fusion — to pour

-grade — to go

-lysis — to break, separate

-meter — to measure

-orrhea — flow, discharge

-partum — birth, labor

-plasia — formation, development

-physis — to grow

-stasis — to stop, control

-trophy — nourishment, development

III. PREFIXES AND TERMINOLOGY

Prefix	Meaning	Terminology	Meaning
a, an	not, without	apnea	_____
		anoxia	_____
ab	away from	abnormal	_____
		abductor[1]	_____

_____

[1] See Appendix A

ad	toward	adductor _____
		adrenal glands[2] _____
ana	up	anabolism _____
		analysis _____
ante	before, forward	ante cibum _____
		ante partum _____
anti	against	antisepsis[3] _____
		antibiotic[4] _____
		antigen[5] _____

In this word, anti stands for antibody.

		antibody _____
		antitoxin _____
auto	self	autogenous _____
bi	two	bifurcation _____
		bilateral _____
brady	slow	bradycardia _____
cata	down	catabolism _____
con	with, together	congenital anomaly[6] _____
		connective _____
contra	against, opposite	contralateral _____
dia	through, complete	diameter _____
		diagnosis[7] _____

[2] See Appendix B
[3] See Appendix C
[4] See Appendix D
[5] See Appendix E
[6] See Appendix F
[7] See Appendix G

		diarrhea _____
		dialysis[8] _____
dys	bad, painful, difficult	dyspnea _____
ec, ecto	out, outside	ectoderm[9] _____
		ectopic pregnancy[10] _____
en, endo	in, within	endoderm _____
		endoscope _____
		endocrine _____
epi	upon, on, above	epithelium _____
eu	good	eupnea _____
ex	out, away from	exophthalmia[11] _____
hemi	half	hemiglossectomy _____
hyper	excessive, above, beyond	hyperplasia[12] _____
		hypertrophy _____
		hyperglycemia _____
hypo	deficient, under	hypodermic _____
		hypoglycemia _____
in	not	insomniac _____
in	in	incision _____
infra	below, inferior	infracardiac _____
inter	between	intercostal _____

[8] See Appendix H
[9] See Appendix I
[10] See Appendix J
[11] See Appendix K
[12] See Appendix L

intra	within	intravenous _____
macro	large	macrocephalia _____
mal	bad	malignant _____
		malaise _____
meso	middle	mesoderm _____
meta	beyond, between, change	metamorphosis _____
		metastasis _____
micro	small	microscope _____
pan	all	pancytopenia _____
para	near, beside, abnormal	parathyroid[13] _____
		paralysis _____
per	through	percutaneous _____
peri	surrounding	pericardium _____
		periosteum _____
polio	gray matter of the brain or spinal cord	polioencephalitis _____
		poliomyelitis _____
poly	many	polymorphonuclear _____
		polyneuritis _____
post	after, behind	post mortem _____
		postnatal _____
pre	before, in front of	precancerous _____
pro	before	prognosis _____

---

[13] See Appendix M

pseudo	false	pseudocyesis _____
retro	behind, back	retroperitoneal _____
		retrograde[14] _____
semi	half	semiconscious _____
sub	under	subcostal _____
supra	above	suprathoracic _____
		suprarenal glands _____
syn, sym	together, with	syndactylism _____
		synthesis _____
		syndrome[15] _____

Before the letters b, p, and m, syn becomes sym.

		symbiosis _____
		symmetry _____
		symphysis[16] _____
tachy	fast	tachypnea _____
trans	across	transfusion _____
ultra	beyond, excess	ultrasonography[17] _____

IV. APPENDICES

Appendix A

Abductors are muscles which draw the limbs **away** from the center of the body, while adductors are muscles which draw the limbs **toward** the center of the body.

---

[14] See Appendix N
[15] See Appendix O
[16] See Appendix P
[17] See Appendix Q

Appendix B

The adrenal glands are endocrine glands located above each kidney. They are sometimes called suprarenal glands (supra = above). They secrete chemicals called hormones which affect the functioning of the body.

Appendix C

Noun suffixes like -sepsis which end in sis can become adjectives by dropping the sis and adding tic. Hence, antisepsis becomes antiseptic. The prefix anti is pronounced an-tuh; the prefix ante is pronounced an-tee.

Appendix D

An antibiotic is an agent which destroys or inhibits the growth of microorganisms (small living things). Penicillin is an example of an antibiotic.

Appendix E

An antigen is a substance usually foreign to the body (such as a poison, virus, or bacterium), which stimulates the production of antibodies. Antibodies are protein substances developed by the body in response to the presence of foreign antigens. For example, the flu virus (antigen) enters the body, causing the production of antibodies in the bloodstream. These antibodies will then attach to and destroy the antigens (viruses) which produced them.

Another example of a familiar antigen-antibody reaction is the Rh condition. A person who is Rh^+ has a protein coating (antigen) on his or her red blood cells (RBC). A person who is Rh^- does not have this factor on his or her RBC.

If an Rh^- woman and an Rh^+ man conceive an embryo, the fetus may be Rh^- or Rh^+. A dangerous condition arises only when the embryo is Rh^+. Figure 5-1 shows the Rh^+ baby growing within an Rh^- mother.

During delivery of the first Rh^+ baby, some of the baby's red blood cells containing antigens may escape into the mother's bloodstream. This sensitizes the mother and causes her to produce antibodies against the new Rh^+ antigens in her blood. Because this occurs at delivery, the first baby is not affected and is normal at birth. Figure 5-2 shows the formation of antibodies by the Rh^- mother in response to the antigens from her baby.

Difficulties arise with the second Rh^+ pregnancy. If the embryo is Rh^+ again, during pregnancy the mother's acquired antibodies will enter the infant's blood stream and attack the infant's red blood cells (Rh^+). The infant's RBC's are destroyed and the infant attempts to compensate for this loss of cells by making many new immature red blood cells (erythroblasts). The infant is born with a condition known as erythroblastosis fetalis. One of the clinical symptoms of erythroblastosis fetalis is jaundice, or yellow skin pigmentation. The jaundice results from the excessive destruction of red blood cells, which causes a substance called bilirubin (chemical pigmentation produced

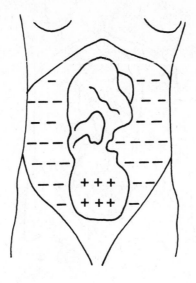

+ = Rh⁺ antigen on   - = Rh⁻ mother
    baby's RBC

Figure 5-1   Rh condition with first pregnancy.

when hemoglobin of red blood cells is broken down) to accumulate in the blood. Figure 5–3 illustrates the destruction of the baby's red blood cells by the antibodies in the mother's bloodstream during the second pregnancy.

To prevent erythroblastosis fetalis, Rh immune globulin is given to the mother after each Rh^+ delivery, abortion, or miscarriage. The globulin destroys Rh^+ cells which have escaped into the mother's circulation, and thus prevents sensitization of the

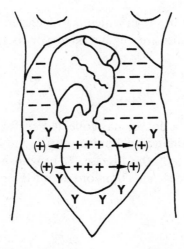

(+) = antigen in mother   Y = antibody made by
      from baby's RBC   mother in response
                                   to foreign Rh⁺
                                   antigen

Figure 5-2   Rh condition with delivery of first pregnancy.

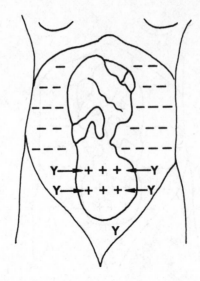

Y = antibodies from
mother which
destroy RBC's
of baby

Figure 5-3   Rh condition with second pregnancy.

mother and formation of Rh$^+$ antibodies so that future babies will not develop erythroblastosis fetalis.

Appendix F

An anomaly is a structure or organ which is irregular in formation (malformation). Examples of congenital anomalies are missing fingers or toes and heart defects.

Appendix G

A **diagnosis** is made when a doctor has collected sufficient information about the patient through physical examination, laboratory tests, and history, and can then make a determination of the nature of the disease. A **prognosis** is usually made after the diagnosis, and indicates the physician's opinions about the probable course or outcome of the disease.

Appendix H

Dialysis literally means "complete separation." A dialysis machine (artificial kidney) can completely separate out from the blood the harmful waste products of the body which are normally removed by the urine.

Appendix I

The **ectoderm**, **endoderm**, and **mesoderm** are the three layers of cells which form in the early stages of growth of the embryo. At this early stage of development, the embryo consists of an outer layer of cells called **ectoderm** (these cells give rise to or specialize into nerve cells and outer skin or epithelial cells in the fetus); a middle layer of cells called **mesoderm** (these cells give rise to connective tissue such as bone, fat, cartilage, muscle, and blood); and an inner layer of cells called **endoderm** (these cells specialize to become the cells of the lining of the digestive organs and glands and of the urinary bladder). Figure 5–4 shows the three layers of cells in the embryo and the major body structures to which they give rise.

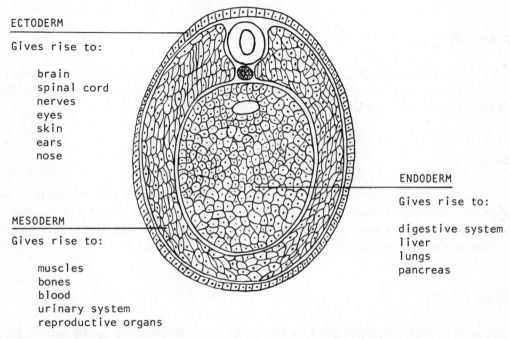

ECTODERM

Gives rise to:

    brain
    spinal cord
    nerves
    eyes
    skin
    ears
    nose

MESODERM

Gives rise to:

    muscles
    bones
    blood
    urinary system
    reproductive organs

ENDODERM

Gives rise to:

    digestive system
    liver
    lungs
    pancreas

Figure 5–4   Ectoderm, endoderm, and mesoderm: The three layers of cells in the embryo which give rise to the major body structures.

Appendix J

In a normal pregnancy, the embryo develops within the uterus. In an ectopic pregnancy, the embryo is implanted outside of the uterus—most commonly it is found in the fallopian tubes, and sometimes in the ovary or abdominal cavity.

Appendix K

Exophthalmia is an abnormal protrusion of the eyeball. It is commonly due to enlargement of the thyroid gland.

Appendix L

Hyperplasia refers to increase in size of an organ by virtue of increase in cell numbers. **Hypertrophy** also means increase in size of an organ or tissue, but in the context of an increase in individual cell size and development.

Appendix M

There are four parathyroid glands located on the dorsal side of the thyroid gland. The parathyroids are endocrine glands which produce a hormone and function entirely separately from the thyroid gland.

Appendix N

In a **retrograde** pyelogram, a contrast medium, or dye, is injected into the tubes of the urinary system (ureters) so that it flows back up into the renal pelvis region of the kidney. X-ray pictures are then taken.

Appendix O

A **syndrome** is a group of signs or symptoms which commonly occur together and indicate a particular disease or abnormal condition. An example of a syndrome is Horner's syndrome, characterized by ptosis of the eyelid, enophthalmos, and a cool, dry face on the affected side due to nerve damage.

Appendix P

A **symphysis** is a type of joint in which the bony surfaces are firmly united by a plate of cartilage. Examples are the junction of the pubic bones of the pelvis, that on the midline in the front of the body, and the sacroiliac joint.

Appendix Q

Ultrasonography is a diagnostic technique using ultrasound waves (inaudible sound waves) to produce an image or photograph of an organ or tissue. The ultrasonic echoes are recorded as they pass through different types of tissue.

V. EXERCISES

A. Test yourself by filling in the meaning of the following prefixes:

1. anti _____   16. infra _____

2. pro _____   17. inter _____

3. meta _____   18. intra _____

4. sub _____   19. hyper _____

5. con _____   20. in _____

6. meso _____   21. ana _____

7. ab _____   22. cata _____

8. peri _____   23. poly _____

9. dys _____   24. pseudo _____

10. para _____   25. mal _____

11. retro _____   26. ultra _____

12. dia _____   27. tachy _____

13. pan _____   28. brady _____

14. ante _____   29. eu _____

15. contra _____   30. auto _____

B. What prefix means the same as:

1. per _____   6. infra _____

2. hemi _____   7. a, an _____

3. contra _____   8. intra _____

4. pre _____   9. ex _____

5. con _____   10. supra _____

C. *Give the meaning of the following terms:*

1. dysplasia _____

2. transcostal _____

3. anomaly _____

4. exocrine _____

5. chondrodystrophy _____

6. antiseptic _____

7. intravenous _____

8. epicardium _____

9. bifurcation _____

10. diarrhea _____

11. amniocentesis _____

12. pseudocyesis _____

D. *Give the meanings of the following suffixes and combining forms:*

1. -stasis	_____	11. lapar/o	_____
2. -meter	_____	12. amni/o	_____
3. -scopy	_____	13. peritone/o	_____
4. -tome	_____	14. gloss/o	_____
5. -orrhea	_____	15. glyc/o	_____
6. -blast	_____	16. pne/o	_____
7. -oid	_____	17. tox/o	_____
8. -emia	_____	18. cost/o	_____
9. -odynia	_____	19. seps/o	_____
10. -ectomy	_____	20. nephr/o	_____

ANSWERS

A.
1. against
2. before
3. beyond, change, between
4. under
5. with, together
6. middle
7. away from
8. surrounding
9. bad, painful, difficult
10. near, beside, abnormal
11. behind
12. through, complete
13. all
14. before
15. against, opposite
16. below
17. between
18. within
19. excessive
20. not, in
21. up
22. down
23. many
24. false
25. bad
26. beyond, excess
27. fast
28. slow
29. good
30. self

B.
1. dia
2. semi
3. anti
4. ante, pro
5. syn
6. sub, hypo
7. in (when it means not)
8. endo
9. ec
10. hyper, epi

C.
1. Bad formation – abnormal tissue development.
2. Across the ribs.
3. Without rule; structure which is unusual or irregular.
4. To separate out – glands which secrete substances **out** into ducts, e.g., tear, sweat, mammary.
5. Poor, bad development of cartilage.
6. Against infection (**sis** becomes **tic** in the adjective form).
7. Pertaining to within a vein.
8. Above the heart.
9. Forking, branching into two.
10. Flow through – water flows through the large bowel instead of being reabsorbed into the body.
11. Surgical puncture of the amnion (the sac in which the embryo develops). This procedure is done to examine the cells of the embryo.
12. False pregnancy.

D.
1. Stopping, controlling.
2. To measure.
3. Process of visual examination.
4. Instrument to cut.
5. Flow, discharge.
6. Embryonic, immature.
7. Resembling.
8. Blood condition.
9. Pain.
10. Removal, excision.
11. Abdominal wall, abdomen.
12. Amnion—sac which envelops the embryo.
13. Peritoneum—membrane around abdominal cavity.
14. Tongue.
15. Sugar.
16. Breathing.
17. Poison.
18. Rib.
19. Infection.
20. Kidney.

REVIEW SHEET 5

Prefixes

a, an	_____	hypo	_____
ab	_____	in	_____
ad	_____	infra	_____
ana	_____	inter	_____
ante	_____	intra	_____
anti	_____	macro	_____
auto	_____	mal	_____
bi	_____	meso	_____
brady	_____	meta	_____
cata	_____	micro	_____
con	_____	pan	_____
contra	_____	para	_____
dia	_____	per	_____
dys	_____	peri	_____
ec, ecto	_____	polio	_____
en, endo	_____	poly	_____
epi	_____	post	_____
eu	_____	pre	_____
ex	_____	pro	_____
hemi	_____	pseudo	_____
hyper	_____	retro	_____

semi _____   tachy _____

sub _____   trans _____

supra _____   ultra _____

syn, sym _____

Combining Forms

amni/o _____   nect/o _____

bol/o _____   norm/o _____

cib/o _____   ophthalm/o _____

cis/o _____   ox/o _____

cost/o _____   pne/o _____

duct/o _____   ren/o _____

furc/o _____   secti/o _____

gloss/o _____   seps/o _____

glyc/o _____   somn/o _____

gnos/o _____   son/o _____

hepat/o _____   the/o _____

later/o _____   thyr/o _____

morph/o _____   tom/o _____

mort/o _____   top/o _____

nat/i _____   tox/o _____

necr/o _____   ven/o _____

Suffixes

-blast _____   -lysis _____

-grade   _____   -plasia   _____

-meter   _____   -fusion   _____

-orrhea   _____   -cyesis   _____

-stasis   _____   -partum   _____

-crine   _____   -physis   _____

-trophy   _____   -drome   _____

CHAPTER 6

DIGESTIVE SYSTEM

In this chapter you will:

Learn the names, locations, and functions of the major organs of the digestive system;

Understand the terms used to describe the major disease processes which affect these organs; and

Learn the combining forms for the organs and structures of the digestive system.

The chapter is divided into the following sections:

I. INTRODUCTION

The digestive system, or gastrointestinal tract, begins with the mouth, where food enters the body, and ends with the anus, where solid waste material leaves the body. The primary functions of the organs of the digestive system are threefold.

First, complex food material which is taken into the mouth (ingestion) must be **digested**, or broken down, mechanically and chemically, as it travels through the gastrointestinal tract. Complex proteins are digested to simpler amino acids; complicated sugars are reduced to simple sugars, such as glucose; and large fat molecules are broken down to fatty acids and triglycerides.

Second, the digested food must be **absorbed** by passage through the walls of the small intestine into the bloodstream so that the valuable energy-carrying nutrients (sugars, amino acids, fatty acids) can travel to all the cells of the body. Within the cells,

93

sugars and fatty acids can be burned in the presence of oxygen (catabolism), thereby releasing the energy stored in the food matter. Amino acids are used by the cells to build large protein molecules (anabolism) necessary for growth and development.

The third function of the gastrointestinal tract is to **eliminate** the solid waste materials which are unable to be absorbed by the small intestine. The solid wastes (feces) are concentrated in the large intestine and finally passed out of the body through the anus.

II. VOCABULARY

These words are used in the chapter and are defined here for you to refer to as you study.

absorption	Passage of nutrients through the wall of the small intestine into the bloodstream.
amino acids	Substances which are the end-products of protein digestion and the building blocks of protein formation.
anastomosis	Creation of a new connection between segments of an organ, as in the surgical joining of the free ends of the large intestine after removal of a diseased portion.
bile	Substance made in the liver and which is necessary for the digestion of fats.
bilirubin	Pigment which is a waste product of hemoglobin destruction. It is excreted from the body in bile.
bowel	Intestine.
buccal cavity	Cheek, or oral, cavity.
calculus	Stone.
cusps	Points.
deglutition	Swallowing.
digestion	Breakdown of complex foods into simpler substances which can pass into the bloodstream.
emulsification	The process of breaking down large fat globules into smaller particles which are able to be digested.

enzyme	A protein which promotes a specific chemical reaction (for example: digestion, or breakdown, of foods).
etiology	Study of the cause of disease.
feces	Solid waste material of digestion excreted through the anus; composed of bacteria, water, epithelial cells, and bile.
flexure	A bending.
glycogen	Starch—the form of sugar storage in the liver.
hiatal hernia	Outpouching of the wall of the stomach upward through the esophageal opening in the diaphragm.
jaundice	Yellow-orange color of skin and tissues.
mastication	Chewing.
melena	Black feces containing blood.
mucosa	Mucous membrane.
orifice	Opening.
papillae	Small projections commonly found on the tongue.
parotid gland	Gland near the ear; a salivary gland.
perforation	An abnormal hole in the side of a hollow organ.
peristalsis	Involuntary contraction and relaxation of the muscles of the digestive tract.
portal system	System of blood vessels which bring nutrient-rich blood to the liver from the abdominal viscera and carry blood away from the liver toward the heart.
rugae	"Wrinkles"—irregular folds, or ridges, located in the stomach wall and on the hard palate.
sphincter	Ring of muscle; tightens and relaxes to act as a valve and allow material to pass from one area to another.

spleen	Oval organ lying posterior and inferior to the stomach in the left upper quadrant (LUQ); forms leukocytes, and filters bacteria and worn-out erythrocytes from the blood.
vagotomy	Incision of the vagus nerve to prevent stimulation of acid flow within the stomach. It is used to treat patients with ulcers.
varix (plural: varices)	Twisted, swollen vein.
vermiform appendix	Wormlike pouch hanging from the first part of the large intestine.
villus (plural: villi)	"Tuft of hair"—tiny projection in the wall of the small intestine through which digested nutrients pass into the bloodstream.

III. ANATOMY OF THE DIGESTIVE SYSTEM

Oral Cavity

The gastrointestinal tract begins with the oral cavity, or mouth. Label Figure 6–1 as you learn the major parts of the oral cavity.

The oral cavity is sometimes called the **buccal** (cheek) **cavity**. The **cheeks** (1) form the walls of the oval-shaped mouth cavity, while the **lips** (2) form the opening to this cavity.

The **hard palate** (3) forms the anterior portion of the roof of the mouth, while the muscular **soft palate** (4) lies posterior to it and separates the mouth from the **pharynx** (throat) (5). **Rugae** (6) are the irregular ridges in the mucous membrane covering the anterior portion of the hard palate. Hanging from the soft palate is a small, soft tissue called the **uvula** (7). It is composed of connective tissue and muscle and aids in the production of sounds and speech. (Uvula means little grape.)

The **tongue** (8) extends across the floor of the oral cavity and is attached by muscles to the mandible (lower jaw bone). It moves food around during **mastication** (chewing) and **deglutition** (swallowing). The tongue is covered with a series of small projections called **papillae** which contain cells (taste buds) sensitive to the chemical nature of food.

The **tonsils** (9) are masses of lymphatic tissue located in depressions of the mucous membranes in the walls of the pharynx. They act as a filter to protect the body from the invasion of microorganisms, and produce lymphocytes, which are white blood cells able to fight disease.

The **gums** (10) are made of fleshy tissue and surround the sockets in which the **teeth** (11) are found. There are 32 permanent teeth, 16 in each jaw bone. There are: 4 incisors (in/cis/or = one who cuts into); 2 cuspids (points), or canine (doglike); 4 premolars, or bicuspids (bi/cusp/id = two points); and 6 molars.

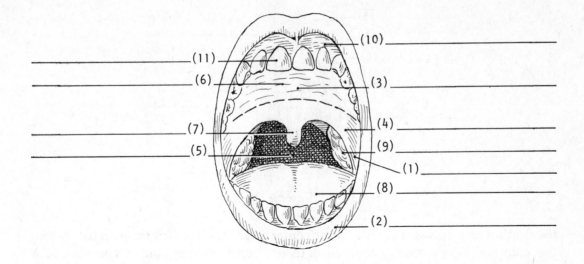

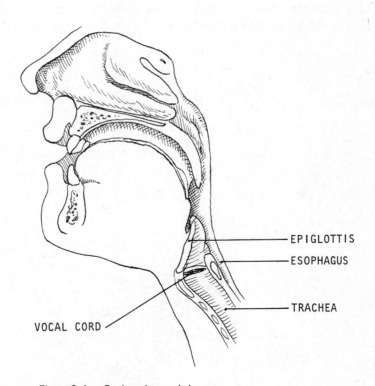

Figure 6-1   Oral cavity and throat.

Figure 6–2 shows the inner anatomy of a tooth. Label it as you read the following. A tooth consists of a **crown** (1), which is above the gum, and a **root** (2), which is embedded in an alveolus, or tooth socket. The outermost protective layer of the crown is called the **enamel** (3). The enamel is a dense, hard, white substance—the hardest substance in the body. Underneath the enamel is a layer which extends throughout the crown and root and is the main bulk of the tooth; it is called the **dentin** (4). Dentin is composed of bony tissue and is covered by a protective layer of **cementum** (5). Below

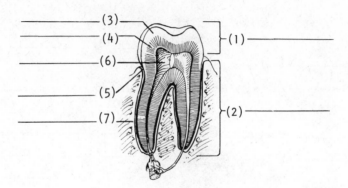

Figure 6-2   Anatomy of a tooth.

the dentin is a soft, vascular layer in the center of the tooth called the **pulp** (6). Within the pulp are blood vessels, connective tissue, nerve endings, and lymph vessels. A **periodontal membrane** (7) surrounds the root and holds the tooth in place.

The three pairs of **salivary glands** pictured in Figure 6–3 are exocrine glands. The salivary glands produce a fluid called **saliva** which contains important digestive enzymes to chemically break down starches into sugar. Saliva is released from the **parotid** (near

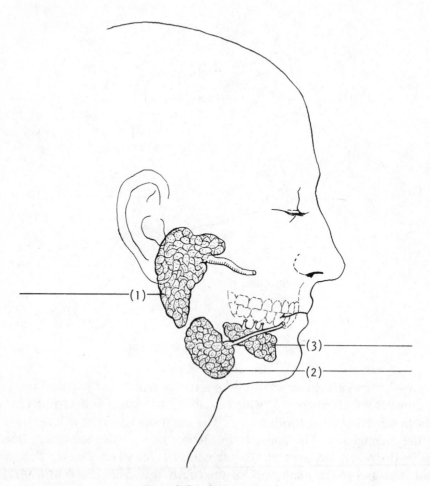

Figure 6-3   Salivary glands.

the ear) glands (1), **submaxillary** (lower jaw) glands (2), and **sublingual** (under the tongue) glands (3), through narrow ducts which carry the saliva into the mouth.

Figure 6–4 traces the passage of food through the digestive system after it leaves the oral cavity. Label the figure as you study the following descriptions of the major organs.

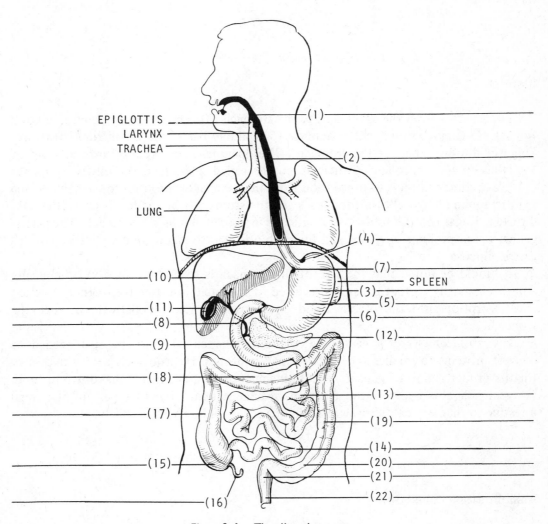

Figure 6–4   The digestive system.

Pharynx

Food passes from the mouth to the **pharynx** (1). The pharynx is a muscular tube lined with a mucous membrane. It serves as a passageway for air from the nasal cavity to the larynx (voice box), as well as for food going from the mouth to the **esophagus** (2). A flap of tissue called the epiglottis (meaning "upon the windpipe") covers the opening to the larynx and prevents food from entering the windpipe (trachea) by closing over the air passageway during deglutition, or swallowing.

Esophagus

The **esophagus** is a 9 to 10 inch muscular tube extending from the pharynx to the stomach. It aids in swallowing and moves food along the gastrointestinal tract. **Peristalsis** is the name of the involuntary, progressive, wavelike contraction of the esophagus and other tubes of the gastrointestinal tract which propel the food through the system.

Stomach

Food passes from the esophagus to the **stomach** (3). The stomach is composed of a **fundus** (4) (upper, round part), a **body** (5) (middle part), and an **antrum** (6) (lower bulge in the distal part of the stomach). The openings allowing food into and out of the stomach are controlled by rings of muscles called **sphincters**. The **cardiac sphincter** (7) relaxes and contracts to move food from the esophagus into the stomach, while the **pyloric sphincter** (8) allows food to leave the stomach when it has been sufficiently digested. **Rugae** are the folds in the mucous membrane lining the stomach. The gastric glands which produce enzymes and hydrochloric acid to digest food are located in this gastric mucosa.

It should be noted that the role of the stomach is to prepare the food chemically and mechanically so that it can be received in the small intestine for further digestion and absorption into the blood. Food does not enter the bloodstream through the stomach.

The stomach secretes gastric juices containing an enzyme (pepsin) needed to convert proteins to smaller substances called peptones. Hydrochloric acid is necessary for the proper action of pepsin. Besides mechanical and chemical breakdown of food, the stomach also controls the ejection of material into the first part of the small intestine so that it is passed only in small quantities and only when ready.

Small Intestine (Small Bowel)

The small intestine, or small bowel, extends from the pyloric sphincter to the first part of the large intestine. It is 20 feet long and has three parts. The **duodenum** (9), the first part, receives food from the stomach, bile from the **liver** (10) and **gallbladder** (11), and pancreatic juice from the **pancreas** (12). Food is digested in the duodenum and passes in peristaltic waves from the duodenum to the second part, the **jejunum** (13), which is about 8 feet long. The jejunum connects with the third section, the **ileum** (14), about 11 feet long, which is attached to the large intestine.

In the wall of the entire small intestine are millions of tiny, finger-like projections called **villi** (singular: villus). It is through the capillary network of the villi that digested foods (simple sugars, amino acids, and fatty acids) pass to enter the bloodstream (absorption). (A schematic cross-section of a villus is pictured in Figure 6–5.)

unfazed or didut faze

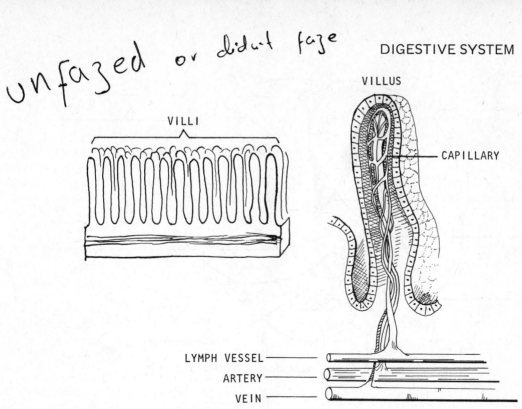

Figure 6-5   Villi in the lining of the small intestine.

Large Intestine (Large Bowel)   (Continue labeling Figure 6-4)

The large intestine extends from the ileum to the anus. It is divided into four parts—cecum, colon, sigmoid colon, and rectum. The **cecum** (15), or first part, is a pouch on the right side which is connected to the ileum by the ileocecal sphincter (ring of muscles). The **vermiform** (wormlike) **appendix** (16) hangs from the cecum; the appendix is a blind alley and has no function. The **colon** is about 5 feet long and has three divisions: The **ascending colon** (17) extends from the cecum to the under surface of the liver where it turns to the left (hepatic flexure) into the **transverse colon** (18); the transverse colon passes horizontally to the left toward the spleen, and as it reaches the splenic region it turns downward (splenic flexure) into the **descending colon** (19). The **sigmoid colon** (20) (resembling an S) is at the distal end of the descending colon and leads into the **rectum** (21). The rectum terminates in the lower opening of the gastrointestinal tract, the **anus** (22).

The large intestine receives the fluid by-products of digestion from the small intestine. Unabsorbed solid material is stored in the colon and water is reabsorbed into the bloodstream while the solid material travels along to eventually be eliminated from the body as **feces**.

Liver, Gallbladder, and Pancreas

Three important accessory organs of the digestive system are the **liver, gallbladder,** and **pancreas**. Although food does not pass through these organs, they play a crucial role in the proper digestion and absorption of nutrients. Label Figure 6–6 as you study the following.

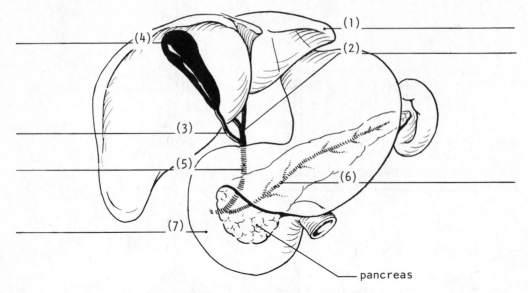

Figure 6–6   Liver, gallbladder, and pancreas.

The liver (1), located in the right upper quadrant (RUQ) of the abdominal cavity, manufactures a thick, yellowish-brown, sometimes greenish, fluid called **bile**. Bile contains cholesterol (a fatty substance), bile acids, and several bile pigments. One of these bile pigments is called **bilirubin**. Bilirubin is a waste product produced when hemoglobin (from destroyed red blood cells) is broken down in the liver. The liver then combines bilirubin with bile and both are excreted through the digestive system in the feces.

Bile is released continuously from the liver and travels down the **hepatic duct** (2) to the **cystic duct** (3). The cystic duct leads to the **gallbladder** (4), a pear-shaped sac under the liver, which stores and concentrates bile for later use. After meals, in response to the presence of foods in the stomach and duodenum, the gallbladder contracts, forcing the bile out the cystic duct and into the **common bile duct** (5), which joins with the **pancreatic duct** (6) just before the entrance to the **duodenum** (7). The duodenum receives a mixture of bile and pancreatic juice.

Bile acts as an emulsifier, with detergent-like effect on the fats in the duodenum. This allows for more successful enzymatic digestive action by the pancreatic juice. Without bile, most of the fat taken into the body would remain undigested.

The liver, besides producing bile, has many other vital and important functions in the body. Some of these are:

1. Keeping the amount of glucose (sugar) in the blood at a normal level. The liver can remove excess glucose from the bloodstream and store it (as a starch called **glycogen**) in the hepatocytes. This process is called glycogenesis. Also, the liver can put sugar back into the bloodstream when the sugar level is dangerously low. This process is called glycogenolysis. Liver cells can also make new sugar from amino acids and other materials, and this process is called gluco/neo/genesis. (Figure 6—7 reviews the role of the liver in the formation and storage of sugar.)

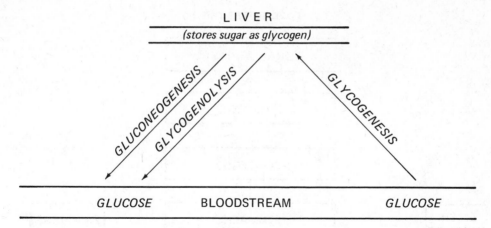

Figure 6–7   The role of the liver in the formation and storage of sugar.

2. Manufacturing protein substances. Two of these protein compounds are prothrombin and fibrinogen, which aid in the clotting of blood. The liver also makes albumin, which is the major circulating protein.
3. Destruction of worn-out red blood cells. The liver clears the body of bilirubin pigment which is produced when hemoglobin is broken down and red blood cells are destroyed.
4. Removal of poisons or toxins from the blood, and formation of antibodies to fight disease.
5. Production of urea, which is a waste product of protein breakdown. Urea enters the bloodstream and travels to the kidney where it is concentrated in urine and eliminated from the body.

The term **portal system** (portal circulation) is used frequently with regard to the liver. Portal system refers to the blood vessels which bring blood filled with nutrients from the intestines to the liver. It also refers to the blood vessels which carry the blood from the liver to the large veins leading to the heart.

The **pancreas** functions as both an exocrine and endocrine organ. As an exocrine organ, it has an important digestive function: It manufactures and secretes pancreatic juice which passes through the pancreatic duct into the duodenum, where it helps to break down all types of foods. One of the enzymes it makes is called **lipase**, which is helpful in digesting fats (lip/o = fat, ase = enzyme). Another is **amylase** (amyl/o = starch), an enzyme which breaks down sugars and starches.

As an endocrine organ, special cells in the pancreas produce a hormone called **insulin**, which enters the bloodstream directly and plays a role in the utilization of sugar by the body.

Figure 6–8 is a flow chart following the pathway of food through the digestive tract.

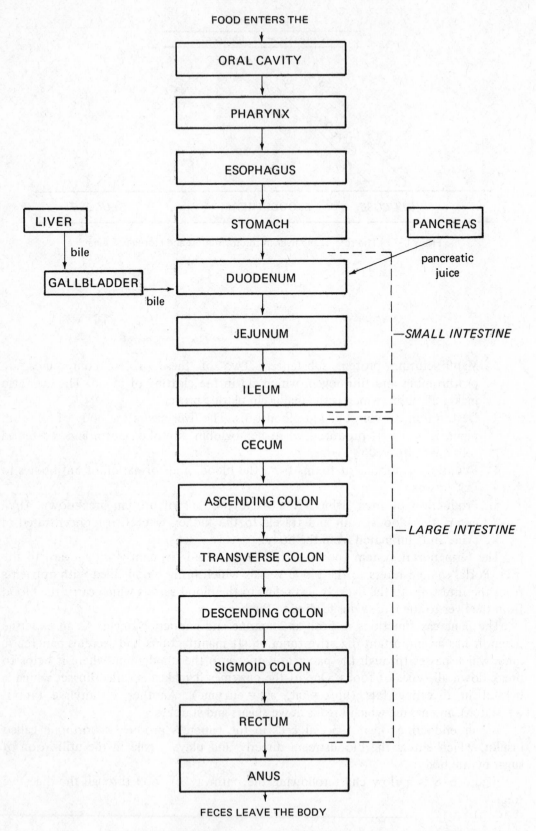

Figure 6–8 Pathway of food through the digestive tract.

IV. COMBINING FORMS AND RELATED TERMINOLOGY

Combining Form	Structure or Substance	Terminology	Meaning
or/o stomat/o	mouth	oral _____	
		stomatitis _____	
bucc/o	cheek	buccal mucosa _____	
labi/o cheil/o	lip	labial _____	
		cheilosis _____	
dent/i odont/o	tooth	dentibuccal _____	
		periodontal _____	
		odontalgia _____	
gingiv/o	gum	gingivitis _____	
lingu/o gloss/o	tongue	lingual _____	
		glossotomy _____	
palat/o	palate	palatoplasty _____	
tonsill/o	tonsil	tonsillectomy _____	
sial/o	saliva	sialolithiasis _____	
		-iasis means abnormal condition and is commonly used with lith/o.	
sialaden/o	salivary glands	sialadenitis _____	
pharyng/o	throat, pharynx	pharyngeal _____	
		Note that the final g is softened by adding an e between the suffix -al and the root—far-in-jē-al.	
esophag/o	esophagus	esophagogastric _____	
		esophageal _____	
gastr/o	stomach	gastrectomy _____	
celi/o	belly, abdomen	celiac _____	

enter/o	small intestine	enterostomy _____
		mesentery _____
		enteric anastomosis _____

An anastomosis is a new surgical connection between segments of an organ. An enteroenterostomy (new opening between two parts of the small intestine) is the same procedure as an enteric anastomosis.

duoden/o	duodenum	duodenal _____
jejun/o	jejunum	jejunostomy _____
ile/o	ileum	ileitis _____
cec/o	cecum	ileocecal sphincter _____
appendic/o append/o	appendix	appendicitis _____
		appendectomy _____
col/o	colon	colostomy _____
sigmoid/o	sigmoid colon	sigmoidoscope _____
rect/o	rectum	rectocele _____
an/o proct/o *(refers to anal and rectal regions)*	anus	anorectal _____
		proctologist _____
hepat/o	liver	hepatomegaly _____
chol/e bil/i	gall, bile	cholelithiasis _____
		biliary _____
cholecyst/o	gallbladder	cholecystectomy _____
choledoch/o	common bile duct	choledochotomy _____
bilirubin/o	bilirubin	hyperbilirubinemia _____
pancreat/o	pancreas	pancreatitis _____
peritone/o	peritoneum	peritoneoscopy _____

splen/o	spleen	splenomegaly _____
herni/o	hernia	herniotomy _____
amyl/o	starch	amylase _____
gluc/o	sugar	gluconeogenesis _____
glyc/o	sugar	hyperglycemia _____
glycogen/o	glycogen	glycogenolysis _____
lip/o	fat	lipolysis _____
steat/o	fat	steatorrhea _____
lith/o	stone	cholelithectomy _____
-ase	enzyme	lipase _____
-iasis	condition	choledocholithiasis _____
-prandial	meal	postprandial _____

V. PATHOLOGY OF THE DIGESTIVE SYSTEM

Although explanations for terms are given, you should consult your medical dictionary for additional information about the disease condition.

anorexia
(an/orexia)

Lack of appetite.

dental caries

Cavities in teeth created by decay of tissue.

aphthous stomatitis
(aphth/ous)

Inflammation of the mouth associated with small ulcers (canker sores).

oral leukoplakia
(leuk/o/plakia)

White plaques or patches on mucous membranes. This is a precancerous lesion which may become malignant.

cirrhosis
(cirrh/osis)

Abnormal condition of tawny, orange-yellow color.

This disease condition is a result of chronic damage to hepatocytes which leads to malfunction of the liver. Alcoholism combined with nutritional deficiency is a common etiological (eti/o = cause) factor, but damage to the liver may be caused by other factors as well, such as infection. Hepatomegaly occurs first, but then the liver becomes smaller and permeated, or filled, with fibrous scar tissue as the hepatocytes die. The portal vein (leading from the abdominal viscera to the liver) becomes obstructed by scarring and destruction of tissue so that blood backs up in the veins of the digestive system organs. Also, **jaundice** (yellow-orange color of the skin and tissues) may occur in late stages because of the inability of the liver to remove red cell breakdown products such as bilirubin from the blood.

esophageal varices   Swollen, twisted veins around the esophagus.

This condition is usually due to portal hypertension (high blood pressure in the portal vessels) which is in turn caused by cirrhosis of the liver. The danger of this condition is the possibility of massive hemorrhage (bursting forth of blood).

jaundice   Yellow-orange coloration of skin and tissues.
 (icterus)

Jaundice can be caused by many different pathological conditions. Gastrointestinal conditions leading to jaundice would involve obstruction of bile passageways (i.e., choledocholithiasis). Hyperbilirubinemia results because bilirubin (a bile pigment) is not excreted from the body and accumulates in the blood. This causes the characteristic appearance of yellowness of skin, whites of the eyes, and body fluids. Bilirubin is formed when red blood cells become old and break down in the liver and spleen. It may also accumulate in the blood and body tissues as a result of excessive hemolysis (erythroblastosis fetalis) or disturbances in functioning of liver cells (cirrhosis).

regurgitation   To flood back. The return of solids and fluids to
 (re/gurgitation)   the mouth from the stomach.

achlorhydria   Lack of hydrochloric acid.
 (a/chlor/hydria)

This gastric condition may be due to carcinoma of the stomach, ulcer, or gastritis.

ulcer   Sore, or lesion (wound), of the mucous membranes
           or skin.

There are many different kinds of ulcers. The kind most commonly associated with the gastrointestinal system is the peptic ulcer, occurring as a gastric or duodenal ulcer. When mucous membrane tissue in the stomach or duodenum becomes injured and necrosed, the digestive juices and acid from the stomach begin to digest the dead tissue. An ulcer is thus formed, which, if not treated, can lead to perforation into the abdominal cavity and bleeding. Some relief from the pain and discomfort of an ulcer can be achieved with vagotomy (cutting the nerve which stimulates acid secretion in the stomach), pyloroplasty (relieving the muscular spasms of the pyloric sphincter which blocks the passage of food from the stomach to duodenum), and bicarbonates, which neutralize the acid in the stomach.

dysentery
(dys/enter/y)

Painful intestines.

Although enter/o is a combining form for the small intestine, dysentery commonly refers to the large intestine (large bowel) and is a colitis. Two forms of dysentery are found: amoebic and bacillary. Amoebic dysentery is caused by a one-celled organism, called an amoeba, which is swallowed in infected food; bacillary dysentery is caused by ingesting a bacilli-type of bacteria called shigella. Both forms of dysentery produce diarrhea and pain.

gallstones

Collection of bile which forms in the gallbladder and bile ducts.

A gallstone is formed when cholesterol, bilirubin, and other components of bile remain in the gallbladder and bind into small, hard stones (calculi). When one of the gallstones becomes lodged in the neck of the gallbladder or in one of the ducts (cystic and common bile duct) which lead from the gallbladder, it dams up the flow of bile. Pressure builds up in the gallbladder, and acute pain is experienced. Infection can then form and spread through the gallbladder and liver. Cholecystectomy is the usual method of treatment. Figure 6–9 shows how gallstones can block the cystic duct and cause pain.

melena
(melen/a)

Black stools, or feces containing blood.

ascites

Abnormal accumulation of fluid in the peritoneal cavity.

Obstruction of the flow of blood in the portal system can lead to back-up of blood and pouring out of fluid from the blood into the peritoneal cavity. Ascites may also result from cirrhosis, tumor, infection, or heart failure. It is sometimes called "dropsy."

diverticula
(divert/i/cul/a)
(singular: diverticulum)

Turning aside, often referring to an abnormal side pocket in a hollow structure such as the intestine.

Common sites of diverticula are the sigmoid colon and the duodenum. Diverticulosis does not display symptoms, but if inflammation occurs diverticulitis results and is associated with pain and tenderness. Diverticulectomy can be performed to relieve the condition. Figure 6–10 illustrates diverticula.

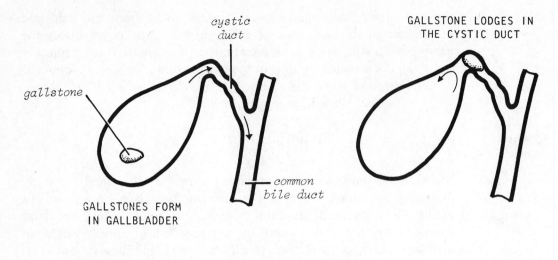

cystic duct

GALLSTONE LODGES IN
THE CYSTIC DUCT

gallstone

common bile duct

GALLSTONES FORM
IN GALLBLADDER

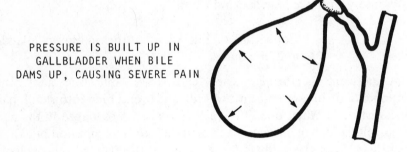

PRESSURE IS BUILT UP IN
GALLBLADDER WHEN BILE
DAMS UP, CAUSING SEVERE PAIN

Figure 6-9   Gallstones.

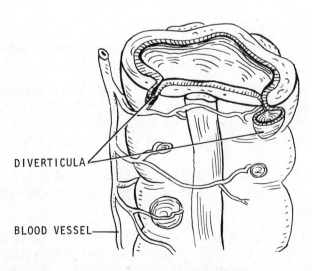

DIVERTICULA

BLOOD VESSEL

Figure 6-10   Diverticula of the large intestine. The mucous lining bulges through the muscular wall to form a diverticulum.

hernia
Protrusion or projection of an organ or part through the wall of the cavity which contains it.

A hernia can occur when a small loop of bowel protrudes through a weak place in the abdominal wall. The loop tends to come down during straining, coughing, or lifting of heavy weights. The danger of a hernia is a loss of blood supply to the herniated intestine and strangulation, and, because of the gangrene and peritonitis which can result, an operation to surgically repair the hernia must be performed.

A **hiatal hernia** is the protrusion of part of the stomach through the esophageal opening of the diaphragm. Figure 6–11 is a diagram of an abdominal hernia and a hiatal hernia.

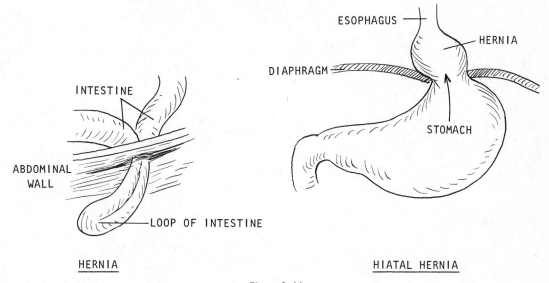

Figure 6–11

intussusception
(in/tus/susception)
Telescoping of the intestines.

This condition commonly occurs in children and usually in the ileocecal region. Part of the ileum slips into the cecum and can lead to strangulation, as in the case of a hernia. Surgery is performed to resect (cut out) the intussusception, and end-to-end anastomosis is done. Figure 6–12 illustrates intussusception.

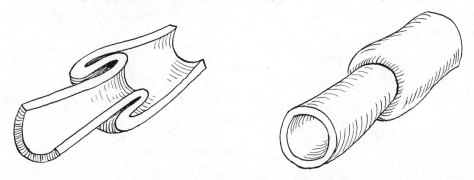

Figure 6–12 Intussusception.

volvulus   Twisting of the intestine upon itself.

This form of intestinal obstruction is marked by a twisting, or torsion, of a loop of the bowel. An operation can be performed to untwist the loop of the intestine and correct the condition. Figure 6–13 illustrates volvulus.

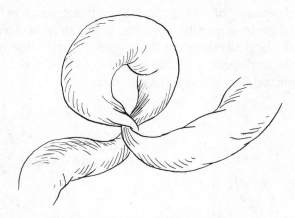

Figure 6–13 Volvulus.

VI. EXERCISES

A. *Match the following terms with their meanings:*

1. deglutition

2. absorption

3. mastication

4. digestion

5. peristalsis

6. excretion

7. anastomosis

8. regurgitation

_____ bringing food back up the gastrointestinal tract.

_____ breakdown of complex substances.

_____ new opening up between two hollow organs or fibers.

_____ contraction and relaxation of muscles to propel food along the gastrointestinal tract.

_____ formation of wastes and removal from the body.

_____ passage of simple nutrients into the bloodstream.

_____ swallowing.

_____ chewing.

B. *Give the location and function of the following structures in the digestive system:*

	Location	Function
1. gallbladder	_____	_____
2. villi	_____	_____
3. parotid gland	_____	_____
4. pyloric sphincter	_____	_____
5. liver	_____	_____
6. pulp	_____	_____
7. pharynx	_____	_____
8. duodenum	_____	_____
9. ileum	_____	_____
10. pancreas	_____	_____

C. *Build medical terms:*

1. Pertaining to under the tongue _____

2. Inflammation of a salivary gland _____

3. Blood conditions of excessive bilirubin _____

4. Pertaining to the throat _____

5. Removal of a tonsil _____

6. Enlargement of the liver and spleen _____

7. Hernia of the rectum _____

8. New opening between the third part of the small intestine and the cecum

    _____

9. Incision into the common bile duct _____

10. Prolapse of the anus and the rectum _____

11. Condition of disease of the small intestine _____

12. Removal of the colon _____

13. Surgical repair of the lips _____

14. Pertaining to the cheek _____

15. Pain in the tooth _____

16. Inflammation of the gums _____

17. Study of the causes of diseases _____

18. After meals _____

D. *Give the meaning of the following medical terms:*

1. gastroscopy _____

2. stomatitis _____

3. celiomyalgia _____

4. colorectostomy _____

5. esophagotomy _____

6. sigmoidopexy _____

7. duodenogram _____

8. sialolithiasis _____

9. cholecystectomy _____

10. pancreatitis _____

E. *Describe the following gastrointestinal disorders:*

1. diverticulosis _____

2. esophageal varices _____

3. intussusception _____

4. cirrhosis _____

_____

5. ulcer _____

6. dysentery _____

_____

7. peritonitis _____

8. hiatal hernia _____

_____

9. volvulus _____

10. pancreatic carcinoma _____

F. *Give the meaning of the following medical symptoms:*

1. melena _____

2. leukoplakia _____

3. anorexia _____

4. steatorrhea _____

5. hypoglycemia _____

6. achlorhydria _____

7. ascites _____

8. jaundice _____

ANSWERS

A. 8
4
7
5
6
2
1
3

Location	Function

B.
1. Sac under the liver.
2. Small intestine.
3. Salivary gland near the ear.
4. Ring of muscle at distal end of the stomach.
5. RUQ of the abdominal cavity.
6. Oral cavity; part of a tooth.
7. Between the oral cavity and the esophagus; throat.
8. First part of the small intestine.
9. Third part of the small intestine.
10. Behind the stomach in the LUQ.

Stores and concentrates bile.
Absorption of food into bloodstream.
Produces saliva which digests starch to sugar.
Controls passage of materials from the stomach to the duodenum.
Produces bile, excretes waste products of hemoglobin destruction, regulates blood sugar.
Soft, inner section of tooth; contains blood vessels and nerves.
Serves as a passageway for food and air.

Digestion and absorption of food.
Absorption of food into the bloodstream through villi.

Produces enzymes to digest food, and also a hormone, insulin, which helps to bring sugar to the cells.

C.
1. subglossal/sublingual
2. sialadenitis
3. hyperbilirubinemia
4. pharyngeal
5. tonsillectomy
6. hepatosplenomegaly
7. rectocele
8. ileocecostomy
9. choledochotomy
10. proctoptosis
11. enteropathy
12. colectomy
13. cheiloplasty
14. buccal
15. odontalgia
16. gingivitis
17. etiology
18. postprandial or postcibal

D.
1. Process of visually examining the stomach.
2. Inflammation of the mouth.
3. Pain in the muscles of the belly, or abdomen.
4. New opening between the colon and rectum; colorectal anastomosis.
5. Incision of the esophagus.
6. Fixation of the sigmoid colon.
7. Record (x-ray) of the duodenum.
8. Condition (abnormal) of having salivary stones.
9. Removal of the gallbladder.
10. Inflammation of the pancreas.

E.
1. Abnormal condition of small outpouchings of the intestinal tract.
2. Swollen, twisted veins in the esophagus.
3. Telescoping of the intestines—one part slipping into the other.
4. Literally, abnormal condition of orange-yellow; atrophy and destruction of liver cells leading to malfunction of liver and jaundice.
5. Sore, or lesion, in digestive system.
6. Painful intestines—usually refers to bacterial or amoebic infection of the gastrointestinal tract with diarrhea as main symptom.
7. Inflammation of the peritoneum (membrane lining the abdominal cavity).
8. Esophageal hernia; protrusion of a loop of the stomach through the esophageal opening in the diaphragm.
9. Abnormal twisting, or torsion, of the intestines.
10. Cancerous tumor of the pancreas.

F.
1. Black stools.
2. White plaques, or patches.
3. Lack of appetite.
4. Flow (excessive) of fat in feces.
5. Low blood sugar.
6. Lack of hydrochloric acid.
7. Collection of fluid in the peritoneal cavity.
8. Orange-yellow condition of the skin, whites of eyes, mucous membranes; due to biliary obstruction, hemolysis, or liver malfunction.

CHAPTER 7

ADDITIONAL SUFFIXES

In this chapter you will:

Learn additional suffixes and use them with the combining forms of the digestive system to build and analyze medical words; and

Review the terminology of the digestive system as you complete exercises in medical terminology.

The chapter is divided into the following sections:

I. Introduction

II. Suffixes

III. Combining Forms

IV. Exercises

I. INTRODUCTION

This chapter will give you practice in word building, while not introducing a large number of new terms. It is designed to review some of the terms already learned and to give you a breather after a long and difficult chapter.

Study the new suffixes in Section II first. Most of them are frequently used with the digestive system combining forms, and you will use them in completing the terminology list in Section III. The exercises include terms previously introduced in the last few chapters, so you may have to refer back as you complete them.

II. SUFFIXES

Suffix	Meaning	Terminology	Meaning
-clysis	irrigation, washing	enteroclysis _____	
-ectasis, -ectasia	stretching, dilation	gastrectasia _____	
		angiectasis _____	
-emesis	vomiting	hyperemesis _____	
-lysis	destruction, breakdown	hemolysis _____	
-orrhaphy	suture	gastrorrhaphy _____	
-orrhagia	bursting forth of blood	gastrorrhagia _____	
-orrhea	flow, discharge	rhinorrhea _____	
-orrhexis	rupture	enterorrhexis _____	
-pepsia	digestion	dyspepsia _____	
-phagia	eating, swallowing	polyphagia _____	
-plasty	surgical repair	pyloroplasty _____	
-ptysis	spitting	hemoptysis _____	
-spasm	sudden, violent, involuntary contraction of muscles	pylorospasm _____ _____	
-stalsis	constriction	peristalsis _____	
-stasis	stopping, controlling	cholestasis _____	
-stenosis	tightening, stricture	pyloric stenosis _____	
-tresia	opening	esophageal atresia _____	

III. COMBINING FORMS

Combining Form	Meaning	Terminology	Meaning
bucc/o	_____	buccal _____	
cec/o	_____	cecotomy _____	
celi/o	_____	celiac artery _____	
cheil/o	_____	cheilostomatoplasty _____	
chol/e	_____	cholelithotomy _____	
cholecyst/o	_____	cholecystojejunostomy _____	
		_____	
choledoch/o	_____	choledochoduodenostomy _____	
		_____	
col/o	_____	colopexy _____	
dent/i	_____	dentalgia _____	
duoden/o	_____	duodenorrhaphy _____	
enter/o	_____	enteroanastomosis _____	
esophag/o	_____	esophageal _____	
gastr/o	_____	gastrospasm _____	
gingiv/o	_____	gingivitis _____	
gloss/o	_____	glossopalatine _____	
glyc/o	_____	glycolysis _____	
hepat/o	_____	hepatocholangioduodenostomy _____	
		_____	
herni/o	_____	herniorrhaphy _____	
		herniorrhexis _____	

jejun/o _____ jejunojejunostomy _____

ile/o _____ ileectomy _____

labi/o _____ labioglossopharyngeal _____

lingu/o _____ lingual _____

lip/o _____ lipolysis _____

lith/o _____ cholecystolithotomy _____

odont/o _____ odontorrhagia _____

or/o _____ oral cavity _____

pancreat/o _____ pancreatogenic _____

proct/o _____ proctoclysis _____

pylor/o _____ pyloroplasty _____

rect/o _____ rectostenosis _____

sial/o _____ sialodochitis _____

splen/o _____ splenorrhagia _____

steat/o _____ steatorrhea _____

stomat/o _____ aphthous stomatitis _____

IV. EXERCISES

A. *Build medical words:*

1. Prolapse of the stomach _____

2. Process of recording (x-ray) the gallbladder _____

3. Irrigation of the rectum _____

4. Vomiting blood _____

5. Stretching of the lymph vessels _____

6. Hemorrhage from a tooth _____

7. Suturing of a hernia _____

8. Anastomosis between the cecum and colon _____

9. Spasm of the pyloric sphincter _____

10. Spitting up blood _____

11. Rupture of the colon _____

12. Removal of the pancreas _____

13. Process of visually examining the anus and rectum _____

14. Inability to swallow _____

15. Stone in the salivary gland _____

B. *Give the meaning of the following medical terms:*

1. enterotomy _____

2. cheilitis _____

3. nephropexy _____

4. abdominocentesis _____

5. osteomalacia _____

6. pyloroplasty _____

7. buccal _____

8. choledochoduodenostomy _____

9. diarrhea _____

10. dyspepsia _____

11. esophagostenosis _____

12. enteroclysis _____

13. gastric atrophy _____

14. herniorrhaphy _____

15. atresia _____

16. jejunoileostomy _____

17. celiac angiography _____

18. ptosis _____

19. emetic _____

20. sialodochotomy _____

C. *Give the meaning of the following digestive system terms:*

1. dysentery _____

2. achlorhydria _____

3. anorexia _____

4. portal cirrhosis _____

_____

5. ascites _____

6. pharyngitis _____

7. periesophageal hernia _____

8. diverticulosis _____

9. cholecystic calculi _____

10. icterus _____

11. melena _____

12. peristalsis _____

13. postprandial _____

14. anastomosis _____

15. deglutition _____

16. mastication _____

D. *Give the suffix for the following:*

1. rupture _____

2. suture _____

3. hemorrhage _____

4. washing, irrigation _____

5. breaking down, _____
   destruction

6. stretching _____

7. prolapse _____

8. narrowing _____

9. hardening _____

10. flow, discharge _____

11. digestion _____

12. eating, _____
    swallowing

13. spitting _____

14. vomiting _____

15. opening _____

16. violent contraction _____
    of muscles

17. fixation _____

18. surgical puncture _____

19. constriction _____

20. stopping, _____
    controlling

21. surgical repair _____

ANSWERS

A. 1. gastroptosis
   Remember, **p** when followed by a consonant (t, n, etc.) in the beginning of a word is **silent** (pneumonia, nū-mō′-ni-a; ptosis, tō′-sis); however, when the **p** is in the middle of a word it is pronounced (gas-trop-tō′-sis).

2. cholecystography	7. herniorrhaphy	12. pancreatectomy
3. rectoclysis	8. cecocolostomy	13. proctoscopy
4. hematemesis	9. pylorospasm	14. aphagia
5. lymphangiectasia	10. hemoptysis	15. sialadenolith
6. odontorrhagia	11. colorrhexis	

B. 1. Incision of the small intestine.
   2. Inflammation of the lips.
   3. Fixation of the kidney.
   4. Surgical puncture of the abdominal cavity.
   5. Softening of bone.
   6. Surgical repair of the pylorus (distal end of the stomach).
   7. Pertaining to the cheek.
   8. New opening between the common bile duct and the duodenum.
   9. "Flow through"; watery stools.
   10. Difficult, bad digestion.
   11. Tightening of the esophagus.
   12. Irrigation of the intestines.

13. Wasting of the stomach (mucous membrane lining of the stomach).
14. Suture of a hernia.
15. No opening.
16. New opening between the jejunum and the ileum (an anastomosis).
17. Process of recording vessels in the belly.
18. Prolapse, sagging.
19. Pertaining to vomiting.
20. Incision into a salivary gland.

C. 1. Painful intestines.
2. Lack of hydrochloric acid in the stomach.
3. No appetite.
4. Literally means "abnormal condition of orange-yellow." Portal refers to the system of blood vessels in the liver. Cirrhosis involves atrophy of liver cells and subsequent destruction leading to impairment of liver function and circulation of blood and bile.
5. An accumulation of fluid in the peritoneal cavity (hydroperitoneum).
6. Inflammation of the throat.
7. Loop of the stomach slips through esophageal hole in the diaphragm; hiatal hernia.
8. Abnormal condition of having small outpouchings of the intestinal tract.
9. Stones in the gallbladder.
10. Yellow; jaundice.
11. Black stools.
12. Constriction and relaxation of the muscles especially around the walls of the digestive system tubes.
13. After meals.
14. New opening between two hollow organs.
15. Swallowing.
16. Chewing.

D. 1. -orrhexis
2. -orrhaphy
3. -orrhagia
4. -clysis
5. -lysis
6. -ectasis
7. -ptosis
8. -stenosis
9. -sclerosis
10. -orrhea
11. -pepsia
12. -phagia
13. -ptysis
14. -emesis
15. -tresia
16. -spasm
17. -pexy
18. -centesis
19. -stalsis
20. -stasis
21. -plasty

REVIEW SHEET 6-7

Combining Forms

amyl/o	_____	gastr/o	_____
an/o	_____	gingiv/o	_____
appendic/o	_____	gloss/o	_____
bil/i	_____	gluc/o	_____
bilirubin/o	_____	glyc/o	_____
bucc/o	_____	glycogen/o	_____
cec/o	_____	hepat/o	_____
celi/o	_____	herni/o	_____
cervic/o	_____	ile/o	_____
cheil/o	_____	jejun/o	_____
chol/e	_____	labi/o	_____
cholecyst/o	_____	lingu/o	_____
choledoch/o	_____	lip/o	_____
cirrh/o	_____	lith/o	_____
col/o	_____	mandibul/o	_____
dent/i	_____	maxill/o	_____
diverticul/o	_____	necr/o	_____
duoden/o	_____	odont/o	_____
enter/o	_____	or/o	_____
esophag/o	_____	palat/o	_____
eti/o	_____	pancreat/o	_____

peritone/o _____

pharyng/o _____

proct/o _____

pylor/o _____

rect/o _____

sial/o _____

sialaden/o _____

sigmoid/o _____

splen/o _____

steat/o _____

stomat/o _____

thorac/o _____

tonsill/o _____

Suffixes

-ase _____

-centesis _____

-clysis _____

-ectasia _____

-ectasis _____

-emesis _____

-iasis _____

-lithiasis _____

-lysis _____

-orrhagia _____

-orrhaphy _____

-orrhea _____

-orrhexis _____

-pepsia _____

-pexy _____

-phagia _____

-plasty _____

-prandial _____

-ptosis _____

-ptysis _____

-spasm _____

-stalsis _____

-stasis _____

-stenosis _____

-tresia _____

Additional Terms

If you have difficulty explaining any of these terms, refer back to the information in Chapters 6 and 7.

absorption _____

achlorhydria _____

amino acids _____

anastomosis _____

anorexia _____

aphthous stomatitis _____

ascites _____

bile _____

bilirubin _____

calculus _____

cirrhosis _____

deglutition _____

dental caries _____

diverticula _____

duodenum _____

emulsification _____

enzyme _____

esophageal varices _____

feces _____

flexure _____

gallstones _____

gastric mucosa _____

glycogen _____

hiatal hernia _____

ileum intussusception _____

jaundice (icterus) _____

jejunum _____

mastication _____

melena _____

oral leukoplakia _____

parotid gland _____

perforation _____

peristalsis _____

portal system _____

regurgitation _____

rugae _____

sphincter _____

spleen _____

ulcer _____

vagotomy _____

villi _____

volvulus _____

CHAPTER 8

URINARY SYSTEM

In this chapter you will:

Learn the location and the function of organs in the urinary system;

Learn the terms for the various pathological conditions of the urinary system;

Be able to use and recognize the combining forms, prefixes, and suffixes of the system; and

Understand the use and interpretation of urinalysis as a diagnostic test.

The chapter is divided into the following sections:

I. INTRODUCTION

You have just learned how food is brought into the bloodstream by the digestive system. In a future chapter you will learn how oxygen is brought into the bloodstream by the respiratory system. Food and oxygen are combined in the cells of the body to produce energy (catabolism). In the process, however, the substance of the food and oxygen is not destroyed. Instead, the small particles of which the food and oxygen are made are actually rearranged into new combinations. These are waste products. When foods like sugars and fats which contain particles of carbon, hydrogen, and oxygen combine with oxygen in cells, the wastes produced are gases called carbon dioxide (carbon and oxygen) and water (hydrogen and oxygen) in the form of vapor. These gases are removed from the body by exhalation through the lungs.

Protein foods are more complicated than sugars and fats. They contain carbon, hydrogen, and oxygen **plus** nitrogen and other elements. The waste that is produced when proteins combine with oxygen is called **nitrogenous waste**, and it is more difficult to excrete (to separate out) from the body than are gases like carbon dioxide and water vapor.

The body cannot efficiently put the nitrogenous waste into a gaseous form and exhale it, so it excretes it in the form of a soluble (dissolved in water) waste substance called **urea**. The major function of the urinary system is to remove urea from the bloodstream so that it does not accumulate in the body and become toxic.

Urea is formed in the liver from ammonia, which in turn is derived from the breakdown of simple proteins (amino acids) in the body cells. The urea is carried in the bloodstream to the kidneys, where it passes with water, salts, and acids out of the bloodstream and into the kidney tubules as **urine**. Urine then travels down the ureters into the bladder and out of the body.

Besides removing urea from the blood, another important function of the kidneys is to maintain the proper balance of water, salts, and acids in the body fluids. The kidney does this by secreting some substances into the urine and holding back other necessary substances in the body.

II. VOCABULARY

acetone	Abnormal breakdown product produced in the body when fats are burned; also called ketone bodies.
acid	A compound which gives off hydrogen particles in solution. Acids have a sour taste and unite with bases (alkaline compounds) to form salts.
albumin	A protein found in the blood.
alkaline (base)	Substance which forms hydroxide particles in solution. Alkaline substances have a bitter taste and unite with acids to form salts.
antidiuretic hormone (ADH)	ADH is secreted by the pituitary gland (endocrine organ at the base of the brain) and stimulates the kidney tubules to reabsorb water. In pathological conditions in which ADH is not secreted (diabetes insipidus), polyuria and polydipsia (excessive thirst) are common symptoms.
calculus	A stone.

cast

Mold, or copy, of an object. Urinary casts are molds of the renal tubules and may be discharged in the urine.

catheter

Tube for giving and withdrawing fluids.

creatinine

Waste product formed from protein metabolism and excreted in the urine.

diabetes insipidus

Pathological condition caused by inadequate secretion of antidiuretic hormone by the pituitary gland. Water is not properly reabsorbed by the kidney tubules, so that polyuria and polydipsia result. Insipidus means tasteless, reflecting that the urine is very dilute and watery—not sweet as in diabetes mellitus.

diabetes mellitus

Malfunction of the pancreas in which the hormone insulin is not secreted in adequate amounts and sugar cannot leave the bloodstream to be used by the cells in the production of energy. Mellitus means sweet. It is diabetes mellitus that is meant when the word diabetes is used by itself.

dialysis

"Complete separation"—artificial filtration of waste materials from the blood. There are two kinds:

hemodialysis—using an artificial kidney machine which filters wastes from the patient's blood.
peritoneal dialysis—removal of waste is accomplished by introducing large volumes of fluid into the peritoneal (abdominal) cavity. Waste substances pass from the blood into the peritoneal fluid. The fluid is then removed and exchanged for "clean" fluid.

enuresis

Bedwetting, or inability to hold back urine.

essential hypertension

High blood pressure of undetermined cause.

excretion

Removal of waste materials from the bloodstream.

insulin

Hormone produced by the pancreas.

ketone bodies

Abnormal breakdown products produced when fats are burned in cells; also called acetone.

meatus

Opening or canal.

micturition	Urination.
nitrogenous wastes	Waste products containing nitrogen; produced when proteins are used in cells. Urea is a nitrogenous waste.
phenylketonuria (PKU)	This condition results from an excessive accumulation in the blood of an amino acid called phenylalanine and is associated with mental deficiency. The infant affected lacks an enzyme which can break down phenylalanine in the blood. Hence, phenylalanine collects in the blood and phenylketones are present in the urine. A PKU test is done at birth to test for the presence of phenylalanine in the blood or phenylketones in the urine. To prevent the damaging effects of this enzyme deficiency, infants with PKU are fed low-phenylalanine diets which prevent accumulation of the substance in the blood.
renin	A substance produced by the kidney which contracts blood vessels, thereby increasing blood pressure.
retention	Holding back; urine retention is the inability of the urinary bladder to empty, or expel urine.
retrograde	Going back in a reverse direction. In a retrograde pyelogram, dye is injected into the urethra and goes back up through the urinary tract so that x-rays can be taken of the urinary system.
secondary hypertension	High blood pressure secondary to other ailments. For example, secondary hypertension may be a result of kidney disease.
specific gravity	A measurement that reflects the amount of wastes and minerals in the urine.
stricture	Narrowing of a passageway due to scarring, muscle spasms, or other causes.
suppuration	Pus formation.
urea	Major nitrogen-containing end-product of protein metabolism which is excreted in the urine.
uric acid	Nitrogenous substance excreted in the urine.

III. ANATOMY OF THE MAJOR ORGANS

The organs of the urinary system are: (See Figure 8–1)

1. Two **kidneys**—bean-shaped organs situated behind the abdominal cavity (retroperitoneal) on either side of the vertebral column in the lumbar region of the spine.

The kidneys are embedded in a cushion of adipose tissue and surrounded by fibrous connective tissue for protection. They are fist-sized and weigh about half a pound each.

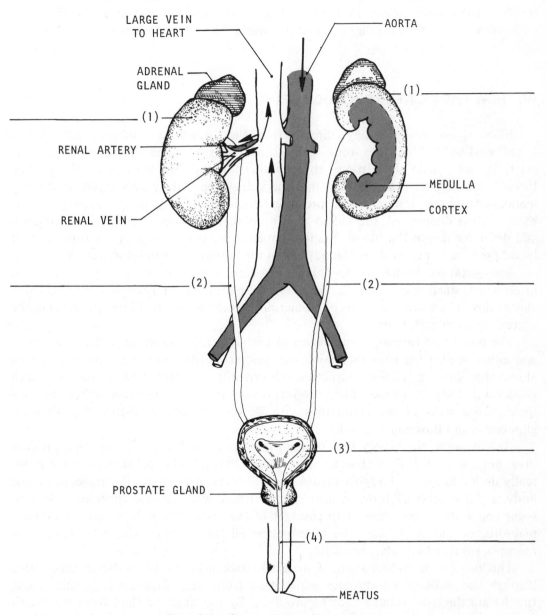

Figure 8–1 Organs of the urinary system.

The kidneys consist of an outer **cortex** region (cortex means bark, as in bark of a tree) and an inner **medulla** region (medulla means marrow or inner portion).

The **aorta** (largest artery in the body) brings waste-filled blood from the heart to the kidneys via the short, thick **renal arteries** which branch into both kidneys. The filtration of waste materials from the blood to form urine takes place within the microscopic tubules of the kidney. The **renal vein** carries blood away from the kidneys to larger veins and then back to the heart.

2. Two **ureters**—muscular tubes lined with mucous membrane. They convey urine in peristaltic waves from the kidney to the urinary bladder.

3. **Urinary bladder**—hollow, muscular, distensible sac in the pelvic cavity. It serves as a temporary reservoir for urine.

4. **Urethra**—membranous tube through which urine is discharged from the urinary bladder. The process of expelling urine through the urethra is called **micturition**. The external opening of the urethra is called the urethral or urinary **meatus**.

IV. HOW THE KIDNEYS PRODUCE URINE

Blood is led to the kidneys directly from the aorta by way of the renal arteries. Each renal artery branches into many small arteries called **arterioles**. Since the arterioles are small, blood passes through them slowly, but constantly. Blood flow through the kidneys is so essential that the kidneys have their own special device for maintaining blood flow. If blood pressure falls in the vessels of the kidney so that blood flow is diminished, the kidney is stimulated to produce a substance called **renin** and discharge it into the blood. Renin stimulates the contraction of arterioles so that blood pressure is increased and blood flow in the kidneys is restored to normal.

Each arteriole in the kidney breaks up into a mass of very tiny, coiled, and intertwined small blood vessels (capillaries) shaped like a little ball and called a **glomerulus**. There are thousands of glomeruli (literally means small ball of wool) in the cortex region of each kidney.

The process of forming urine begins in the glomerulus as water, salts, sugar, urea, and other wastes (such as **creatinine** and **uric acid**) **filter** out from the thin-walled glomerulus into a cuplike structure (**Bowman's capsule**) which encloses each glomerulus. Large molecules, like proteins, remain in the bloodstream and cannot pass through the walls of the glomerulus into Bowman's capsule. Figure 8–2 shows a glomerulus and Bowman's capsule.

At this point, the kidney has filtered out of the blood not only the waste product urea, but also a great deal of water, sugar, and salts and other substances that it is not really desirable for the body to discard. It would certainly not be advantageous for the body if the process of forming urine stopped here and valuable substances, such as sugar and water, were allowed to pass out of the body. The kidney must, therefore, **reabsorb**, or put back, into the bloodstream all the materials the body needs (for example, sugar, most water, and salts).

This process of reabsorption of materials back into the bloodstream takes place through the walls of the tubules which lead from each Bowman's capsule. These tubules are the **renal tubules** (See Figure 8–3). By the time the fluid from Bowman's capsule has passed through the tubules, reabsorption has taken place and the fluid has

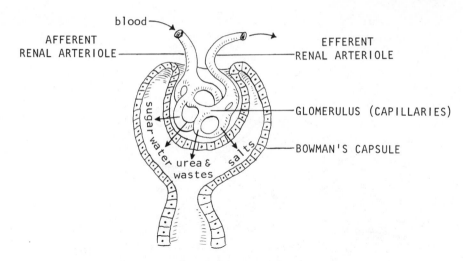

Figure 8–2   Glomerulus and Bowman's capsule.

become a relatively concentrated solution carrying only wastes and some water. Approximately 50 gallons of water filter out of the glomerulus each day, and 99 per cent of this is reabsorbed through the renal tubules back into the blood.

In addition, acids and other substances which the body does not need are **secreted** into the distal renal tubules from the bloodstream. Figure 8–3 shows the renal tubules and the capillary blood vessels which surround them to accept valuable materials back into the blood.

The distal renal tubules, carrying urine (composed of 95 per cent water, plus 5 per cent urea, creatinine, acids, and salts, and some bile pigments), merge to form the **renal pelvis**, a space that fills most of the medulla of the kidney. Cuplike divisions of the renal pelvis which receive urine from the tubules are called **calyces** (singular: calyx).

The renal pelvis narrows into the **ureter** which carries the urine to the **bladder** where the urine is temporarily stored. The exit area of the bladder to the urethra is closed by sphincters which do not permit urine to leave the bladder. As the bladder fills up, however, there is a point at which muscular contractions of the walls of the bladder begin and pressure is placed on the base of the urethra, which causes the desire to urinate. This continues until urination takes place. Figure 8–4 shows the renal pelvis, calyces, and ureter leading from the renal pelvis.

Study the flow diagram in Figure 8–5 to trace the process of forming urine and expelling it from the body.

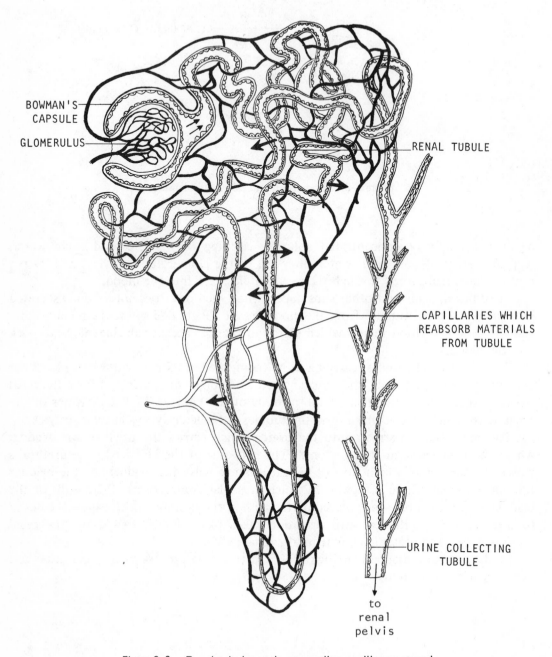

BOWMAN'S
CAPSULE

GLOMERULUS

RENAL TUBULE

CAPILLARIES WHICH
REABSORB MATERIALS
FROM TUBULE

URINE COLLECTING
TUBULE

to
renal
pelvis

Figure 8–3   Renal tubules and surrounding capillary network.

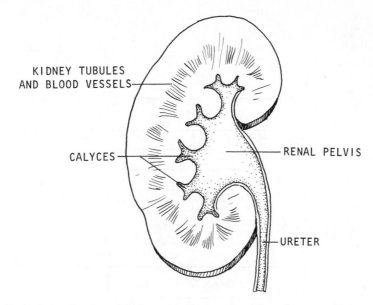

KIDNEY TUBULES
AND BLOOD VESSELS

CALYCES

RENAL PELVIS

URETER

Figure 8–4   Section of kidney showing renal pelvis, calyces, and ureter.

V. COMBINING FORMS AND TERMINOLOGY

Combining Form	Meaning	Terminology	Meaning
cortic/o	cortex *(outer section of kidney)*	cortical _____ _____	
glomerul/o	glomerulus *(collection of capillaries)*	glomerular _____ _____	
medull/o	medulla *(inner section of kidney)*	medullary _____ _____	
nephr/o	kidney	paranephric _____	
		nephroptosis _____	
		nephrorrhaphy _____	
		nephromegaly _____	
		nephrohypertrophy _____	
		nephrectomy _____	

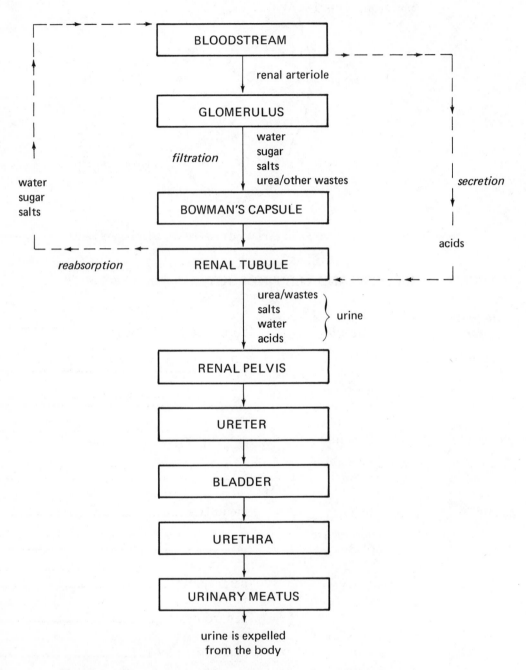

Figure 8–5   Flow diagram of the process of forming and expelling urine.

nephrolithotomy _____

nephrosclerosis _____

nephropexy _____

nephrotomography _____

_____

ren/o   kidney   renal ischemia _____

renal transplantation _____

_____

renal calculus _____

renal dialysis _____
(see vocabulary list)

_____

pyel/o   renal pelvis   intravenous pyelogram (IVP) _____

_____

retrograde pyelogram _____

_____

pyelostomy _____

pyelolithotomy _____

pyeloplasty _____

cali/o   calyx, calyces   caliectasis _____

ur/o   urine (urea),   uremia _____
                       urinary tract

urogram _____

diuresis _____
Caffeine, alcohol, and urea can act as diuretics.

		enuresis _____
		antidiuretic hormone _____
		(see vocabulary list)
		_____
		urostasis _____
azot/o	urea, nitrogen	azotemia _____
ureter/o	ureter	ureterolithotomy _____
		ureterostomy _____
		ureterectomy _____
		ureteral spasm _____
		ureterocystostomy _____
		_____
cyst/o	urinary bladder	cystitis _____
		nephrocystanastomosis _____
		_____
		cystourethrography _____
		_____
		cystoendoscopy _____
vesic/o	urinary bladder	vesicourethral junction _____
		_____
urethr/o	urethra	urethritis _____
		urethrospasm _____
dips/o	thirst	polydipsia _____
-uria	urination, urine	dysuria _____
		anuria _____

glycosuria _____

polyuria _____

phenylketonuria _____
(see vocabulary list)

_____

albumin/o	protein	albuminuria _____
		(proteinuria)
py/o	pus	pyuria _____
noct/i	night	nocturia _____
olig/o	scanty	oliguria _____
bacteri/o	bacteria	bacteriuria _____

VI. URINALYSIS

Urinalysis is an examination of urine to determine the presence of abnormal elements. It may also reveal the presence of diabetes mellitus, although diabetes mellitus is not a renal disease. (Diabetes mellitus is a disease of the endocrine gland cells within the pancreas.)

The following are some of the tests made in a urinalysis:

1. **Color**—Normal urine color is yellow or amber. The intensity of the color depends on the amount of water contained in the urine. A smoky red or brown color of urine is due to the presence of large amounts of blood.

2. **Reaction**—This is a test of the acidity or alkalinity of urine. Normal urine is slightly acid. However, in infections of the bladder the reaction of the urine may be alkaline because of the actions of bacteria within the urine which decompose the urea and release ammonia.

3. **Albumin**—Albumin is a protein normally found in the bloodstream and not in the urine. If it is detected in the urine (albuminuria), it may indicate an inflammation in the urinary tract or a leak in the glomerular membrane which allows albumin to enter the tubules and pass into the urine.

4. **Sugar**—Sugar is not normally found in the urine. In most cases when it does appear it indicates diabetes mellitus. In diabetes mellitus, because of malfunction of the pancreas, the hormone insulin is lacking in the bloodstream. The blood sugar level becomes very high because without insulin sugar cannot leave the blood to enter the cells. As sugar-filled blood passes through the kidney, the kidney tubules cannot reabsorb the high levels of sugar and sugar "spills over" into the urine (glycosuria).

5. **Specific gravity**—The specific gravity of urine reflects the amount of wastes, minerals, and solids in the urine. The urine of patients with diabetes mellitus has a higher than normal specific gravity because of the presence of sugar. In kidney diseases such as nephritis, the specific gravity of urine is low because water is unable to be reabsorbed by the tubules, and this dilutes the wastes and minerals in the urine.

6. **Ketone bodies** (acetone)—Ketone bodies are abnormal breakdown products from fat catabolism in cells. They accumulate in the blood and urine when fat, instead of sugar, is used as fuel. In diabetes mellitus, lack of insulin prevents sugar from reaching the body cells, and cells must use up their available fat for energy. Acetonuria (ketonuria) is a symptom, then, of diabetes mellitus.

Ketone bodies are quite dangerous if they accumulate in the body. Their presence can increase the acidity of the blood to the point at which the patient goes into coma (unconsciousness) and dies.

7. **Casts**—These are fibrous, or protein, materials which are thrown off into the urine in kidney disease. There are many forms of casts, determined by the material of which they are made. The casts are molded to the shape of the part of the kidney in which they are formed. There are pus casts, waxy casts, fatty casts, epithelial casts, blood casts, and so forth. Figure 8–6 illustrates some types of urinary casts.

8. **Pus**—Pyuria gives a cloudy, or turbid, appearance. Large numbers of polymorphonuclear leukocytes are present as well. Pyuria may be caused by infection in the kidney (pyelonephritis), cystitis, or stone in the kidney or bladder.

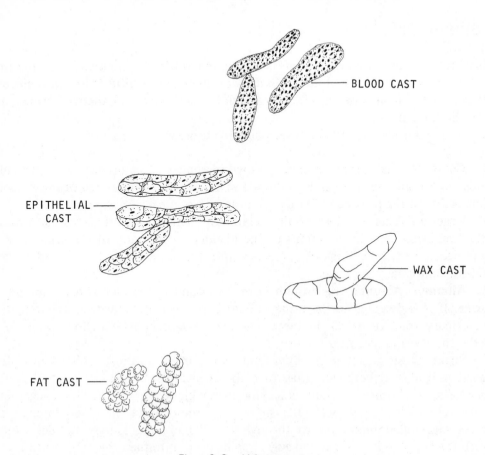

Figure 8–6   Urinary casts.

VII. PATHOLOGICAL TERMINOLOGY

glomerulonephritis   Inflammation of the kidney glomerulus.

This disease, also known as Bright's disease, affects both kidneys and causes destruction of the glomerular capillary walls. Protein, which normally is held in the bloodstream when blood passes through the glomerulus, now seeps through inflamed capillary walls and enters the urine (albuminuria). Other complications of the disease are elevated blood pressure and progressive renal failure (loss of kidney function) with retention of urea in the bloodstream (uremia). This may be fatal. Treatment of glomerulonephritis consists of drugs to control the inflammation, and dialysis or kidney transplant if uremia occurs.

pyelonephritis   Inflammation of the renal pelvis of the kidney.

This is the most common type of renal disease. It is caused by bacterial infection. Many small abscesses form in the kidney and these open out into the renal pelvis. Pyuria is found in urinalysis. If a large amount of kidney tissue is destroyed, the patient may develop renal failure and die of uremia. Treatment consists of antibiotics and surgical correction of any underlying obstruction to urine flow.

hypertension   Elevated blood pressure.

This condition may be the result of kidney disease (secondary hypertension) or may result from no apparent cause (essential hypertension). In the former case, blood flow within the kidney is decreased, owing to obstruction of a renal artery or kidney damage, and may result in the release of a substance called renin from the kidney. Renin can increase arterial blood pressure permanently. In essential hypertension, because of high blood pressure over many years, the arteriole walls become narrow and thickened (arteriosclerosis). The glomeruli then do not receive enough oxygen and they become ischemic, leading to atrophy and necrosis of kidney tissue.

nephrolithiasis   Condition of kidney stones.

Renal calculi (stones) are usually composed of uric acid or calcium salts. They form in the renal pelvis or the bladder, and their cause is relatively unknown. Poor diet, infection, and tumor of the parathyroid glands (which regulate calcium metabolism) may contribute to the formation of calculi. The result of nephrolithiasis may be obstruction of the kidney, ureter, or bladder, leading to increasing pressure behind the stone, which can contribute to hydronephrosis. If infection accompanies the blockage, pyelonephrosis may develop, as well as dilation of the renal pelvis and bladder. Treatment consists of relief of pain, medicine to relax the muscle of the tubes so that the stone may pass out, and intake of fluids to increase the urine flow. Surgical nephrolithotomy, pyelolithotomy, cystolithotomy, or ureterolithotomy may be indicated.

hydronephrosis
Enlargement and distention of the kidney due to block of urine outflow.

This condition can be caused by renal calculi, tumors, stricture of the ureter(s), or hypertrophy of the prostate (a gland at the base of the bladder in males). Surgical removal of obstruction may be indicated.

polycystic kidney
Multiple fluid-filled sacs (cysts) are formed within and upon the kidney.

This condition is also known as congenital cystic kidney. Small cysts may be present at birth or develop in the middle years of life, leading to nephromegaly. The cysts contain water, but may also include blood. Hemorrhage from renal vessels may occur and result in hematuria. A downhill clinical course includes hypertension, renal dysfunction, and uremia.

hypernephroma
Renal carcinoma occurring in adulthood.

This is the major cancerous tumor of the kidneys. It often metastasizes to the bone, blood, and lungs.

urinary retention
Blockage in the passage of urine from the bladder.

This condition can lead to enlargement of the bladder, infection, and kidney disease if left uncorrected.

Wilms' tumor
Tumor of the kidney occurring in childhood.

The tumor may be treated with surgery, radiation, and chemotherapy (drug treatment). There is a high percentage of cure with this tumor if it is treated before metastasis has occurred.

VIII. EXERCISES

A. Give the meaning of the following:

1. nephrorrhaphy _____

2. glomerulonephritis _____

3. nephrosis _____

4. renal ectopia _____

5. nephrolithiasis _____

6. pyeloplasty _____

7. nephrectomy _____

8. bilateral cortical renal necrosis _____

_____

9. renal hyperplasia _____

10. ureterosigmoidostomy _____

_____

B. *Build medical terms:*

1. Condition (abnormal) of water in the kidney _____

2. Bursting forth of blood from the kidney _____

3. Incision of the urinary bladder _____

4. Enlargement of the kidney _____

5. Painful urination _____

6. Pus in the urine _____

7. Dilation of the renal pelvis _____

8. Condition of hardening (of arteries) in the kidney _____

_____

9. Fixation of the kidney _____

10. Pain in the urethra _____

C. *Give the meaning of the following terms:*

1. hypoproteinemia _____

2. albuminuria _____

3. renal calculi _____

4. essential hypertension _____

5. uremia _____

6. hematuria _____

7. pyelonephritis _____

8. micturition _____

9. Wilms' tumor _____

10. caliectasis _____

11. polydipsia _____

12. antidiuretic hormone _____

_____

13. phenylketonuria _____

14. casts _____

15. ketonuria _____

16. Bowman's capsule _____

17. dialysis _____

_____

18. renal ischemia _____

19. oliguria _____

20. specific gravity _____

_____

D. *Give the names of the major structures that are involved in the urinary process from the point at which blood enters the glomerulus from the renal arterioles in the cortex of the kidney:*

1. _____*glomerulus*_____   4. _____

2. _____   5. _____

3. _____   6. _____

7. _____   8. _____

E. *Give the meaning of the following combining forms:*

1. noct/i   _____   6. pyel/o   _____

2. albumin/o _____   7. py/o   _____

3. vesic/o   _____   8. azot/o   _____

4. cortic/o   _____   9. olig/o   _____

5. cali/o   _____   10. cyst/o   _____

ANSWERS

A. 1. Suture of the kidney.
2. Inflammation of the glomerulus and the kidney.
3. Abnormal condition of the kidney.
4. Displacement of the kidney.
5. Abnormal condition of kidney stones.
6. Surgical repair of the renal pelvis.
7. Removal of the kidney.
8. Death of the cortex region in both kidneys.
9. Excessive development, or growth, of the kidney(s).
10. New opening between the ureter and the sigmoid colon (anastomosis).

B. 1. hydronephrosis
2. nephrorrhagia
3. cystotomy
4. nephromegaly
5. dysuria
6. pyuria
7. pyelectasis
8. nephrosclerosis
9. nephropexy
10. urethralgia or urethrodynia

C. 1. Deficient protein in the blood; common in glomerulonephritis.
2. Albumin (protein) in the urine.
3. Stones in the kidney.
4. High blood pressure in the kidney due to no apparent cause.
5. Urine (urea) in the blood.
6. Blood in the urine.
7. Inflammation of the renal pelvis and kidney.
8. Urination.
9. Malignant tumor of the kidney, occurring in childhood.
10. Dilation of the calyces of the renal pelvis.
11. Excessive thirst.
12. Hormone secreted by the pituitary gland in the brain; causes the kidney tubules to hold back water and produce less urine.
13. Phenylketones in the urine.
14. Molds of parts of the urinary system; they are found in the urine and named for the substance of which they are composed.
15. Acetone or ketone bodies in the urine.
16. Capsule under each glomerulus; collects filtered materials from the blood.
17. Literally means "complete separation"–it is a method of removing the toxic materials from the blood when the kidneys have failed.

18. Condition of holding back blood from the cells of the kidney.
19. Scanty urine flow.
20. A determination of the amount of wastes, minerals, and solids in the urine.

D.
1. glomerulus
2. Bowman's capsule
3. renal tubules
4. renal pelvis
5. ureter
6. bladder
7. urethra
8. urinary meatus

E.
1. night
2. protein
3. bladder
4. cortex (outer section)
5. calyces
6. renal pelvis
7. pus
8. urea, nitrogen
9. scanty
10. urinary bladder

REVIEW SHEET 8

Combining Forms

albumin/o	_____	necr/o	_____
azot/o	_____	nephr/o	_____
bacteri/o	_____	noct/i	_____
cali/o	_____	olig/o	_____
cortic/o	_____	py/o	_____
cyst/o	_____	pyel/o	_____
dips/o	_____	ren/o	_____
glomerul/o	_____	tox/o	_____
glyc/o	_____	ur/o	_____
glycos/o	_____	ureter/o	_____
hydr/o	_____	urethr/o	_____
medull/o	_____	vesic/o	_____

Suffixes

-cele	_____	-orrhagia	_____
-ectasis	_____	-orrhaphy	_____
-lithiasis	_____	-orrhea	_____
-lithotomy	_____	-orrhexis	_____
-lysis	_____	-ostomy	_____
-megaly	_____	-otomy	_____
-ole	_____	-pexy	_____

-ptosis _____   -stasis _____

-sclerosis _____   -ule _____

-spasm _____   -uria _____

Prefixes

a, an _____   en _____

anti _____   poly _____

dia _____   retro _____

dys _____

Match the urinary system structure in Column I with its location or function in Column II:

Column I	Column II

1. urethra   _____   Tiny structure surrounding each glomerulus; receives filtered materials from blood.

2. cortex

3. Bowman's capsule   _____   Tubes carrying urine from kidney to urinary bladder.

4. calyces   _____   Tubules leading from Bowman's capsule. Urine is formed there as water, sugar, and salts are reabsorbed into the bloodstream.

5. renal pelvis

6. glomerulus

7. medulla   _____   Inner (middle) region of the kidney.

8. renal tubules   _____   Muscular sac which serves as a reservoir for urine.

9. urinary bladder   _____   Cuplike divisions of the renal pelvis which receive urine from the renal tubules.

10. ureters

        _____   Tube carrying urine from the bladder to the outside of the body.

        _____   Central urine-collecting basin in the kidney which narrows into the ureter.

_____   Collection of capillaries through which materials from the blood are filtered into Bowman's capsule.

_____   Outer region of the kidney.

Additional Terms

acetone _____

albumin _____

antidiuretic hormone (ADH) _____

calculus _____

cast _____

catheter _____

creatinine _____

diabetes insipidus _____

diabetes mellitus _____

enuresis _____

essential hypertension _____

excretion _____

hemodialysis _____

hypernephroma _____

intravenous pyelogram (IVP) _____

ketone bodies _____

meatus _____

micturition _____

nitrogenous wastes _____

peritoneal dialysis _____

phenylketonuria (PKU) _____

polycystic kidney _____

renin _____

retention _____

retrograde pyelogram _____

secondary hypertension _____

specific gravity _____

stricture _____

suppuration _____

urea _____

uric acid _____

Wilms' tumor _____

CHAPTER 9

FEMALE REPRODUCTIVE SYSTEM

In this chapter you will:

Learn the terms to describe the structures which are part of the female reproductive system;

Understand how these structures and their various hormones function in the processes of menstruation and pregnancy;

Be able to use the new combining forms, suffixes, and prefixes related to the female reproductive system to build medical terms; and

Learn the terms and descriptions for some of the major diseases of the female reproductive system.

The chapter is divided into the following sections:

I. INTRODUCTION

Sexual reproduction is the union of the female sex cell (ovum) and the male sex cell (sperm) which results in the creation of a new individual. The ovum and sperm cell are specialized cells differing primarily from normal body cells in one important way.

153

Each sex cell (also called a **gamete**) contains exactly half the number of chromosomes that a normal body cell contains. When the ovum and sperm cell unite, the cell produced receives half of its genetic material from its female parent, and half from its male parent; thus it contains a full, normal complement of hereditary material.

Sex cells are produced in special organs called **gonads** in the male and female. The female gonads are the **ovaries**, and the male gonads are the **testes**. The union (also called **fertilization**) of the male and female sex cells in humans takes place within the female body. **Copulation** (meaning "to couple") is the act whereby the male deposits sperm cells within the duct in the female through which an ovum (egg cell) emerges. If fertilization takes place, the new cell formed begins a nine-month period of development within the **uterus** (womb) of the female.

This chapter discusses the terminology related to the female reproductive system, and the next is devoted to the male reproductive system.

The female reproductive system consists of organs which produce ova and provide a place for the growth of the embryo. In addition, the female reproductive organs supply important hormones that contribute to the development of female secondary sex characteristics (body hair, breast development, structural changes in bones and fat).

Ova are produced by the ovary from the onset of **puberty** (beginning of the fertile period when secondary sex characteristics develop) to **menopause** (cessation of fertility and diminishing of hormone production). If fertilization occurs at any time during the years between puberty and menopause, the fertilized egg may grow and develop within the uterus. Various hormones are secreted from the ovary and from a blood-vessel-filled organ (**placenta**) which grows in the wall of the uterus during pregnancy. If fertilization does not occur, hormone changes result in the shedding of the uterine lining, ând bleeding, or **menstruation**, occurs. The interactions of hormones in pregnancy and menstruation will be discussed in detail in a later section of this chapter.

The names of the hormones which play important roles in the processes of menstruation and pregnancy, and in the development of secondary sex characteristics, are **estrogen** and **progesterone**. Other hormones which govern the functions of the ovary, breast, and uterus are secreted by the anterior lobe of the pituitary gland, which is located behind the bridge of the nose in the anterior portion of the brain.

II. VOCABULARY

amnion	Membrane which lies closest to developing embryo.
anteflexion	A turning forward. The uterus is normally ante-flexed.
Bartholin's glands	Small glands at the vaginal orifice which secrete lubricating fluid into the vagina.
areola	Dark-pigmented area around the nipple of the breast.
cauterization	The process of burning tissue in order to stop bleeding or remove diseased tissue.

chorion	Outermost layer of the two protective layers which surround the embryo.
clitoris	Organ of sensitive erectile tissue anterior to the urinary opening.
contraception	Any method used to prevent fertilization of the egg and, thus, pregnancy.
corpus luteum (yellow body)	Glandular tissue formed in the ovary within the empty egg sac; produces the hormone progesterone.
cul-de-sac	Region of the abdomen midway between the rectum and uterus.
curettage	Scraping a surface using a spoon-shaped instrument called a curette.
dilation	A widening and opening of a channel or tube; dilatation.
egg cell	Ovum; female sex cell.
embryo	Stage in prenatal development from fertilization of the egg through its second month.
estrogen	Hormone produced by the ovaries; responsible for secondary sex characteristics and development of reproductive organs.
fallopian tubes	Hornlike tubes through which the egg travels into the uterus.
fertilization	Union of sperm and egg cell.
fetus	Developing individual from third month to birth.
fimbriae	Finger-like ends of the fallopian tube near the ovary.
follicle-stimulating hormone (FSH)	Hormone produced by the anterior lobe of the pituitary gland; stimulates maturation of the egg in ovary.
gamete	Sex cell; sperm or egg cell.
genitalia	Internal and external reproductive organs.

gonads	Organs in male and female which produce sex cells; testes and ovaries.
graafian follicle	Sac within the ovary which contains the ovum and produces a hormone (estrogen).
human chorionic gonadotropin (HCG)	A hormone produced by the placenta during pregnancy; its presence in the bloodstream is the basis for a positive pregnancy test.
intrauterine device (IUD)	A mechanical device inserted into the uterus and used as a means of contraception.
labia	Lips; the labia majora and labia minora are the lips surrounding the vaginal and urethral orifices.
ligament	Band of connective tissue.
luteinizing hormone (LH)	Hormone produced by the anterior lobe of the pituitary gland. It promotes the growth and functioning of the corpus luteum in the ovary.
menopause	End of the fertile period in the female; associated with diminishing hormone production.
menstruation (menses = month)	A periodic (monthly) shedding of the lining of the uterus, associated with bleeding and, for some, abdominal cramps.
mucinous	Full of mucin (a protein substance in mucus).
negative feedback	Signals sent back to the place of origin of substances so as to reduce production.
orifice	An opening.
ovaries	Pair of almond-shaped organs in the lower abdomen; they produce ova and hormones associated with female reproduction and secondary sex characteristics.
ovulation	Rupture of the graafian follicle and release of ovum into the fallopian tube.
ovum (plural: ova)	Egg cell.
Pap smear	Test to detect cancerous changes in cells of the uterus and cervix.

parturition	Act of giving birth.
perineum	Area between the anus and vagina in the female.
placenta	Spongelike vascular organ which develops during pregnancy in the uterine wall and serves as a communication between the bloodstream of the fetus and that of the mother. The placenta also secretes hormones which are important in sustaining pregnancy.
progesterone	Hormone produced by the corpus luteum and the placenta; important in sustaining pregnancy.
puberty	Beginning of the fertile period in males and females when secondary sex characteristics develop.
serous	Pertaining to serum.
sinus	A cavity.
spermatozoon	Sperm cell.
sperm cell	Male reproductive cell.
uterus	Pear-shaped muscular organ in pelvic cavity in which embryo develops; also called the womb.
vulva	External genitalia of the female, including the lips of the vagina and perineum.

III. MAJOR ORGANS OF THE FEMALE REPRODUCTIVE SYSTEM

Uterus, Ovaries, and Associated Organs

Figures 9–1 and 9–2 should be labeled as you read and study the following paragraphs.

Figure 9–1 is a lateral view of the female reproductive organs and shows their relationship to the other organs in the pelvic cavity. The **ovaries** (1) (only one ovary is shown in this lateral view) are a pair of small almond-shaped organs located in the lower abdomen. The **fallopian tubes** (2) (only one is shown in this view) lead from each ovary to the **uterus** (3), which is a muscular organ situated between the urinary bladder and the rectum and midway between the sacrum and the pubic bone. The uterus is normally in a position of anteflexion (bent forward). Midway between the uterus and the rectum is a region in the abdominal cavity known as the **cul-de-sac** (4). This region is often examined for the presence of cancerous growths.

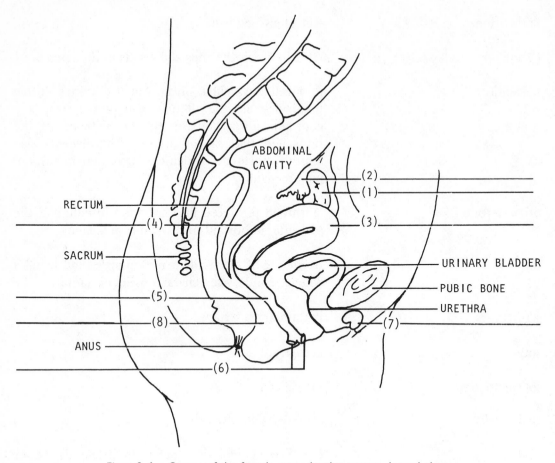

Figure 9-1 Organs of the female reproductive system, lateral view.

The **vagina** (5) is a muscular tube extending from the uterus to the exterior of the body. **Bartholin's glands** (6) are two small, rounded glands on either side of the vaginal orifice. These glands produce a mucous secretion which lubricates the vagina. The **clitoris** (7) is an organ of sensitive, erectile tissue located anterior to the vaginal orifice and in front of the urethral meatus. The clitoris is homologous with the penis in the male.

The region between the vaginal orifice and the anus is called the **perineum** (8). This region, at the floor of the pelvic cavity, may be torn in childbirth, resulting in damage to the urinary meatus and the anus. To avoid a perineal tear, the obstetrician often cuts the perineum before delivery.

Figure 9–2 is an anterior view of the female reproductive system. The **ovaries** (1) are held in place on either side of the uterus by the **utero-ovarian ligaments** (2) and are protected by a surrounding mass of fat.

Within each ovary are thousands of small sacs called **graafian follicles** (3). Each graafian follicle contains an **ovum** (4). When an ovum is mature, the graafian follicle ruptures to the surface and the ovum leaves the ovary. The release of the ovum from the ovary is called **ovulation**. The ruptured follicle fills first with blood, and then with a yellow fatlike material. It is then called the **corpus luteum** (5) (meaning "yellow body").

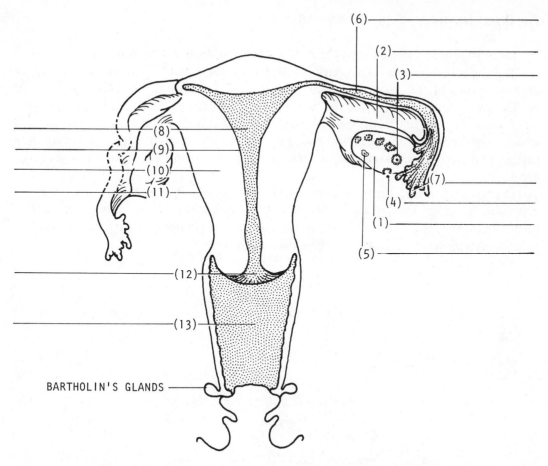

Figure 9-2 Organs of the female reproductive system, anterior view.

Near each ovary is a duct, about 5½ inches long, called a **fallopian tube** (6). The egg, after its release from the ovary, is caught up by the finger-like ends of the fallopian tube. These ends are called **fimbriae** (7). The tube itself is lined with small hairs which, through their motion, sweep the ovum along. It usually takes the ovum about five days to pass through the fallopian tube.

It is within the fallopian tube that fertilization takes place if any sperm cells are around. If copulation takes place near the time of ovulation and no contraception is used, there is a likelihood that sperm cells will be in the fallopian tube when the egg cell is passing through. If copulation has not taken place, the ovum remains unfertilized and, after a day or two of waiting, dies.

The fallopian tubes, one on either side, lead into the **uterus** (8), a pear-shaped organ with muscular walls and a mucous membrane lining filled with a rich supply of blood vessels. The specialized epithelial mucosa of the uterus is called the **endometrium** (9); the middle, muscular layer is the **myometrium** (10); and the outer, membranous tissue layer is the **perimetrium** (11).

The narrow, lower portion of the uterus is called the **cervix** (12) (meaning "neck"). The cervical opening leads into a 3-inch-long tube called the **vagina** (13), which opens to the outside of the body. The external genitalia (reproductive organs) of the female are called the **vulva**. This includes two sets of vaginal lips (**labia majora** and **labia minora**), clitoris, perineum, and the vaginal and urethral orifices.

The Breast *(Accessory Organ of Reproduction)*

Label Figure 9–3 as you read the following description of breast structures.

The breasts are two mammary (milk-producing) glands located in the upper anterior region of the chest. They are composed of **glandular tissue** (1) which develops in response to hormones from the ovaries during puberty. The breasts also contain **fatty tissue** (2), special **lactiferous** (milk-carrying) **ducts** (3), and **sinuses** (cavities) (4) which carry milk to the opening, or nipple. The breast nipple is called the **mammary papilla** (5), and the dark-pigmented area around the mammary papilla is called the **areola** (6).

During pregnancy, the hormones from the ovaries and the placenta stimulate glandular tissue in the breasts to their full development. After parturition (giving birth), hormones from the pituitary gland and adrenal glands stimulate the production of milk (lactation) and its ejection from the breast.

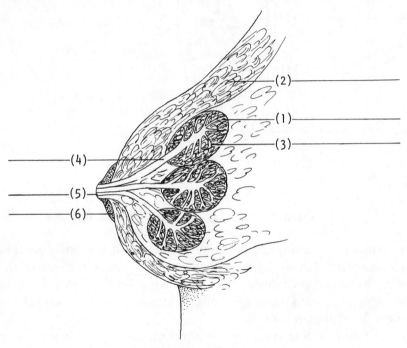

Figure 9–3   The breast.

IV. TERMINOLOGY OF MENSTRUATION AND PREGNANCY

Menstrual Cycle

The menstrual cycle is divided into 28 days. These days can be grouped into four time periods, which are useful in describing the events of the cycle. The time periods are:

Days 1–5
(Menstrual Period)

These are the days during which bloody fluid containing disintegrated endometrial cells, glandular secretions, and blood cells is discharged through the vagina.

Days 6–13
(Postmenstrual Period)

After the menstrual period is ended, the lining of the uterus begins to repair itself as the hormone estrogen is released by the maturing graafian follicle in the ovaries. This is also the period of the growth of the ovum in the graafian follicle.

Days 13–14
(Ovulatory Period)

On about the 14th day of the cycle, the graafian follicle ruptures (ovulation) and the egg leaves the ovary to travel slowly down the fallopian tube.

Days 15–28
(Premenstrual Period)

The empty graafian follicle fills with a yellow material and becomes known as the **corpus luteum**. The corpus luteum functions as an endocrine organ and secretes two hormones, **estrogen** and **progesterone**, into the bloodstream. These hormones build up the lining of the uterus in anticipation of fertilization of the egg and pregnancy.

If fertilization does **not** occur, the corpus luteum in the ovary stops producing progesterone and estrogen and regresses. The fall in levels of progesterone and estrogen leads to the breakdown of the uterine endometrium and a new menstrual cycle begins (days 1–5).

Pregnancy

If fertilization does occur in the fallopian tube, the fertilized egg travels to the uterus and implants in the uterine endometrium. The corpus luteum in the ovary continues to produce progesterone and estrogen which support the vascular and muscular development of the uterine lining.

The **placenta**, which is the organ of communication between the mother and embryo, now forms within the uterine wall. The placenta is derived from maternal endometrium and partly from the **chorion**, a membrane which surrounds the developing embryo. The **amnion** is the innermost of the embryonic membranes, and it holds the fetus suspended in an amniotic cavity surrounded by a fluid called the **amniotic fluid**. At no time during pregnancy do the maternal blood and fetal blood mix, but important nutrients, oxygen, and waste products are exchanged as the maternal and fetal circulations pass in close proximity to each other within the placenta.

From the third month of pregnancy onward, the placenta produces its own hormone, **human chorionic gonadotropin** (HCG), which stimulates the ovary to continue to produce progesterone and estrogen.

Figure 9–4 shows the embryo, its placenta, and the membranes which surround it in the uterus.

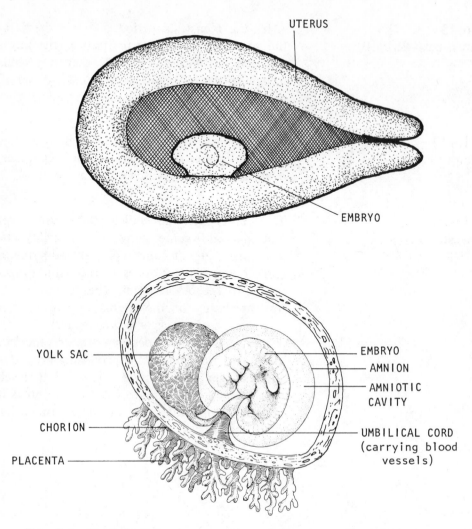

Figure 9-4   The embryo, its placenta, and membranes surrounding it in the uterus.

V. HORMONAL INTERACTIONS

As we have seen in the previous discussion of the menstrual cycle and pregnancy, the building up and breaking down of the lining of the uterus is dependent on the level of hormones from the ovary (estrogen and progesterone). These hormones from the ovary, however, are under the influence of other hormones from the anterior lobe of the pituitary gland.

One hormone from the anterior lobe of the pituitary gland is called **follicle-stimulating hormone (FSH)**. FSH travels from the pituitary gland, through the bloodstream, to the ovary, where it stimulates the graafian follicle to ripen and the ova to mature. In addition, FSH stimulates the graafian follicles to produce the hormone estrogen.

Estrogen, released into the bloodstream from the ovaries, travels back to the anterior lobe of the pituitary gland and causes that organ to produce another hormone called **luteinizing hormone (LH)**. LH in the bloodstream encourages the release of the egg from the follicle (ovulation) and promotes the formation and maintenance of the corpus luteum, which begins to produce estrogen and progesterone after ovulation.

If pregnancy occurs, the corpus luteum is maintained and the level of progesterone and estrogen in the bloodstream increases under the influence of **human chorionic gonadotropin (HCG)**, a hormone produced by the placenta. The **high level** of estrogen and progesterone in the bloodstream "turns off" the secretion of FSH by the anterior lobe of the pituitary. This effect (high levels of chemicals limiting the level of another chemical) is called **negative feedback**. Without FSH secretion, ovulation ceases and new eggs are not released during pregnancy.

Birth control pills, which contain varying levels of estrogen and progesterone, produce a condition which mimics pregnancy. These hormones thus block FSH secretion, and ovulation is suppressed. Another contraceptive mechanism, the intrauterine device (IUD), is a coil which is placed in the uterus, preventing implantation of the fertilized egg.

If pregnancy does not occur, the ovum dies and no placenta is formed. Hormone secretions (estrogen and progesterone) by the corpus luteum abruptly fall, stimulating increased FSH production, and a new ovulation begins.

Study Figure 9–5 to review the interactions of hormones in menstruation and pregnancy.

VI. COMBINING FORMS AND TERMINOLOGY

Combining Form	Meaning	Terminology	Meaning
oophor/o	ovary	oophorectomy	_____
		oophoropexy	_____
		oophoritis	_____
oo/o	egg	oocyte	_____
ovari/o	ovary	ovariorrhexis	_____
ov/o	egg	ovum	_____
		ovogenesis	_____
		ovulation	_____
salping/o	fallopian tubes, oviducts	salpingostomy	_____
		salpingitis	_____

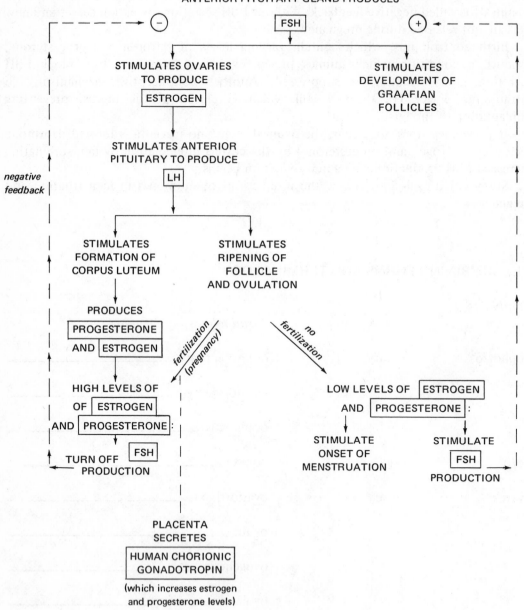

PITUITARY HORMONES ARE:
FSH = FOLLICLE-STIMULATING HORMONE
LH = LUTEINIZING HORMONE

OVARIAN HORMONES ARE:
ESTROGEN
PROGESTERONE

ANTERIOR PITUITARY GLAND PRODUCES

FSH

STIMULATES OVARIES TO PRODUCE

ESTROGEN

STIMULATES DEVELOPMENT OF GRAAFIAN FOLLICLES

STIMULATES ANTERIOR PITUITARY TO PRODUCE

LH

negative feedback

STIMULATES FORMATION OF CORPUS LUTEUM

STIMULATES RIPENING OF FOLLICLE AND OVULATION

PRODUCES

PROGESTERONE
AND ESTROGEN

fertilization (pregnancy)

no fertilization

HIGH LEVELS OF OF ESTROGEN
AND PROGESTERONE :

TURN OFF PRODUCTION FSH

LOW LEVELS OF ESTROGEN
AND PROGESTERONE :

STIMULATE ONSET OF MENSTRUATION

STIMULATE FSH PRODUCTION

PLACENTA SECRETES

HUMAN CHORIONIC GONADOTROPIN

(which increases estrogen and progesterone levels)

Figure 9–5   Interaction of hormones in menstruation and pregnancy.

		salpingocele _____
		salpingo-oophorectomy _____
-salpinx *(as a suffix)*	fallopian tubes	pyosalpinx _____
		hematosalpinx _____
		hydrosalpinx _____
hyster/o	uterus, womb	hysterectomy _____
		hysterorrhexis _____
		hysteropexy _____
		panhysterosalpingo-oophorectomy _____
		_____
uter/o	uterus	uterine _____
metr/o, metri/o	uterus	metrorrhagia _____
		endometriosis _____
		pyometrium _____
my/o	muscle	myometrium _____
cervic/o	cervix, neck	cervicitis _____
		endocervicitis _____
bartholin/o	Bartholin's glands	bartholinitis _____
vagin/o	vagina	vaginal _____
		vaginitis _____
colp/o	vagina	colporrhaphy _____
		colposcope _____
		colpohysterectomy _____
culd/o	cul-de-sac	culdoscopy _____

perine/o	perineum	colpo<u>perine</u>oplasty _____
		_____
episi/o	vulva	<u>episi</u>otomy _____
vulv/o	vulva	<u>vulv</u>outerine _____
		<u>vulv</u>ovaginitis _____
men/o	menses, menstruation	a<u>men</u>orrhea _____
		dys<u>men</u>orrhea _____
		<u>men</u>orrhagia _____
		oligo<u>men</u>orrhea _____
chori/o	chorion	<u>chori</u>ocarcinoma _____
amni/o	amnion	<u>amni</u>ocentesis _____
		<u>amni</u>otic fluid _____
mamm/o	breast	<u>mamm</u>ary _____
mast/o	breast	<u>mast</u>ectomy _____
lact/o	milk	<u>lact</u>ation _____
gravid/o	pregnancy	<u>gravid</u>ism _____
		grav. 1, 2, 3, 4 _____
-para	to bear, bring forth, live births	uni<u>para</u> (para 1) _____
		multi<u>para</u> _____
		nulli<u>para</u> (para 0) _____
		bi<u>para</u> (para 2) _____
-tocia	labor, birth	dys<u>tocia</u> _____
		brady<u>tocia</u> _____
-cyesis	pregnancy	pseudo<u>cyesis</u> _____

-arche   beginning   men<u>arche</u> _____

VI. PATHOLOGICAL CONDITIONS

endocervicitis   Inflammation of the inner lining of the cervix.

The mucous membrane lining the cervix (endocervix) is the site of chronic inflammation in this condition. Because the lining of the cervix is not swept away each month, as is the endometrium of the uterus during menstruation, it can be the location of infection for long periods of time. Two different classes of bacteria may be responsible for the infection: staphylococci, streptococci, or other pyogenic bacteria; and gonococci, which are the cause of gonorrhea.

If the cervix is injured during delivery of the fetus, chronic bacterial infection may result. Cervical erosions, or ulcers, may form from endocervicitis, and this is characterized by the appearance of raw, red patches on the cervical mucosa. Leukorrhea, which is the discharge of white or yellow mucoid substance, is a symptom of endocervicitis and cervical erosion. Because this lesion may prove to be a precancerous lesion, it is treated with antibiotics and the erosion is removed by electrocauterization (burning to remove diseased tissue).

ectopic pregnancy   Pregnancy which is not in the uterus.

Ninety-five per cent of ectopic pregnancies occur in the fallopian tubes. Other sites of implantation may be the ligaments surrounding the uterus or the surface of the ovary. Chronic salpingitis and benign tubal tumors may be other factors leading to ectopic implantation. Ectopic pregnancies usually terminate by rupture of the placenta and its detachment from the walls of the fallopian tube, with massive hemorrhage into the tube (hematosalpinx). Surgery is indicated to remove the fetus and perform a salpingectomy.

ovarian cysts   Collections of fluid or solid material within a sac in the ovary.

Ovarian cysts may be of two types: One type is formed from graafian follicles and is called a follicular cyst; another type is called a cystadenoma and is really a benign tumor. Resection of ovarian cystadenomas is advisable because it is difficult to distinguish benign from malignant cystic tumors without pathological examination.

cystadenocarcinoma of the ovary   Malignant tumor of the ovary.

This tumor is often discovered as a large, round mass which is composed of tumor cells lining large fluid-filled spaces. The tumor may be **serous** (producing a clear, thin fluid resembling serum), or may be **mucinous** (producing a thick, mucoid fluid resembling mucus).

breast carcinoma   Malignant tumor of the breast.

      This tumor may spread to the skin, chest wall, and commonly to the lymph nodes located in the axilla (armpits) adjacent to the affected breast. From the lymph nodes it may spread to any of the other body organs, including bone, liver, lung, or brain. The tumor is usually removed for purposes of diagnosis and as a primary means of treatment. There is considerable controversy about what type of operation is indicated. For small lumps in the breast with no lymph node enlargement detected, a **lumpectomy** is performed. This involves removal of the lump and some adjacent tissue. Other surgeons prefer to perform a **simple mastectomy**, which is removal of all the breast tissue but not of lymph nodes. Probably the most common operation performed is the **radical mastectomy**, in which the breast, pectoral (chest) muscles, and the contents of the axilla are removed completely. The latter operation provides more complete information about the extent of spread of the tumor and aids in the planning of further therapy. For example, if the tumor is found in the axillary lymph nodes, then further therapy with drugs or radiation or both is indicated and cure of the patient is still possible.

pelvic inflammatory disease   Inflammation in the pelvic region.
  (P.I.D.)

      This general condition is usually used to refer to salpingitis, but many physicians use it to include other problems, such as cervicitis, endometritis, and oophoritis. Symptoms are vaginal discharge, pain in the LLQ and RLQ in early stages, and dysmenorrhea, metrorrhagia, and severe tenderness on palpation (process of examining by touch). The etiology of P.I.D. is commonly gonococcal infection. Penicillin is the preferred therapeutic agent.

fibroids   Benign tumors in the uterus.

      Fibroids are composed of fibrous tissue and muscle. If they grow too large and cause symptoms such as metrorrhagia, pelvic pain, or menorrhagia, hysterectomy or myomectomy is indicated.

carcinoma of the uterus and   Malignant tumor of the uterus and cervix.
cervix

      Early detection is important in this malignant pathological condition. Smears made from the cervix can show the presence of exfoliated cancer cells. Exfoliation refers to the scraping off of tissue (folio = leaf). The cells are examined under the microscope and evidence of cellular change is noted (in size and shape, nuclei, and cytoplasmic growth). This test is called the Papanicolaou test, or Pap smear.

dilation and curettage (D & C)   Dilating and scraping the lining of the uterus.

> This is not a pathological condition, but is a procedure which may be done following abortion to remove fragments of retained placenta; to correct menstrual irregularity; to remove growths such as polyps; or to diagnose cancer of the uterus or fallopian tubes. Dilation is first accomplished by inserting a series of probes of increasing size into the cervix; the uterus is then scraped with a curette, which is a metal loop on the end of a long, thin handle.

VII. EXERCISES

A. *Build medical words:*

1. Muscular layer of the uterus _____

2. Rupture of the uterus _____

3. Fixation of an ovary _____

4. Suture of the area between the anus and vagina _____

5. Bursting forth of blood during menses _____

6. Abnormal condition of the inner lining of the uterus _____

    _____

7. Inflammation of fallopian tubes (both sides) _____

8. Pus in the uterine tubes _____

9. Removal of the uterus, fallopian tubes, and ovaries _____

    _____

10. Suture of the vagina and the vulva _____

11. Incision of the cervix _____

12. Slow delivery or labor _____

13. Inflammation of the breast _____

14. Pertaining to producing milk _____

15. False pregnancy _____

16. Beginning of menstruation _____

17. Inflammation of the inner lining of the cervix _____

18. Scanty menstrual flow _____

19. Egg cell _____

20. New opening in the fallopian tubes _____

B. *Give the meaning of the following:*

1. D & C _____

2. graafian follicle _____

3. para II _____

4. P.I.D. _____

5. fibroids _____

6. LH _____

   _____

7. grav. III _____

8. cystadenoma _____

9. ectopic pregnancy _____

10. FSH _____

    _____

11. placenta _____

    _____

12. estrogen _____

    _____

13. HCG _____

14. culdocentesis _____

15. gonads _____

16. radical mastectomy _____

17. anteflexion _____

18. areola _____

19. gamete _____

20. clitoris _____

C. *Match the process with its correct meaning:*

1. parturition   _____   Burning to seal tissue.

2. micturition   _____   Monthly discharge of blood, regulated by
                                  hormones.
3. deglutition
                      _____   Urination.
4. fertilization
                      _____   Giving birth.
5. cauterization
                      _____   Producing milk.
6. menstruation
                      _____   Swallowing.
7. lactation
                      _____   Union of egg and sperm.

D. *Match the structure with its location:*

1. fimbriae   _____   Innermost membrane layer of embryo.

2. Bartholin's glands _____   Ovarian opening of fallopian tubes.

3. chorion   _____   Middle layer of tissue in uterus.

4. corpus luteum   _____   Outermost membrane layer surrounding
                                  embryo connected to placenta.
5. myometrium
                      _____   Within the ovary.
6. amnion
                      _____   On each side of the vaginal meatus.
7. perineum
                      _____   Area between the vulva and the anus.

ANSWERS

A.
1. myometrium
2. hysterorrhexis
3. oophoropexy
4. perineorrhaphy
5. menorrhagia
6. endometriosis (parts of the endometrium are found in various sites in the pelvic cavity)
7. bilateral salpingitis
8. pyosalpinx
9. hysterosalpingo-oophorectomy
10. colpoepisiorrhaphy
11. cervicotomy
12. bradytocia
13. mastitis
14. lactogenic
15. pseudocyesis
16. menarche (pronounced men-ar'kē)·
17. endocervicitis
18. oligomenorrhea
19. oocyte
20. salpingostomy

B.
1. Dilation and curettage (scraping).
2. Sac in the ovary in which the ovum grows and matures.
3. Woman having given birth to two live infants.
4. Pelvic inflammatory disease.
5. Resembling fibers; benign tumor in the uterus or breast.
6. **Luteinizing hormone**; produced by the anterior pituitary gland, and stimulates the graafian follicle (in the ovary) to rupture and ovulation to occur. (Also, this hormone stimulates the formation and continuation of the corpus luteum in the ovary.)
7. Woman who has had three pregnancies.
8. Glandular tumor containing cysts or sacs of fluid—usually benign.
9. Implantation of the embryo in a place other than uterine wall, e.g., fallopian tubes, ovary, ligaments.
10. **Follicle-stimulating hormone**; produced by the anterior lobe of the pituitary gland; stimulates the ovaries to produce estrogen and the ovum to ripen in the graafian follicle.
11. Structure within the uterus, composed of blood vessels, which provides the necessary communication between mother and fetus for food and oxygen and waste removal.
12. Hormone produced by the ovaries which is responsible for secondary sex characteristics in females and for the building up and sustaining of the endometrium and placenta during pregnancy.
13. **Human chorionic gonadotropin**; a hormone produced by the placenta during pregnancy.
14. Surgical puncture of the cul-de-sac.
15. Organs in the male and female which produce sex cells (sperm and egg).
16. Removal of breast, pectoral muscles, and contents of the axilla for breast carcinoma.
17. Forward bending; the normal position of the uterus in the pelvic cavity.
18. Dark-pigmented area around the nipple of the breast.
19. Sperm or egg cell.
20. Sensitive, erectile tissue of the external female genitalia.

C. 5
6
2
1
7
3
4

D. 6
1
5
3
4
2
7

REVIEW SHEET 9

Combining Forms

amni/o	_____	metr/o	_____
bartholin/o	_____	metri/o	_____
cervic/o	_____	my/o	_____
chori/o	_____	olig/o	_____
colp/o	_____	oo/o	_____
culd/o	_____	oophor/o	_____
episi/o	_____	ov/o	_____
fibr/o	_____	ovari/o	_____
fibros/o	_____	perine/o	_____
gravid/o	_____	peritone/o	_____
gynec/o	_____	py/o	_____
hyster/o	_____	salping/o	_____
lact/o	_____	uter/o	_____
mamm/o	_____	vagin/o	_____
mast/o	_____	vulv/o	_____
men/o	_____		

Suffixes

_____ bursting forth of blood.

_____ surgical repair.

_____ suture.

_____ prolapse.

_____ dilation, dilatation.

_____ narrowing, tightening.

_____ flow, discharge.   _____ hernia.

_____ rupture.   _____ to bear, to bring forth.

_____ incision.   _____ labor, birth.

_____ new opening.   _____ pregnancy.

_____ fixation, put in place.   _____ fallopian tube.

Prefixes

uni   _____   nulli   _____

bi   _____   endo   _____

brady   _____   pan   _____

dys   _____   peri   _____

multi   _____   pseudo   _____

Additional Terms

amnion   _____

areola   _____

chorion   _____

corpus luteum   _____

cul-de-sac   _____

embryo   _____

estrogen   _____

fetus   _____

follicle-stimulating hormone (FSH)   _____

gamete   _____

genitalia   _____

gonads _____

graafian follicle _____

grav. 0, 1, 2, 3, etc. _____

human chorionic gonadotropin (HCG) _____

intrauterine device (IUD) _____

luteinizing hormone (LH) _____

menarche _____

menopause _____

negative feedback _____

ovum _____

para 0, 1, 2, 3, etc. _____

placenta _____

progesterone _____

puberty _____

Match the female genital organ in Column I with its location or function in Column II:

Column I	Column II
1. ovaries	_____ Finger-like ends of the fallopian tube near the ovary.
2. vagina	_____ Lips surrounding the vaginal and urethral orifices.
3. fallopian tubes	
4. uterus	_____ The female gonads; located in the lower abdomen.
5. perineum	_____ Muscular organ between the urinary bladder and rectum.
6. fimbriae	
7. clitoris	_____ Secrete a lubricating fluid into the vagina.

8. labia majora and minora _____ Muscular tube extending from the uterus to the exterior of the body.

9. Bartholin's glands

_____ Sensitive erectile tissue anterior to the urethral orifice.

_____ Hornlike tubes through which the egg travels to the uterus.

_____ Area in the female between the anus and vagina.

Match the process in Column I with its meaning in Column II:

Column I	*Column II*
1. curettage	_____ Giving birth.
2. ovulation	_____ Burning tissue to stop bleeding or remove diseased tissue.
3. parturition	_____ Union of egg and sperm cell.
4. menstruation	_____ Widening or opening of a canal or tube.
5. contraception	_____ Release of egg cell from ovary.
6. fertilization	_____ Scraping a surface.
7. cauterization	_____ Monthly shedding of the lining of the uterus.
8. dilation	_____ Preventing the union of egg and sperm, and thus pregnancy.

CHAPTER 10

MALE REPRODUCTIVE SYSTEM

In this chapter you will:

Learn the location and function of the organs of the male reproductive system;

Gain knowledge of the combining forms used to describe the structures of the system; and

Understand the terms which describe the major pathological conditions of the male reproductive system.

The chapter is divided into the following sections:

   I. Introduction

  II. Vocabulary

 III. Anatomy of the Male Reproductive System

 IV. Combining Forms and Terminology

  V. Pathological Conditions

 VI. Exercises

I. INTRODUCTION

The male sex cell, the **spermatozoon** (sperm cell), is extremely tiny and microscopic—in volume, only one-third the size of an erythrocyte, and less than 1/100,000th the size of the female ovum. It is a relatively uncomplicated cell, composed of a head region, which contains nuclear hereditary material, and a tail region, consisting of a **flagellum** (hairlike process) that makes the sperm motile, somewhat resembling a tadpole. The sperm cell contains relatively little food and cytoplasm, for it need live only long enough to travel from its point of release from the male to where the egg cell lies within the female (fallopian tube). Only one spermatozoon of approximately 100 million sperm cells which may be released during a single **ejaculation** (ejection of sperm and fluid from the male urethra) can penetrate a

177

single ovum. The union of ovum and sperm is called fertilization, and the fertilized egg is the beginning of a new individual.

If more than one egg is passing down the fallopian tube when sperm are present, multiple fertilizations are possible, and twins, triplets, quadruplets, and so forth, may occur. Twins resulting from the fertilization of separate ova by separate sperm cells are called **fraternal twins**. Fraternal twins have individual patterns of inheritance and resemble each other no more than ordinary brothers and sisters.

Identical twins are formed from the fertilization of a single egg cell by a single sperm. As the fertilized egg cell divides and forms many cells, it somehow comes apart and each part continues separately to undergo further division, each producing an embryo. Identical twins are always of the same sex and very similar in form and feature.

The organs of the male reproductive system are designed to produce and release billions of spermatozoa throughout the lifetime of a male from puberty onward. In addition, the male reproductive system secretes a hormone called **testosterone**. Testosterone is responsible for the production of the bodily characteristics of the male (such as beard, pubic hair, voice deepening) and also for the proper development and maintenance of accessory male sexual organs (prostate gland and seminal vesicles) which secrete fluids to insure the lubrication and viability of sperm.

II. VOCABULARY

bulbourethral glands	Cowper's glands; two glands near the male urethra. Their secretion lubricates the urethra.
circumcision	Surgical removal of the foreskin.
Cowper's glands	Glands which secrete a fluid (part of semen) into the urethra.
ejaculation	Ejection of sperm and fluid from the urethra.
epididymis	"Upon a twin"—the tubes which are located on top of each testis; they carry and store the sperm cells before they enter the vas deferens.
flagellum	Hairlike process on a sperm cell which makes it motile.
foreskin	Flap of tissue covering the glans penis.
fraternal twins	Twins resulting from two separate egg cells which were fertilized by two separate sperm cells.
glans penis	Sensitive tip of the penis (male organ of copulation).

identical twins	Twins resulting from one fertilized egg which comes apart early in development, each part continuing to grow separately into a complete individual.
interstitial tissue	Tissue which lies between the essential parts of an organ. In the testes these are the glandular cells which produce the hormone testosterone.
parenchymal tissue	The essential parts of an organ. In the testes these are the seminiferous tubules which produce sperm.
prepuce	Foreskin; tissue covering the glans penis.
prostate gland	Gland at the base of the urinary bladder which secretes a fluid into the urethra during ejaculation.
semen	Spermatozoa and fluid.
seminal vesicles	Glands which secrete a fluid into the vas deferens.
seminiferous tubules	Narrow, coiled tubules in the testes which produce sperm; parenchymal tissue of the testes.
spermatozoa	Sperm cells.
sterilization	Any procedure rendering an individual incapable of reproduction; vasectomy, castration, and salpingectomy are examples.
testosterone	Hormone secreted by the interstitial tissue of the testes which is responsible for male sex characteristics.
vas deferens	Narrow tube which carries sperm from the epididymis to the urethra.

III. ANATOMY OF THE MALE REPRODUCTIVE SYSTEM

Label Figure 10–1 as you study the following description of the anatomy of the male reproductive system.

The male gonads consist of a pair of **testes** (singular: testis), also called **testicles** (1), which develop in the kidney region of the body before descending during embryonic development into the **scrotum** (2), a sac enclosing the testes on the outside of the body.

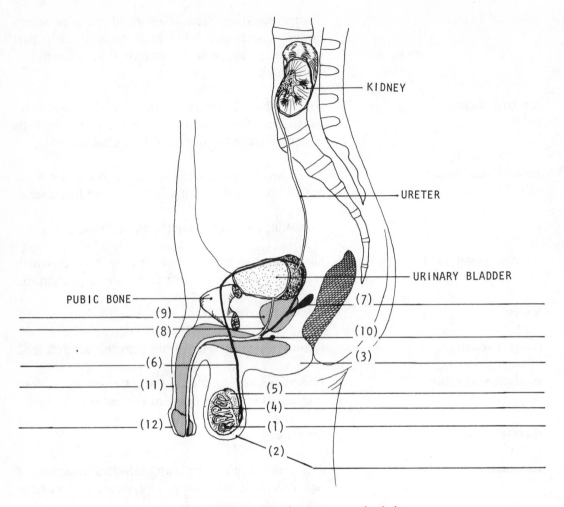

KIDNEY

URETER

URINARY BLADDER

PUBIC BONE

(9)
(8)
(6)
(11)
(12)

(7)
(10)
(3)
(5)
(4)
(1)
(2)

Figure 10-1 Male reproductive system, sagittal view.

The scrotum, lying between the thighs, exposes the testes to a lower temperature than they would have to endure if they were enclosed within the body. This lower temperature is necessary for the adequate maturation and development of sperm. Lying between the anus and the scrotum, at the floor of the pelvic cavity in the male, is the **perineum** (3), which is analogous to the perineal region in the female.

The interior of a testis is composed of a large mass of narrow, coiled tubules called the **seminiferous tubules** (4). These tubules contain cells which manufacture spermatozoa. The seminiferous tubules are the **parenchymal tissue** of the testis, which means that they perform the essential, active work of the organ. Other cells in the testis, called **interstitial tissue**, lie between the parenchymal tissue and, while they do not produce sperm, as do the parenchymal cells, they manufacture an important male hormone, **testosterone**.

As they are formed, sperm cells move through the seminiferous tubules and are collected in ducts which lead to a large tube at the upper part of each testis. This is the **epididymis** (5). The spermatozoa become motile in the epididymis and are temporarily stored there. The epididymis runs down the length of the testicle and then turns upward again and becomes a narrow, straight tube called the **vas deferens** (6). The vas deferens is about 2 feet long and carries the sperm up into the pelvic region, around the urinary bladder, and then down toward the urethra. It is the vas deferens that is cut or tied off when a sterilization procedure called a **vasectomy** is performed.

The **seminal vesicles** (7) are glands which are located at the base of the bladder and open into the vas deferens as it joins the **urethra** (8). The seminal vesicles secrete a thick, yellowish substance that nourishes the sperm cells and forms much of the volume of ejaculated semen. **Semen** is a combination of fluid and spermatozoa which is ejected from the body through the urethra. In the male, as opposed to the female, the genital opening combines with the urinary (urethral) opening.

At the region where the vas deferens enters the urethra, and almost encircling the upper end of the urethra, is the **prostate gland** (9). The prostate gland secretes a thick fluid which, as part of semen, aids the motility of the sperm. This gland is also supplied with muscular tissue which aids in the expulsion of sperm during ejaculation. **Cowper's glands (bulbourethral glands)** (10) are just below the prostate gland and also secrete fluid into the urethra.

The urethra passes through the **penis** (11) to the outside of the body. The penis is composed of erectile tissue and at its tip expands to form a soft, sensitive region called the **glans penis** (12). Ordinarily, a fold of skin called the **foreskin (prepuce)** covers the glans penis. Circumcision is the process whereby the foreskin is removed, leaving the glans penis visible at all times.

The flow diagram in Figure 10–2 traces the path of spermatozoa from their formation in the seminiferous tubules of the testes to the outside of the body.

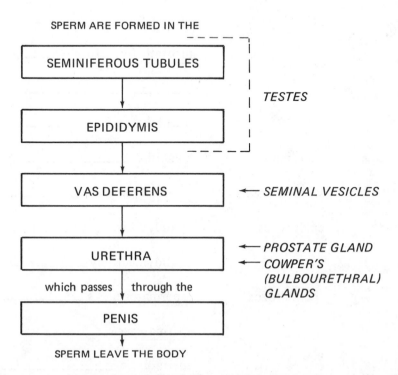

Figure 10–2 The passage of sperm from the seminiferous tubules in the testes to the outside of the body.

IV. COMBINING FORMS AND TERMINOLOGY

Combining Form	Meaning	Terminology	Meaning
test/o	testis, testicle	testosterone _____	
		testicular _____	
orchid/o, orchi/o, orch/o	testis	orchitis _____	
		orchidectomy _____ (castration)	
		orchotomy _____	
		orchidopexy _____	
		anorchism _____	
vas/o	vessel, duct (referring to the vas deferens)	vasectomy _____ After vasectomy, semen without spermatozoa is produced; potency and libido (sexual desire) are not impaired.	
prostat/o	prostate gland	prostatitis _____	
		prostatic hypertrophy _____ _____	
		prostatectomy _____	
balan/o	glans penis	balanitis _____	
vesicul/o	seminal vessels	vesiculectomy _____	
epididym/o	epididymis	epididymitis _____	
		epididymectomy _____	
sperm/o spermat/o	spermatozoa	aspermatogenesis _____	
		spermaturia _____	
		spermolytic _____	

Noun suffixes ending in -sis, like -lysis, form adjectives by dropping the -sis and adding -tic.

zo/o	animal life	azoospermia _____
andr/o	male	androgen _____
cry/o	cold	cryogenic _____
crypt/o	hidden	cryptorchism _____

V. PATHOLOGICAL CONDITIONS

cryptorchism

Undescended testicles.

This condition can be corrected by surgically bringing the testicles down into the scrotal sac. Sterility is thus prevented.

phimosis

Narrowing of the opening of the foreskin over the glans penis.

This condition prevents the retraction of the foreskin over the glans penis, interfering with urination and leading to infection. Treatment is circumcision.

hypospadias or **hypospadia**

Congenital opening of the male urethra on the undersurface of the penis.

hydrocele

Hernia of fluid in the testes or the tubes leading from the testes.

varicocele

Enlarged, herniated, swollen veins near the testes.

benign prostatic hypertrophy

An overgrowth of the glandular tissue of the prostate.

This is a common occurrence in men over 60 years old. The effects of the prostatic enlargement are urinary obstruction and inability to empty the bladder completely. Both of these conditions can lead to urinary retention and infection, with cystitis, hydronephrosis, pyelonephritis, and ureterectasis. Without treatment, this condition can become fatal if renal failure or septicemia develops. Surgical treatment is prostatectomy, and it can be done in several ways. Transurethral prostatectomy (also called transurethral resection, or T.U.R.), using an endoscope and cauterization device, is one method. Other endoscopes have cryogenic devices attached and the prostate is removed by freezing the tissue. The gland may also be removed through the perineum or from an opening in the bladder from above.

adenocarcinoma of the prostate   Malignant tumor of the prostate.

This is the most common cause of cancer in men over 50 years of age (not including skin cancer). Radical (complete) prostatectomy by perineal, retropubic, or transsacral route is performed. Radiotherapy and chemotherapy are other methods used to treat metastases of the tumor.

testicular cancers   Malignant tumors of the testes.

This type of cancer represents about 1 per cent of all cancer in males. There are several types of tumors, classified according to the type of tissue which is involved. Some of the types are:

seminoma – a tumor of embryonic cells which have not differentiated into cells of male or female type.

teratocarcinoma – a tumor composed of embryonic tissue which has differentiated into bone, hair, teeth, cartilage, and skin cells. All these types of tissue are found in the tumor. (The combining form terat/o means monster.)

choriocarcinoma – a highly malignant tumor composed of chorionic (placental) type tissue.

Tumors of the testes are commonly treated with surgery (orchiectomy) and radiotherapy.

VI. EXERCISES

A. Build medical words:

1. Inflammation of the testes _____

2. Removal of the tubules which carry the spermatozoa to the vas deferens

   _____

3. Excessive development of the prostate gland _____

4. Condition of hidden testes _____

5. Condition of production of sperm cells _____

6. Excision (partial) of the vas deferens _____

7. Excision of the prostate and seminal vesicles _____

8. Condition of scanty sperm _____

9. Discharge from the glans penis _____

10. Sperm in the urine _____

B. *Give the meaning of the following:*

1. hypospadias _____

2. parenchymal _____

3. seminiferous tubules _____

4. cryogenic _____

5. interstitial _____

6. testosterone _____

   _____

7. phimosis _____

8. azoospermia _____

9. seminoma _____

10. teratocarcinoma _____

C. *Review exercise. Give the meaning of the following:*

1. -stasis _____   11. -ectasis _____

2. -sclerosis _____   12. -centesis _____

3. -stenosis _____   13. -genesis _____

4. -orrhexis _____   14. culd/o _____

5. -orrhagia _____   15. oophor/o _____

6. -ptosis _____   16. salping/o _____

7. -plasia _____   17. hyster/o _____

8. -phagia _____   18. metr/o _____

9. -orrhaphy _____   19. colp/o _____

10. -pexy _____   20. mast/o _____

ANSWERS

A.
1. orchitis
2. epididymectomy
3. prostatic hypertrophy
4. cryptorchism
5. spermatogenesis
6. vasectomy
7. prostatovesiculectomy
8. oligospermia
9. balanorrhea
10. spermaturia

B.
1. Congenital anomaly in which the urethra opens on the underside of the penis.
2. The distinctive tissue or cells of an organ; glomerulus and tubules of the kidney, seminiferous tubules of the testes.
3. The tubules in the testes which make sperm cells.
4. Pertaining to producing cold or low temperatures.
5. The cells which lie between the distinctive cells of an organ; in the testes, these cells are glandular and produce a hormone, testosterone.
6. A hormone made by the interstitial cells of the testes and responsible for secondary sex characteristics.
7. A narrowing, or stenosis, of the foreskin on the glans penis.
8. Lack of spermatozoa in the semen.
9. Malignant tumor of the testes composed of undifferentiated embryonic tissue.
10. Malignant tumor of the testes composed of differentiated tissue such as bone, hair, skin, teeth, cartilage.

C.
1. stopping, controlling
2. hardening
3. narrowing
4. rupture
5. hemorrhage
6. prolapse
7. formation
8. eating, swallowing
9. suture
10. fixation
11. widening
12. surgical puncture
13. beginning, producing
14. cul-de-sac
15. ovary
16. fallopian tube
17. uterus
18. uterus
19. vagina
20. breast

REVIEW SHEET 10

Combining Forms

andr/o	_____	prostat/o	_____
balan/o	_____	sperm/o	_____
cry/o	_____	spermat/o	_____
crypt/o	_____	test/o	_____
epididym/o	_____	vas/o	_____
orchid/o	_____	vesicul/o	_____
orchi/o	_____	zo/o	_____
orch/o	_____		

Suffixes

-ectomy	_____	-pexy	_____
-genic	_____	-trophy	_____
-lysis	_____	-uria	_____
-otomy	_____		

Additional Terms

adenocarcinoma of the prostate _____

benign prostatic hypertrophy _____

circumcision _____

choriocarcinoma _____

ejaculation _____

flagellum _____

foreskin

_____

fraternal twins

_____

glans penis

_____

hydrocele

_____

hypospadias

_____

identical twins

_____

interstitial tissue

_____

parenchymal tissue

_____

phimosis

_____

prepuce

_____

semen

_____

seminoma

_____

sterilization

_____

teratocarcinoma

_____

testicular cancers

_____

testosterone

_____

varicocele

_____

Match the male reproductive structure in Column I with its description in Column II:

Column I	*Column II*
1. bulbourethral glands (Cowper's)	_____ Tubes above each testis; carry and store sperm.
2. testes	_____ Gland surrounding the urethra at the base of the urinary bladder; secretes a fluid into the urethra during ejaculation.
3. scrotum	
4. vas deferens	_____ Parenchymal tissue of the testes; produces sperm.

5. epididymis   _____ Sperm cell.

6. seminal vesicles   _____ Male organ of copulation.

7. prostate gland   _____ Male gonads; produce sperm and male sex hormones.

8. penis

     _____ Pair of glands which secrete a fluid into the vas deferens.

9. seminiferous tubules

10. spermatozoon   _____ Sac on outside of the body enclosing the testes.

     _____ Tube carrying sperm from the epididymis to the urethra.

     _____ Pair of glands near the male urethra which secrete a fluid into the urethra.

CHAPTER 11

THE NERVOUS SYSTEM

In this chapter you will:

Learn the names, locations, and functions of the major organs and parts of the nervous system;

Understand the terminology used to describe some of the pathological conditions which can affect the system; and

Analyze and use the combining forms and suffixes which describe the anatomy, physiology, and pathology of the nervous system.

The chapter is divided into the following sections:

I. INTRODUCTION

The nervous system is one of the most complex of all human body systems. More than 10 billion nerve cells are operating constantly all over the body to coordinate the activities we do consciously and voluntarily, as well as those that occur unconsciously or involuntarily. We speak, we move muscles, we hear, we taste, we see, we think, our glands secrete hormones, we respond to danger, pain, temperature, touch, we have memory, association, discrimination—all of these composing a small number of the many activities controlled by our nervous system.

Nerve cells collected into bundles called nerves carry electrical messages all over the body. External stimuli, as well as internal chemicals such as acetylcholine, activate the cell membranes of nerve cells so as to release stored electrical energy within the cells. This energy when released and passed through the length of the nerve cell is called the nervous impulse. External receptors, like sense organs, as well as internal receptors in muscles and blood vessels receive and transmit impulses to the complex network of nerve cells in the brain and spinal cord. Within this central part of the nervous system, impulses are recognized, interpreted, and finally relayed to other nerve cells which extend out to all parts of the body, such as muscles, glands, and internal organs.

II. VOCABULARY

acetylcholine	Chemical which is released at the spaces between individual nerve cells and between nerve cells and other tissue cells. Acetylcholine aids in the transmission of nerve impulses.
afferent nerves	Nerves which carry impulses toward the brain and spinal cord from sensory receptors, for example, the skin, the eye, and the ear.
arachnoid membrane	Middle layer of the three membranes which surround the brain and spinal cord.
astrocytes	Type of neuroglial cells; the connective, supporting tissue of the nervous system.
autonomic nervous system	Consists of nerves which carry impulses from the brain and spinal cord to muscles, glands, and other body organs. These nerves control involuntary body functions.
axon	Microscopic fiber which carries the nervous impulse along a nerve cell.
cauda equina	"Horse tail"—a fan of nervous fibers formed below the second lumbar vertebra in the spinal column.
cell body	Part of a nerve cell which contains the cell nucleus.
central nervous system (CNS)	The brain and the spinal cord.
cerebellum	Posterior part of the brain. It is responsible for coordinating muscle movements and maintaining balance.

cerebral cortex	Outer region of the cerebrum; also called the "gray matter" of the brain.
cerebrospinal fluid (CSF)	Liquid which circulates throughout the brain and spinal cord.
cerebrum	Largest part of the brain; responsible for voluntary muscular activity, vision, speech, taste, hearing, thought, memory, and many other functions.
convolutions	Elevated portions of the cerebral cortex; also called gyri.
dendrites	Microscopic branching fibers of a nerve cell which are the first parts to receive the nervous impulse.
dura mater	Outermost of the three membranes surrounding the brain and spinal cord.
efferent nerves	Nerves, outside of the brain and spinal cord, which carry impulses away from the central nervous system to the muscles, glands, and organs of the body.
embolism	A sudden blocking of a vessel by a clot.
epinephrine	Hormone produced by the adrenal glands in times of stress. Epinephrine stimulates the heart, constricts blood vessels to increase blood pressure, and opens airways to make breathing easier.
fissures	Depressions, or grooves, in the surface of the cerebral cortex; also called sulci.
ganglion (plural: ganglia)	"Knot"—collection of many nerve cell bodies outside the brain and spinal cord.
gyri	Elevations in the surface of the cerebral cortex; also called convolutions.
hypothalamus	Portion of middle part of the brain which lies beneath the thalamus and controls sleep, water balance, temperature regulation, and the secretions from the pituitary gland.
lumbar puncture (LP)	Insertion of a needle into the lumbar region of the spinal cord to remove cerebrospinal fluid for diagnostic purposes.

medulla oblongata	Part of the brain just above the spinal cord; controls breathing and heartbeat.
meninges	Three protective membranes which surround the brain and spinal cord.
microglial cells	Type of supporting and connective cells within the nervous system; one of the neuroglial cells.
motor	Pertaining to movement.
myelin sheath	Tissue which surrounds the axon of some nerve fibers.
neurilemma	Membranous covering around the myelin sheath of nerve cells outside the brain and spinal cord.
neuroglia	Nerve cells which do not carry impulses but which are supportive and connective in function within the nervous system. Examples are astrocytes, microglial cells, and oligodendroglia.
neuron	A nerve cell. Its function is to carry impulses throughout the body.
nerve	Macroscopic structure consisting of axons and dendrites in bundles like strands of rope.
parasympathetic nerves	Involuntary, autonomic nerves which help regulate body functions like heart rate and respiration.
peripheral nervous system	Nerves outside of the brain and spinal cord; cranial and spinal nerves and autonomic nerves.
pia mater	Thin, delicate, inner membrane of the meninges.
plexus (plural: plexuses)	A large network of nerves.
pons	"Bridge"—part of the brain where nerve tracts cross as they proceed to the spinal cord.
receptor	An organ which receives a nervous stimulation and passes it on to nerves within the body. For example, the skin, ears, eyes, and taste buds are receptors.
sensory	Pertaining to sensation, feeling.

spinal nerves	Peripheral nerves carrying impulses between the spinal cord and the abdomen, chest, and extremities.
spinal puncture	Insertion of a needle into the lumbar region of the spinal cord to remove fluid; also called lumbar puncture.
stimulus	An agent capable of initiating a response from a living tissue.
sulci	Depressions in the surface of the cerebral cortex; also called fissures.
sympathetic nerves	Autonomic nerves which influence body functions involuntarily in times of stress.
synapse	The space between neurons through which the nervous impulse "jumps" from one nerve cell to another.
terminal end fibers	Branching fibers of the neuron which lead the nervous impulse away from the axon and toward the synapse.
thalamus	Portion of the middle part of the brain which receives impulses from receptors and relays them to other parts of the brain and body.
ventricles of the brain	Canals in the interior of the brain which are filled with cerebrospinal fluid.

III. GENERAL STRUCTURE OF THE NERVOUS SYSTEM

The nervous system can be classified into two major divisions: the **central nervous system (CNS)** and the **peripheral nervous system.** The central nervous system consists of the **brain** and **spinal cord**. The peripheral nervous system consists of 12 pairs of **cranial nerves**, which carry impulses between the brain and the head and neck, and 31 pairs of **spinal nerves**, which carry messages between the spinal cord and the chest, abdomen, and extremities. Figure 11–1 illustrates these parts of the central and peripheral nervous systems.

In addition to the spinal and cranial nerves (whose functions are mainly voluntary and involved with sensations of smell, taste, sight, hearing, and muscle movements), the peripheral nervous system consists of a large group of nerves which function involuntarily or automatically without conscious control. These peripheral nerves are those of the **autonomic nervous system.** This system of nerve fibers carries impulses

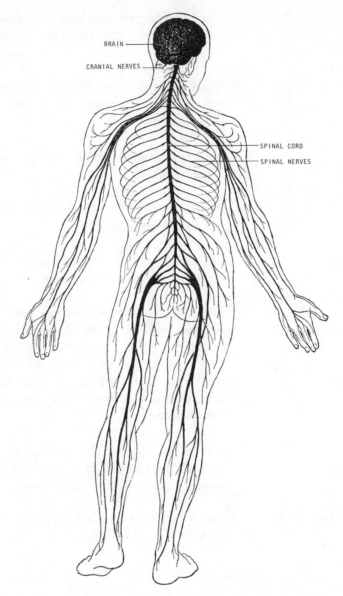

BRAIN

CRANIAL NERVES

SPINAL CORD

SPINAL NERVES

Figure 11-1 The central nervous system, consisting of the brain and the spinal cord. Cranial and spinal nerves (part of the peripheral nervous system) carry impulses to and from the brain and spinal cord.

from the central nervous system to the glands, heart, blood vessels, and the involuntary muscles found in the walls of tubes like the intestines and hollow organs like the stomach and urinary bladder. These nerves are called **efferent**, since they carry impulses away from the central nervous system.

Some of the autonomic nerves are called **sympathetic** nerves and others are called **parasympathetic** nerves. The sympathetic nerves stimulate your body in times of stress and crisis, i.e., increase heart rate and forcefulness, dilate airways so more oxygen can enter, increase blood pressure, stimulate the adrenal glands to secrete epinephrine (adrenalin), and inhibit intestinal contractions so that digestion is slower. The parasympathetic nerves normally act as a balance for the sympathetic nerves.

Parasympathetic nerves slow down heart rate, contract the pupils of the eye, lower blood pressure, stimulate peristalsis to clear the rectum, and increase the quantity of secretions like saliva.

Ganglia (singular: ganglion), which are collections of nerve tissue outside the brain and spinal cord, and plexuses (singular: plexus), which are larger networks of nerves, are prevalent in the autonomic nervous system. Consult your dictionary and note the numerous and widespread distribution of ganglia and plexuses throughout the body.

Figure 11–2 summarizes the major divisions of the nervous system.

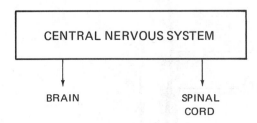

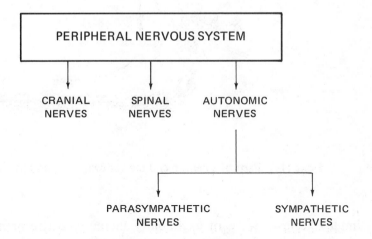

GANGLIA AND PLEXUSES ARE FOUND IN THE PERIPHERAL NERVOUS SYSTEM, ESPECIALLY ALONG THE SYMPATHETIC NERVES

Figure 11–2 Divisions of the nervous system.

IV. NEURONS AND NERVES

A neuron is an individual nerve cell, a microscopic structure. Impulses are passed along the parts of a nerve cell in a definite manner and direction. The parts of a neuron are pictured in Figure 11–3; label it as you study the following.

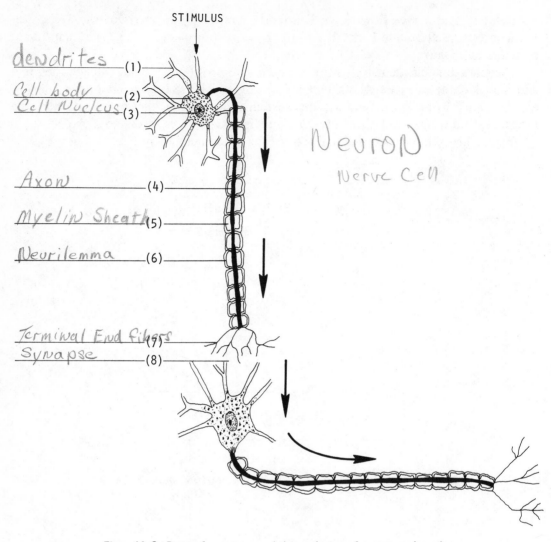

STIMULUS

dendrites (1)
Cell body (2)
Cell Nucleus (3)

Neuron
Nerve Cell

Axon (4)
Myelin Sheath (5)
Neurilemma (6)

Terminal End fibers (7)
Synapse (8)

Figure 11-3 Parts of a neuron and the pathway of a nervous impulse.

A **stimulus** begins a wave of excitability in the receptive branching fibers of the neuron which are called **dendrites** (1). A change in the electrical charge of the dendrite membranes is thus begun and the nervous impulse wave moves along the dendrites like the movement of falling tenpins. The impulse, traveling in only one direction, next reaches the **cell body** (2) which contains the **cell nucleus** (3). Extending from the cell body is the **axon** (4) which carries the impulse away from the cell body. Axons may be covered with a fatty tissue sheath called a **myelin sheath** (5). The myelin sheath gives a white appearance to the nerve fiber; hence the term "white matter," as in parts of the spinal cord, white matter of the brain, and most peripheral nerves. The "gray matter" of the brain and spinal cord refers to collections of cell bodies and dendrites which appear gray because they are not covered by a myelin sheath.

Another axon covering, called the **neurilemma** (6), is a membranous sheath which is outside the myelin sheath on the nerve cells of peripheral nerves. The nervous impulse passes through the axon to leave the cell via the **terminal end fibers** (7) of the neuron. The space where the nervous impulse jumps from one neuron to another is called the **synapse** (8).

While a neuron is a microscopic structure within the nervous system, a **nerve** is macroscopic, able to be seen with the naked eye. A nerve consists of a bundle of dendrites and axons which travel together like strands of rope. Peripheral nerves which carry impulses to the brain and spinal cord from stimulus receptors like the skin, eye, ear, and nose are called **afferent** nerves; those which carry impulses from the CNS to organs which produce responses, for example, muscles and glands, are called **efferent** nerves.

Neurons and nerves are the parenchymal tissue of the nervous system; that is, they do the essential work of the system by conducting impulses throughout the body. The interstitial tissue of the nervous system consists of other cells called **neuroglia**. Neuroglial cells are supportive and connective in function, as well as phagocytic, and are able to help the nervous system ward off infection and injury. Neuroglial cells do not transmit impulses.

There are three types of neuroglial cells. **Astrocytes** (astroglia), as their name suggests, are starlike, and are believed to be responsible for transporting water and salts between capillaries and nerve cells. They are the cells which compose brain tumors (gliomas). **Microglial cells (microglia)** are very small and have many branching processes. These cells are phagocytes. **Oligodendroglia,** as their name implies, possess few dendrites, and their function is unknown. Figure 11–4 pictures the several different kinds of neuroglia.

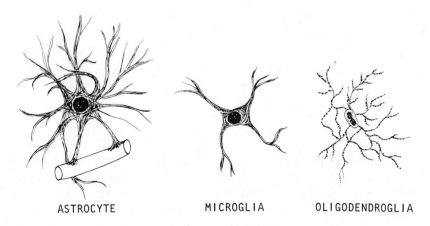

ASTROCYTE   MICROGLIA   OLIGODENDROGLIA

Figure 11–4 Neuroglial cells—the supporting and connective cells of the nervous system.

V. THE BRAIN

The brain is the primary center for regulating and coordinating body activities. It has many different parts, all of which control different aspects of body functions.

The largest part of the brain is the **cerebrum.** The outer nervous tissue of the cerebrum, known as the **cerebral cortex,** is arranged in folds to form elevated portions known as **convolutions** (also called **gyri**) and depressions or grooves known as **fissures** (also called **sulci**).

The cerebrum has many functions. All thought, judgment, memory, association, and discrimination take place within it. In addition, sensory impulses are received through afferent cranial nerves, and when registered in the cortex are the basis for perception. Efferent cranial nerves carry motor impulses from the brain to muscles and glands, and these produce movement and activity. Figure 11–5 shows the location of some of the centers in the cerebral cortex which control speech, vision, smell, and movement.

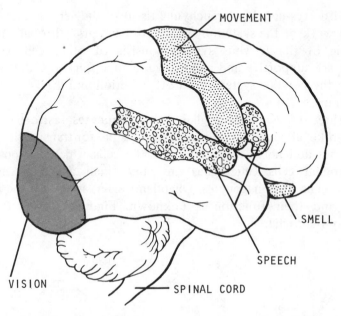

Figure 11-5 Some of the centers in the cerebral cortex—those controlling speech, vision, smell, and movement.

Within the middle region of the cerebrum are spaces, or canals, called **ventricles** (pictured in Figure 11–6). They contain a watery fluid which flows throughout the brain and around the spinal cord. This fluid is called **cerebrospinal fluid (CSF)** and protects the brain and spinal cord from shock as might a cushion. It is usually clear and colorless, and contains lymphocytes, sugar, chlorides, and some protein. Spinal fluid can be withdrawn for diagnosis or relief of pressure on the brain; this is called a **spinal puncture** or **lumbar puncture (LP)**. A hollow needle is inserted in the lumbar region of the spinal column below the region where the nervous tissue of the spinal cord ends, and fluid is withdrawn.

Two other important parts of the brain, the **thalamus** and **hypothalamus**, are below the cerebrum in the interbrain and midbrain. The thalamus monitors the sensory stimuli we receive by suppressing some and magnifying others. The hypothalamus (below the thalamus) contains neurons which control body temperature, sleep, appetite, and emotions such as fear and pleasure. The hypothalamus also regulates the release of hormones from the pituitary gland at the base of the brain and integrates the activities of the sympathetic and parasympathetic nervous systems.

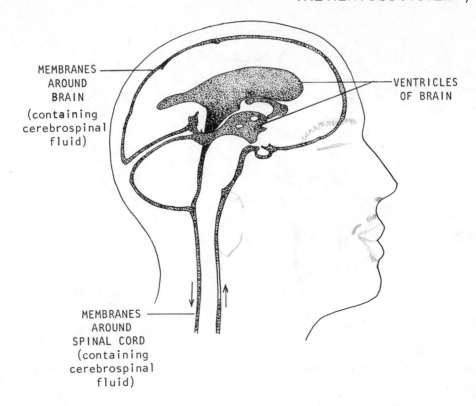

Figure 11-6 Circulation of cerebrospinal fluid in brain and spinal cord.

The following structures within the brain lie below the posterior portion of the cerebrum and connect the cerebrum with the spinal cord: the cerebellum, pons, and medulla oblongata.

The **cerebellum** is located beneath the posterior part of the cerebrum. Its function is to aid in the coordination of voluntary movements and to maintain balance and muscular tone.

The **pons** is a part of the brain which literally means "bridge." It contains nerve fiber tracts which connect the cerebellum and cerebrum with the rest of the brain. Nerve tracts "cross over" in the pons. For example, nerve cells which control the left side of the body are found in the right half of the brain. These cells send out axons which cross over to the opposite side of the brain in the pons and then down the spinal cord. Thus, damage to one side of the brain will cause paralysis on the opposite side of the body.

The **medulla oblongata**, located at the base of the brain, contains important vital centers which regulate internal activity of the body. These are:

1. Respiratory center which controls muscles of respiration in response to chemical or other stimuli;
2. Cardiac center which tends to slow heart rate so it will not beat too rapidly to be effective; and
3. Vasomotor center which affects (constricts or dilates) the muscles in the blood vessel walls thus influencing blood pressure.

Figure 11-7 shows the locations of the thalamus, hypothalamus, cerebellum, pons, and medulla oblongata.

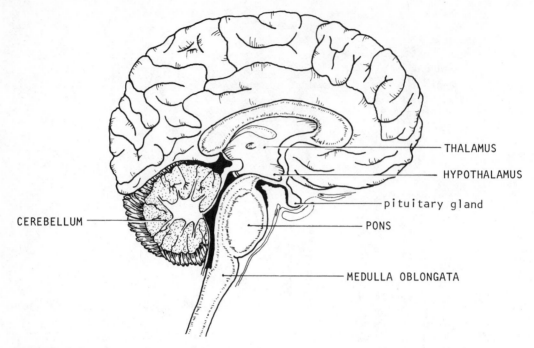

CEREBELLUM

THALAMUS

HYPOTHALAMUS

pituitary gland

PONS

MEDULLA OBLONGATA

Figure 11-7 Parts of the brain: thalamus, hypothalamus, cerebellum, pons, and medulla oblongata.

VI. SPINAL CORD AND MENINGES

Spinal Cord

The **spinal cord** is a column of nervous tissue extending from the medulla oblongata to the second lumbar vertebra within the vertebral column. It ends as the **cauda equina** (horse tail), a fan of nerve fibers found below the second lumbar vertebra of the spinal column. It carries all the nerves which affect the limbs and lower part of the body, and is the pathway for impulses going to and from the brain. A cross-section of the spinal cord (shown in Figure 11–8) reveals an inner section of gray matter (containing cell bodies and dendrites of peripheral nerves) and an outer region of white matter (containing the nerve fiber tracts with myelin sheaths) conducting impulses to and from the brain.

Meninges

The **meninges** are three layers of connective tissue membranes that surround the brain and spinal cord. Label Figure 11–9 as you study the following description of the meninges.

The outermost membrane of the meninges is called the **dura mater** (1). It is a thick and tough membrane and contains channels for blood to come into the brain tissue. The **subdural space** (2) is a space below the dura membrane and contains many blood

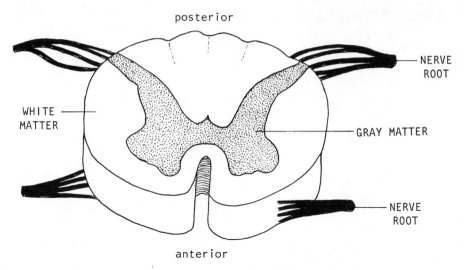

Figure 11–8   Transverse section of the spinal cord.

vessels. The second layer around the brain and spinal cord is called the **arachnoid membrane** (3). The arachnoid ("spider-like") membrane is loosely attached to the other meninges by weblike fibers so there is a space for fluid between the fibers and the third membrane. This space is called the **subarachnoid space** (4), and it contains the cerebrospinal fluid. (**Myelography** is the process of injecting dye, or sometimes air, into the cerebrospinal fluid and recording its passage through the subarachnoid space by x-ray.)

The third layer of the meninges, closest to the brain and spinal cord, is called the **pia mater** (5). It is made of delicate ("pia") connective tissue with a rich supply of blood vessels.

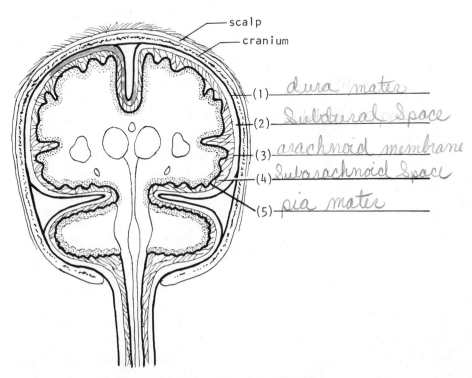

Figure 11–9   The layers of the meninges.

VII. COMBINING FORMS AND TERMINOLOGY

Combining Form	Meaning	Terminology	Meaning
neur/o	nerve	neurotomy	_Cutting the nerve_
		neuralgia	_nerve pain_
		polyneuritis	_inflamation of many nerve_
		neuroanastomosis	
		neuroblastoma	
		neurorrhaphy	
		neurasthenia	
		neurectopia	
		neuropathogenesis	
gangli/o ganglion/o	ganglion ("knot" of nerve cell bodies)	ganglionectomy	
		ganglionitis	
		pharyngeal ganglion	
plex/o	network, especially of nerves	plexal	
		cervical plexus	
		lumbosacral plexus	
cerebr/o	brain, cerebrum	cerebromalacia	
		cerebrospinal	
		cerebral angiography	
encephal/o	brain	encephalitis	
		electroencephalogram (EEG)	

		encephalopathy _____
		anencephaly _____
cerebell/o	cerebellum	cerebellar _____
		cerebellospinal _____
pont/o	pons	cerebellopontine _____
thalam/o	thalamus	thalamotomy _____
ventricul/o	ventricles of the brain	ventriculography _____

Cerebrospinal fluid is removed and replaced by air, which outlines the ventricles on an x-ray film.

myel/o	spinal cord	myelography _____
		myelatrophy _____
		myelocele _____
		myelitis _____
		myelodysplasia _____
mening/o meningi/o	membranes, meninges	meningioma _____
		meningococcus _____
		meningeal _____
		meningomyelocele _____
		meningoencephalitis _____
dur/o	dura mater	subdural hematoma _____
		extradural hematoma _____
algesi/o	excessive sensitivity to pain	analgesia _____
		_____
atel/o	incomplete	atelomyelia _____
brachi/o	arm	brachial plexus _____

| coccyg/o | coccyx, or tail bone | coccygeal plexus _____ |
| esthesi/o | feeling, nervous sensation | anesthesia _____ |

This term applies to a lack of nervous sensation—for example, absence of sense of touch or pain.

		dysesthesia _____
		hypesthesia _____
		hyperesthesia _____
gli/o	"glue," parts of the nervous system that support and connect	neuroglial _____
		oligodendroglia _____
blephar/o	eyelid	blepharoptosis _____
kinesi/o	movement	kinesiology _____
		hyperkinesis _____
my/o	muscle	myoneural _____
tax/o	order, coordination	ataxia _____
phas/o	speech	dysphasia _____
		aphasia _____

Aphasias are of several varieties, such as: motor (ability to formulate but not execute or coordinate the muscles which are necessary for speech); and sensory (ability to see and hear and execute speech, but inability to understand speech or read language).

| polio- | gray—referring to the gray matter of the brain and spinal cord | poliomyelitis _____ |
| -asthenia | lack of strength | neurasthenia _____ |

-paresis	slight paralysis	hemiparesis _____

Affects either right or left side (half) of the body.

-plegia   paralysis, palsy   hemiplegia _____

(loss or impairment of the ability to move parts of the body)

Affects right or left half of the body.

paraplegia _____

Affects the lower extremities.

quadriplegia _____

Affects all four extremities.

VIII. PATHOLOGICAL CONDITIONS

cerebrovascular accident (CVA)   Damage to the brain caused by a disorder within the blood vessels of the cerebrum.

This condition, also known as a stroke or apoplexy, is the result of a localized area of ischemia in the brain. This may be caused by:

1. **Thrombosis**—blood clot in the arteries leading to the brain resulting in occlusion (blocking) of the vessel. This is the most common type of stroke, and may lead to paralysis.

2. **Embolism**—a piece of clot breaks off from its place of origin and occludes a cerebral artery. This type of stroke occurs very suddenly.

3. **Hemorrhage**—this is the result of the degeneration of cerebral arteries. With advancing age, arteriosclerosis, and high blood pressure, cerebral arteries may burst. The result is damage to nerve cells, usually in the motor region of the cerebrum. The patient is usually hemiplegic and aphasic. If the hemorrhage is small, the blood is reabsorbed and the patient can make a good recovery with only slight disability. In a younger patient cerebral hemorrhage is usually due to mechanical injury associated with skull fracture, or bursting of an arterial aneurysm (a weakness in the vessel wall which balloons and eventually bursts).

coma   A deep sleep or unconsciousness due to surgery or illness.

epilepsy   Sudden transient disturbances of brain function.

A neurological disorder involving abnormal recurrent firing of nerve impulses within the brain. Grand (large) mal seizures are characterized by severe convulsions and unconsciousness. Petit (small) mal seizures consist of a momentary lapse of consciousness.

hydrocephalus Abnormal accumulation of fluid in the brain.

If circulation of cerebrospinal fluid in the brain or spinal cord is impaired, fluid may accumulate under pressure in the ventricles of the brain. Characteristic features are enlarged head and small face. To relieve pressure on the brain and treat this condition, a catheter is placed from the ventricle of the brain to the venous blood in the chest or heart so that the CSF is continually drained away from the brain.

meningitis Inflammation of the meninges.

This condition may be caused by bacterial or viral infection of the subarachnoid space of the meninges.

multiple sclerosis Demyelination and destruction of nerve fibers throughout the central nervous system.

A chronic disease of the nervous system characterized by progressive demyelination (de = lack of) of the myelin sheath around the axon of a neuron and hardening of the gray and white matter of the brain and spinal cord. The nerve fibers degenerate and are replaced by scar tissue.

myasthenia gravis Muscle weakness marked by progressive paralysis.

Loss of muscle strength due to lack of a chemical in the myoneural region. Nerve impulses fail to induce normal muscle contraction. It may affect any muscle of the body, but especially those of the face, lips, tongue, throat, and neck. Blepharoptosis may be a symptom.

Parkinson's disease Degeneration of nerves in brain and spinal cord leading to tremors, weakness of muscles, and slowness of movement.

A degenerative disease of the CNS which is characterized by rigidity, tremor of fingers and hands, and flexion of the body so that the head is bent and the patient is in a forward-leaning posture. The lesion is in the midbrain, caused by virus, infection, or arteriosclerosis. Drugs like L-dopa are used to treat the condition by increasing the neurotransmission.

spina bifida Defective closure of the vertebral column through which the spinal cord or meninges may or may not protrude.

This is a congenital anomaly, and it can take several forms. In all forms there is a defect in the spinal column due to imperfect joining of the vertebrae, usually in the lumbosacral region. In **spina bifida occulta** there is no protrusion of the intraspinal contents. If the spinal defect is accompanied by the protrusion of the meninges to the surface of the body to form a saclike structure containing CSF, the condition is called

spina bifida with meningocele. In some cases, the neural tissue protrudes to the surface with the meninges, and this is called **spina bifida with myelomeningocele.** Spina bifida may involve hydrocephalus, paralysis of lower limbs, and lack of control of bladder and rectum. Treatment varies with the individual case; surgery may be indicated to remove the meningocele or myelomeningocele. Figure 11–10 illustrates a meningocele with spina bifida.

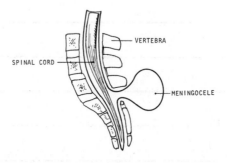

Figure 11–10   Spina bifida with meningocele.

syncope	Fainting; sudden loss of consciousness.
subdural hematoma	Collection of blood in the subdural space.
tumors of the brain	Abnormal growths of brain tissue and meninges.

Most of the primary intracranial tumors arise from neuroglial cells or the meninges. Those that arise from neuroglia are called **gliomas**, and those from the meninges are **meningiomas.**

Gliomas are highly malignant tumors which, however, almost never metastasize. The most common type of glioma is an **astrocytoma**, which occurs most often in childhood in the cerebellum. Others are **glioblastomas**, which occur mainly in the cerebrum of adults, and **medulloblastomas**, which are derived from cerebellar embryonic cells and are common in childhood. Gliomas may be removed surgically, and radiotherapy may be used if the tumor is surgically inaccessible and nonresectable.

Meningiomas nearly always occur in adults and are usually benign and surrounded by a capsule. They usually arise from cells in the pia-arachnoid region and can be removed completely by surgery.

IX. EXERCISES

A. Identify:

1. middle meningeal membrane _____

2. sulci _____

3. ganglion _____

4. dendrites _____

5. pons _____

6. plexus _____

7. medulla oblongata _____

8. efferent neuron _____

9. cerebellum _____

10. dura mater _____

11. synapse _____

12. peripheral nervous system _____

13. neuroglia _____

14. axon _____

15. embolism _____

16. astrocyte _____

17. acetylcholine _____

18. autonomic nervous system _____

B. Build medical words:

1. Incomplete brain _____

2. No coordination _____

3. Inflammation of the meninges _____

4. Hardening of the spinal cord _____

5. Suture of a nerve _____

6. Excessive movement _____

7. One who specializes in the study of rendering one feelingless _____

_____

8. Pertaining to the network of nerves in the arm _____

9. No strength in muscles _____

10. Difficult speech _____

11. Slight paralysis _____

12. Incision into the thalamus _____

13. Tumor of the membranes surrounding the brain and spinal cord _____

_____

14. Hernia of the spinal cord _____

15. Pertaining to the cerebellum and pons _____

C. *Give the meaning of the following:*

1. hyperesthesia _____

2. gyri _____

3. paraplegia _____

4. sympathectomy _____

5. glioma _____

6. hypothalamus _____

7. myelogram _____

8. lumbar puncture _____

9. subdural hematoma _____

10. apoplexy _____

11. multiple sclerosis _____

12. analgesia _____

13. polioencephalitis _____

14. spina bifida _____

15. syncope _____

16. hypesthesia _____

17. leukoencephalopathy _____

18. myoneural _____

19. coma _____

20. aphasia _____

D. *Give the meaning of the following medical abbreviations:*

1. LP _____

2. EKG _____

3. CVA _____

4. CNS _____

5. CSF _____

6. EEG _____

ANSWERS

A. 1. Arachnoid membrane.
  2. Depressions or grooves in the cerebral cortex.
  3. Mass or knot of nerve cells.
  4. Branching fibers that conduct impulses to the cell body of a neuron.
  5. Portion of the brain that connects cerebellum to other brain parts.
  6. Nerve network.
  7. Posterior part of the brain; contains vital centers of regulation.
  8. Nerve cell that conducts impulse away from CNS to effector.

9. Portion of the brain which controls balance and coordination.
10. Tough outer membrane surrounding the brain and spinal cord.
11. Connection between two neurons for passage of impulse.
12. Part of the nervous system that consists of nerves outside the brain and spinal cord.
13. "Nerve glue," i.e., interstitial nerve cells which are supportive; aid in nourishment and fighting disease.
14. Part of a neuron which conducts impulse away from cell body.
15. Floating clot or other material occluding a blood vessel.
16. Type of neuroglial cell; aids in nourishment of neurons. They are frequently gliomas.
17. Body chemical released at the synapse which aids in the transmission of nervous impulse.
18. Involuntary, peripheral nerves which direct functions not under conscious control.

B.
1. atelencephalia
2. ataxia
3. meningitis
4. myelosclerosis
5. neurorrhaphy
6. hyperkinesia
7. anesthesiologist
8. brachial plexus
9. myasthenia
10. dysphasia
11. paresis
12. thalamotomy
13. meningioma
14. myelocele
15. cerebellopontine

C.
1. Excessive feeling.
2. Elevations in the cerebral cortex.
3. Abnormal paralysis—lower half of the body.
4. Removal of a sympathetic nerve.
5. Tumor of "glue"—composed of neuroglial cells, highly malignant.
6. Part of brain which is under the thalamus; controls sleep, temperature, and pituitary gland.
7. Record (x-ray) of the spinal cord.
8. Puncture into the lumbar spinal cord to remove cerebrospinal fluid.
9. Excessive blood flow from the space under the dura mater.
10. Cerebrovascular accident—a stroke.
11. Hardening of nervous tissue of brain and spinal cord leading to paralysis.
12. Lack of excessive sensitivity to pain.
13. Inflammation of the gray matter of the brain.
14. Congenital defect of imperfect closure of spinal column.
15. Fainting.
16. Diminished pain sensation.
17. Disease of the white matter of the brain.
18. Pertaining to muscles and nerves.
19. Lack of consciousness; deep sleep.
20. Inability to speak.

D.
1. lumbar puncture
2. electrocardiogram
3. cerebrovascular accident
4. central nervous system
5. cerebrospinal fluid
6. electroencephalogram

REVIEW SHEET 11

Combining Forms

algesi/o	_____	ganglion/o	_____
angi/o	_____	gli/o	_____
atel/o	_____	hydr/o	_____
blephar/o	_____	kinesi/o	_____
brachi/o	_____	lumb/o	_____
cerebell/o	_____	mening/o	_____
cerebr/o	_____	meningi/o	_____
cervic/o	_____	my/o	_____
coccyg/o	_____	myel/o	_____
crani/o	_____	neur/o	_____
cry/o	_____	plex/o	_____
dur/o	_____	pont/o	_____
encephal/o	_____	tax/o	_____
erythr/o	_____	thalam/o	_____
esthesi/o	_____	vas/o	_____
gangli/o	_____	ventricul/o	_____

Prefixes

a, an	_____	hyper	_____
dys	_____	hypo	_____
hemi	_____	macro	_____

micro _____   quadri _____

polio _____

Suffixes

Give the suffix: *Give the meaning:*

_____ embryonic   -phasia _____

_____ hernia   -phagia _____

_____ hardening   -plasia _____

_____ flow; discharge   -malacia _____

_____ suture   -ectopia _____

_____ paralysis   -poiesis _____

_____ slight paralysis   -kinesia _____

_____ lack of strength   -algesia _____

_____ pain   -taxia _____

_____ berry-shaped   -esthesia _____
             (bacteria)

Give the medical terms for the following:

_____ nerve cell.

_____ thin, delicate innermost membrane of the meninges.

_____ insertion of a needle into the lumbar region of the spinal cord to remove fluid.

_____ organ which receives a nervous impulse from a stimulus and passes it on to nerves within the body.

_____ space between nerve cells through which a nervous impulse travels.

_____ nerves carrying impulses between the brain and the head and neck.

_____ middle meningeal membrane; "spider-like."

_____ tough, outermost meningeal membrane.

_____ nerves which only carry impulses **away** from the brain and spinal cord to glands, muscles, and organs.

_____ nerves which only carry impulses **toward** the brain and spinal cord from receptors such as the sense organs.

Match the part of the nervous system in Column I with a description of its location or function in Column II:

Column I	Column II
1. pons	_____ Network of nerves.
2. cerebellum	_____ Part of the middle region of the brain; below the thalamus and controlling sleep, temperature, and water balance.
3. cerebrum	
4. meninges	_____ Knot of nerve cell bodies outside the brain and spinal cord.
5. thalamus	
	_____ Interstitial connective tissue of the nervous system.
6. medulla oblongata	
7. ganglion	_____ Posterior part of the brain; controls co-ordination of muscle movements and balance.
8. plexus	
9. neuroglia	_____ Largest part of the brain; controls voluntary movement, vision, speech, taste, hearing, and so forth.
10. hypothalamus	
	_____ Part of the brain where nerve fiber tracts cross; superior to the medulla oblongata.
	_____ Protective membranes surrounding the brain and spinal cord.
	_____ Part of the middle region of the brain; relays impulses from receptors like sense organs to other parts of the brain.

Additional Terms

acetylcholine   _____

apoplexy   _____

astrocytes   _____

autonomic nervous system   _____

axon   _____

cauda equina   _____

central nervous system   _____

cerebral cortex   _____

cerebrospinal fluid   _____

cerebrovascular accident   _____

coma   _____

convolutions (gyri)   _____

dendrites   _____

epilepsy   _____

fissures (sulci)   _____

glioma   _____

hydrocephalus   _____

meningioma   _____

microglial cells   _____

multiple sclerosis   _____

myasthenia gravis   _____

myelin sheath   _____

neurilemma   _____

nerve

_____

parasympathetic nerves

_____

Parkinson's disease

_____

spina bifida

_____

stroke

_____

sympathetic nerves

_____

syncope

_____

ventricles of the brain

_____

CHAPTER 12

CARDIOVASCULAR SYSTEM

In this chapter you will:

Learn the terms which describe the anatomy, physiology, and major pathological conditions affecting the heart and blood vessels;

Be able to trace the pathway of blood through the heart and associated blood vessels; and

Build and analyze medical terms and combining forms which relate to the cardiovascular system.

This chapter is divided into the following sections:

I. INTRODUCTION

In previous chapters we have discussed the diverse and important functions of many organs of the body. These functions include conduction of nervous impulses, production of hormones and reproductive cells, excretion of waste materials, and digestion and absorption of food substances into the bloodstream. In order to perform these functions reliably and efficiently, the body organs are powered by a unique energy source. The cells of each organ receive energy from the food substances which reach them after being taken into the body. Food contains stored (potential) energy which can be converted into the energy of movement and work. This conversion of stored energy into the active energy of work occurs when food and oxygen combine in cells during the chemical process of catabolism. It is obvious then that each cell of each organ is dependent on a constant supply of food and oxygen in order to receive sufficient energy to work well.

How does the body assure that oxygen and food will be delivered to all its cells? The cardiovascular system, consisting of a fluid called blood, vessels to carry the blood, and a hollow, muscular pump called the heart, transports food and oxygen to all organs and cells of the body. Blood vessels in the lungs absorb the oxygen which has been inhaled from the air, and blood vessels in the small intestine absorb food substances from the digestive tract. In addition, blood vessels carry cellular waste materials such as carbon dioxide and urea, and transport these substances to the lungs and kidneys, respectively, where they can be eliminated from the body.

The heart and blood vessels and the terminology related to their anatomy, physiology, and disease conditions will be explored in this chapter. The nature of blood and another body fluid called lymph will be discussed in a later chapter.

II. VOCABULARY

aneurysm	Local widening (dilation) of an artery.
angina pectoris	Chest pain.
aorta	Largest artery in the body.
arrhythmias	Abnormal heart rhythms.
arteriosclerosis	A process which causes stiffening or hardening of the walls of arteries.
artery	Largest type of blood vessel; carries blood away from the heart to all parts of the body.
atherosclerosis	A form of hardening of arteries (arteriosclerosis) in which lipids (fats) collect in the walls of blood vessels causing blockage, or occlusions (closures).
atria (singular: atrium)	Two upper chambers of the heart.
atrioventricular node (A-V node)	Specialized tissue between the upper and lower chambers of the heart which conducts an electrical impulse through the heart to cause it to beat.

bundle of His

Specialized conductive tissue in the wall between the ventricles (lower chambers of the heart) which stimulates them to contract and force blood out of the heart.

capillary

Smallest blood vessel which surrounds the tissue cells. Materials pass to and from the bloodstream through the thin capillary walls.

carbon dioxide (CO_2)

A gas released as a waste product of catabolism in the cells.

cardiac catheterization

Introducing a catheter (tube) into the heart and blood vessels for diagnostic purposes.

coronary arteries

Referring to the blood vessels which supply blood to the heart.

deoxygenated

Deficient in oxygen.

diastole

Relaxation phase of the heartbeat.

digitalis

A drug helpful in increasing the strength and regularity of heartbeat; effective in overcoming heart failure and irregular heart rhythm.

emboli (singular: embolus)

"To cast within"—floating clots or other material carried in the bloodstream.

fibrillation

Random, irregular contractions of heart muscle.

flutter

Rapid but regular contractions of the heart muscle.

hypertension

High blood pressure in the arteries.

idiopathic

Referring to a disease process which has no defined course and is of unknown causation. (idi/o = self, to one's own)

infarction

Area of tissue which dies due to lack of blood supply (ischemia).

ischemia

Insufficient blood flow to a tissue.

mitral valve

A valve found between the left upper chamber (atrium) and left lower chamber (ventricle) of the heart. This is also called the bicuspid valve.

murmur	Abnormal sound in the heart.
nitroglycerin	Drug used in angina pectoris to relieve pain by opening coronary arteries and increasing blood flow to the heart muscle.
occlusion	Closure of a blood vessel.
pacemaker	Sensitive tissue in the right atrium which begins the heartbeat; also called the sinoatrial node.
patent	Open.
pericardium	Saclike membrane surrounding the heart.
petechiae	Small, pinpoint hemorrhages.
pulmonary circulation	Flow of blood from the heart to the lungs and back again to the heart.
pulmonary artery	Artery carrying blood from the heart to the lungs. It is the only artery in the body which carries deoxygenated blood.
pulmonary vein	Vein carrying blood from the lungs to the heart. It is the only vein in the body that carries oxygenated blood.
septum (plural: septa)	A partition; in the cardiovascular system, a partition between the right and left sides of the heart.
sinoatrial node (S-A node)	Specialized tissue in the right atrium which generates an electrical impulse that sets off the heartbeat. It is also called the pacemaker.
sphygmomanometer	Instrument to measure blood pressure.
systemic circulation	Flow of blood from the cells of the body to the heart and then back out from the heart to the cells.
systole	Active, contractive phase of heartbeat.
transaminase	Enzyme liberated from myocardial cells during an infarction (heart attack).
tricuspid valve	Having three leaflets, or cusps; the valve located between the right atrium and right ventricle.

valve	A structure in veins or in the heart which temporarily closes an opening so that blood will flow only in one direction.
vegetations	Abnormal outgrowths on a structure—especially the valves of the heart.
vein	Thin-walled vessel which carries waste-filled, deoxygenated blood from the tissues toward the heart.
venae cavae (singular: vena cava)	Two largest veins in the body. The superior and inferior venae cavae empty into the right atrium of the heart.
ventricles	Lower and larger chambers of the heart.

III. BLOOD VESSELS AND THE CIRCULATION OF BLOOD

Blood Vessels

There are three major types of blood vessels in the body. These are called arteries, veins, and capillaries.

Arteries are the large blood vessels which lead blood away from the heart. Their walls are made of connective tissue, elastic fibers, and an innermost layer of epithelial cells. Because arteries carry blood away from the heart, they must be strong enough to withstand the high pressure of the pumping action of the heart. Their elastic walls allow them to expand as the heartbeat forces blood into the arterial system throughout the body. Smaller branches of arteries are called **arterioles**. Arterioles are thinner than arteries and carry the blood to the tiniest of blood vessels, the capillaries.

Capillaries have walls which are only one epithelial cell in thickness. These delicate, microscopic vessels carry nutrient-rich, oxygenated blood from the arteries and arterioles to the body cells. Their walls are thin enough to allow passage of oxygen and nutrients out of the bloodstream and into the tissue fluid surrounding the cells. Once inside the cells, the nutrients are burned in the presence of oxygen (catabolism) to release needed energy within the cell. At the same time, waste products such as carbon dioxide and water pass out of the cells and into the thin-walled capillaries. The waste-filled blood then flows back to the heart in small veins called **venules** which branch to form larger vessels called veins.

Veins are thinner-walled than arteries. They conduct waste-filled blood toward the heart from the tissues. Veins have little elastic tissue and less connective tissue than arteries, and blood pressure in veins is extremely low as compared to pressure in arteries. In order to keep blood moving back toward the heart, veins have valves which prevent the backflow of blood and keep the blood moving in one direction. Muscular action also helps the movement of blood in veins. Figure 12–1 illustrates the

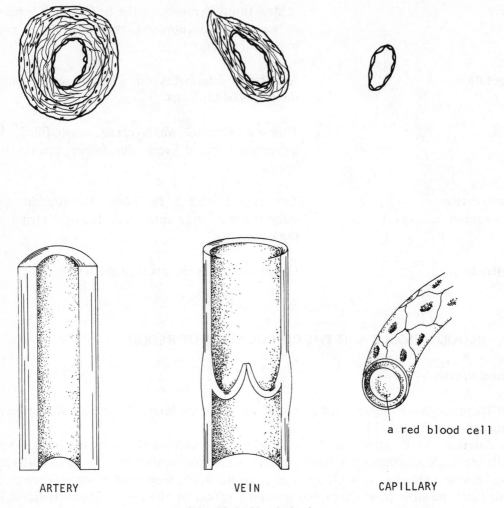

a red blood cell

ARTERY   VEIN   CAPILLARY

Figure 12–1 Blood vessels.

differences in blood vessel sizes. Figure 12–2 is a chart which reviews the major characteristics of the blood vessels.

Circulation of Blood

Arteries, arterioles, veins, venules, and capillaries, together with the heart, form a circulatory system for the flow of blood. Figure 12–3 is a schematic representation of this circulatory system. Refer to it as you read the following paragraphs.

Blood deficient in oxygen (**deoxygenated**) flows through two large veins, the **venae cavae** (1), on its way from the tissue capillaries to the heart. The blood became deoxygenated at the tissue capillaries when oxygen left the blood and entered the body cells.

Deoxygenated blood enters the **right side of the heart** (2) and travels through that side and into the **pulmonary artery** (3), a vessel which divides in two, one branch

ARTERIES	VEINS	CAPILLARIES
Carry blood away from the heart	Carry blood toward the heart	Carry blood between arteries and veins
Thick walls	Thin walls	Walls are only one cell layer thick
Elastic tissue in walls	Little elastic tissue	No elastic tissue
Carry oxygenated blood	Carry deoxygenated blood	Carry oxygenated and deoxygenated blood
	Contain valves to prevent backflow of blood	

Figure 12-2   Characteristics of arteries, veins, and capillaries.

leading to the left lung, the other to the right lung. The arteries continue dividing and subdividing within the **lungs** (4), forming smaller and smaller vessels (arterioles) and finally reaching the lung capillaries. The pulmonary artery is unusual in that it is the only artery in the body which carries deoxygenated blood.

While passing through the lung (pulmonary) capillaries, blood absorbs the oxygen which entered the body during inhalation. The newly oxygenated blood next immediately returns to the heart through the **pulmonary vein** (5). The pulmonary vein is unusual in that it is the only vein in the body which carries oxygen-rich (**oxygenated**) blood. The circulation of blood through the vessels from the heart to the lungs and then back to the heart again is known as the **pulmonary circulation**.

Oxygen-rich blood enters the **left side of the heart** (6) from the pulmonary veins. The muscles in the left side of the heart pump the blood out of the heart through the largest single artery in the body, the **aorta** (7). The aorta moves up at first (ascending aorta) but then arches over dorsally and runs downward (descending aorta) just in front of the vertebral column. The aorta divides into numerous branches called **arteries** (8) which carry the oxygenated blood to all parts of the body. The names of some of these arterial branches will be familiar to you: brachiocephalic, intercostal, esophageal, celiac, renal, and iliac arteries.

The relatively large arterial vessels branch further to form the smaller **arterioles** (9). The arterioles, still containing oxygenated blood, branch into smaller tissue **capillaries** (10), which are near the body cells. Oxygen leaves the blood as it passes through the thin capillary walls to enter the body cells. There, involved in complicated chemical processes, it combines with food to release needed energy.

One waste product of these chemical processes is carbon dioxide (CO_2). CO_2 is produced in the cell but is harmful to the cell if it remains. It must thus pass out of the cells and into the capillary bloodstream, at the same time that oxygen is entering the cell. As the blood makes its way back from the tissue capillaries toward the heart in **venules** (11) and **veins** (12), it is full of CO_2 and deoxygenated.

The circuit is thus completed when deoxygenated blood enters the heart from the venae cavae. This circulation of blood from the body organs (except the lungs) to the heart and back again is called the **systemic circulation**.

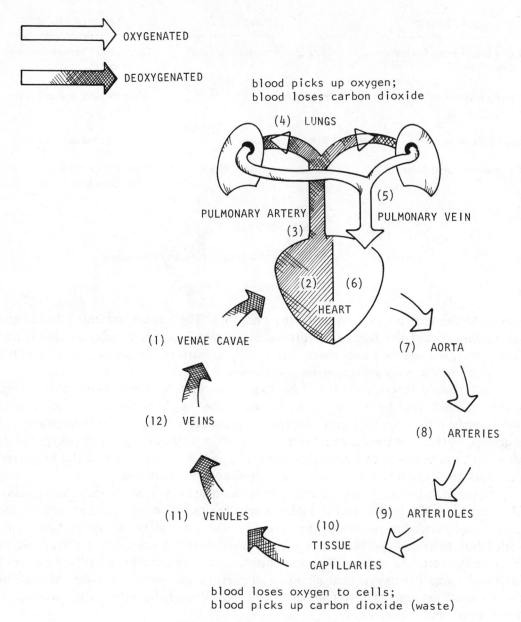

OXYGENATED

DEOXYGENATED

blood picks up oxygen;
blood loses carbon dioxide

(4) LUNGS

PULMONARY ARTERY
(3)

(5)
PULMONARY VEIN

(2) (6)
HEART

(1) VENAE CAVAE

(7) AORTA

(12) VEINS

(8) ARTERIES

(11) VENULES

(9) ARTERIOLES

(10)
TISSUE
CAPILLARIES

blood loses oxygen to cells;
blood picks up carbon dioxide (waste)

Figure 12-3 Circuit of blood flow.

IV. ANATOMY OF THE HEART

The human heart weighs less than a pound, is roughly the size of the human fist, and lies in the thoracic cavity, just behind the breastbone and between the lungs.

The heart is a pump, consisting of four chambers: two upper chambers called **atria** (singular: atrium), and two lower chambers called **ventricles**. It is actually a double pump, bound into one organ and synchronized very carefully. All the blood passes through each pump in a definite pattern. Pump station number one, on the right side of the heart, sends deoxygenated blood to the lungs, where the blood picks up oxygen and releases its carbon dioxide. The newly oxygenated blood returns to the left side of the heart to pump station number two and does not mix with the deoxygenated blood in pump station number one. Pump station number two then forces the oxygenated blood out to all parts of the body. At the body tissues, the blood loses its oxygen and upon returning to the heart, to pump station number one, deoxygenated blood is sent out to the lungs to begin the cycle anew.

Label Figure 12–4 as you learn the names of the parts of the heart and the vessels which carry blood to and from it.

Deoxygenated blood enters the heart through the two largest veins in the body, the **venae cavae**. The **superior vena cava** (1) drains blood from the upper portion of the body, while the **inferior vena cava** (2) carries blood from the lower part of the body.

The venae cavae bring deoxygenated blood which has passed through all of the body to the **right atrium** (3), the thin-walled upper right chamber of the heart. The right atrium contracts to force blood through the **tricuspid valve** (4) (cusps are the flaps of the valves) into the **right ventricle** (5), which is the lower right chamber of the heart. The cusps of the tricuspid valve form a one-way passageway designed to keep the blood flowing only in one direction. As the right ventricle contracts to pump deoxygenated blood to the lungs through the **pulmonary artery** (6), the tricuspid valve stays shut, thus preventing blood from pushing back into the right atrium.

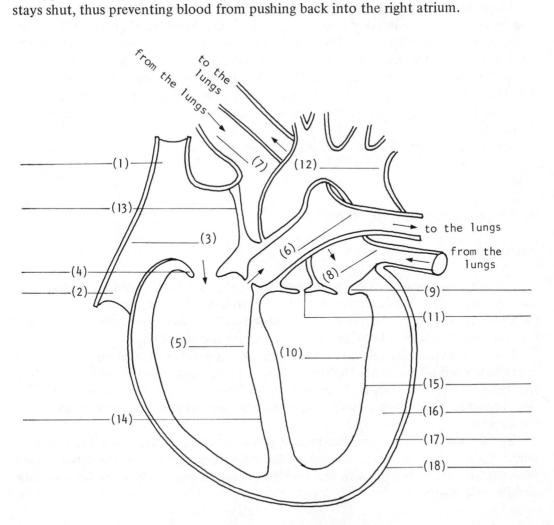

Figure 12–4 Flow of blood through the heart.

The deoxygenated blood which enters the lung capillaries from the pulmonary artery soon loses its large quantity of carbon dioxide into the lung tissue and the carbon dioxide is expelled. At the same time, oxygen enters the capillaries of the lungs and is brought back to the heart within the **pulmonary vein** (7). The newly oxygenated blood enters the **left atrium** (8) of the heart from the pulmonary vein. The walls of the left atrium contract to force blood through the **mitral valve** (9) into the **left ventricle** (10).

The left ventricle has the thickest walls of all four heart chambers (twice the thickness of the right ventricle). It must pump blood with great force so that the blood travels through arteries to all parts of the body. The blood is pumped out of the left ventricle through the **aortic valve** (11) and into the **aorta** (12), which branches to carry blood all over the body. The aortic valve prevents the return of aortic blood to the left ventricle once it has been pumped out.

The four chambers of the heart are separated by partitions called **septa** (singular: septum). The **interatrial septum** (13) separates the two upper chambers (atria), and the **interventricular septum** (14) is a muscular wall which comes between the two lower chambers (ventricles).

The heart wall is composed of three layers. The **endocardium** (15) is a smooth layer of cells which lines the interior of the heart, and also is the material of which the valves of the heart are formed. The **myocardium** (16) is the middle, muscular layer of the heart wall and is the thickest layer. The **epicardium** (17) is a thin layer and forms the outermost layer of the heart wall. The **pericardium** (18) is a delicate, double-folded membrane which surrounds the heart like a sac. It is attached to the breastbone in front and to the diaphragm below, while an inner portion of the membrane adheres to the heart.

Figure 12–5 traces the flow of blood through the heart.

V. PHYSIOLOGY OF THE HEART

Heartbeat

There are two phases of the heartbeat. These phases are called **diastole** (relaxation) and **systole** (contraction). During diastole, the atria of the heart fill with blood from the venae cavae and the pulmonary vein. At the end of diastole, the atria contract and force blood into the ventricles through the tricuspid and mitral valves.

Systole begins as diastole ends. The ventricles, now filled with blood, contract and pump blood out of the heart. The right ventricle pumps blood to the pulmonary artery and lungs, and the left ventricle pumps blood into the aorta and its branches. The mitral and tricuspid valves close during systole to prevent the flow of blood back into the atria.

Systole, then, is the active contraction phase of the heartbeat, when the ventricles pump blood out of the heart. Diastole is the relaxation phase of the heartbeat, when the atria and ventricles fill with blood. Figure 12–6 shows the heart in both systolic and diastolic phases.

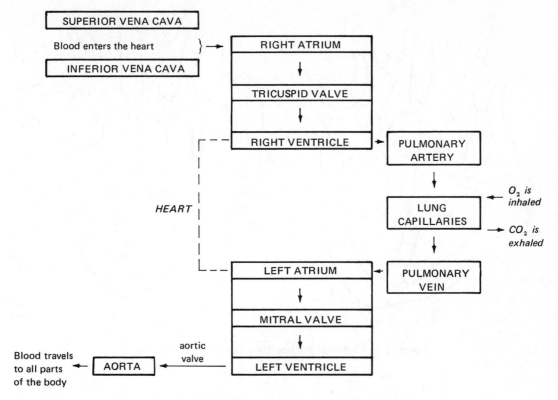

Figure 12–5 Pathway of blood through the heart.

Conduction System of the Heart

What keeps the heart at its perfect rhythm? Although the heart does have nerves which can affect its rate, they are not primarily responsible for its beat. It is known that the heart starts beating in the embryo before it is supplied with nerves, and it will continue to beat in experimental animals even when the nerve supply is cut.

Primary responsibility for initiating the heartbeat (systole and diastole) rests with a small region of specialized muscle tissue in the posterior portion of the right atrium, where an electrical impulse originates. This region of the right atrium is called the **sinoatrial node (S-A node)**. The S-A node is also called the **pacemaker** of the heart. The current of electricity generated by the pacemaker causes the walls of the atria to contract and force blood into the ventricles (ending diastole).

Almost like ripples in a pond of water when a stone is thrown, the wave of electricity passes from the pacemaker to another region of the myocardium. This region is at the posterior portion of the interatrial septum and is called the **atrioventricular node (A-V node)**. The A-V node immediately sends the excitation wave along to a region deep in the ventricle wall, called the **bundle of His**. From there the electrical wave passes to all parts of the ventricles and stimulates them to contract (systole), pumping blood from the heart. A short rest period follows (diastole), and then the pacemaker begins the wave of excitation across the heart again. Figure 12–7 shows the location of the S-A node, the A-V node, and the bundle of His.

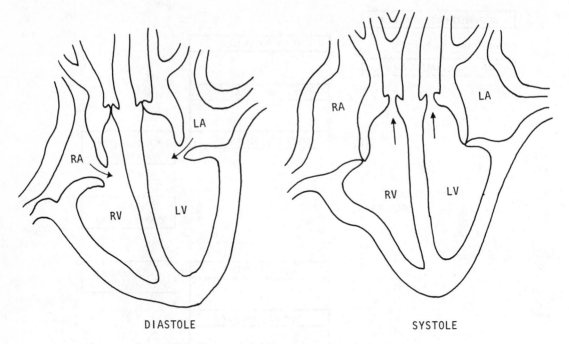

Figure 12-6 Phases of the heartbeat: diastole and systole.

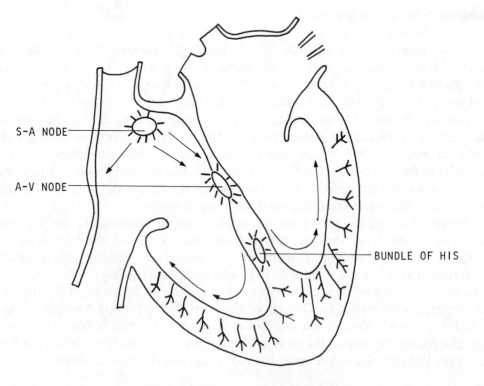

Figure 12-7 Conduction system of the heart.

The record used to detect these electrical changes in heart muscle as the heart beats is called an **electrocardiogram (EKG or ECG)**. The normal EKG shows five waves, or deflections, which represent the electrical changes as a wave of excitation spreads through the heart. The deflections are called P, Q, R, S, and T waves. The P wave occurs as the atria contract and the electrical impulse passes from the S-A node to the A-V node. The Q, R, and S waves represent the spread of excitation through the bundle of His and the ventricle wall (during systole). The T wave represents the electrical recovery and relaxation of the ventricles. Figure 12–8 illustrates P, Q, R, S, and T waves in a normal electrocardiogram.

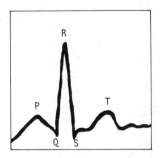

Figure 12–8 An electrocardiogram.

P wave = spread of excitation wave over the atria

QRS wave = spread of excitation wave over the ventricle

T wave = electrical recovery and relaxation of the ventricles

Nervous Control of the Heart

The heartbeat can be regulated by nervous impulses from the autonomic nervous system (parasympathetic and sympathetic nerves). The parasympathetic nerve supply to the heart is distributed mainly to the S-A and A-V nodes and causes a fall in the heart rate. Massive parasympathetic stimulation (the vagus nerve is the major nerve involved) can stop the heart for several seconds.

Sympathetic nerves lead to all areas of the heart, but especially to the ventricular muscle. Sympathetic stimulation increases heart rate and can even strengthen the force of the ventricular contraction. This is felt, for example, during exercise and periods of emotional distress.

Figure 12–9 shows the parasympathetic and sympathetic nerve supply to the heart.

VI. BLOOD PRESSURE

Blood pressure is the force which the blood exerts on the arterial walls. This pressure is measured by a device called a **sphygmomanometer.**

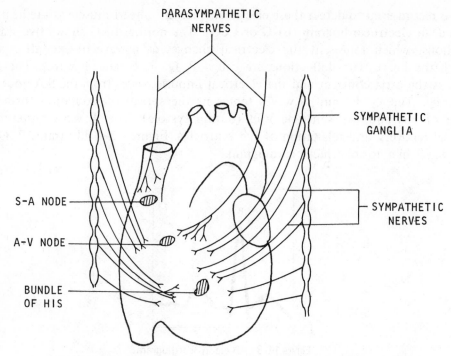

Figure 12-9 The parasympathetic and sympathetic nerve supply to the heart.

The sphygmomanometer consists of a rubber bag inside a cloth cuff which is wrapped around the upper arm, just above the elbow. The rubber bag is inflated with air by means of a rubber bulb. As the bag is pumped up, the pressure within it increases and is measured on a recording device attached to the cuff.

The vessels in the upper arm are compressed by the air pressure in the bag. When there is sufficient air pressure in the bag to stop the flow of blood in the main artery of the arm (brachial artery), the pulse in the lower arm (where the observer is listening with a stethoscope) obviously drops.

Air is then allowed to escape from the bag and the pressure is lowered slowly, allowing the blood to begin to make its way through the gradually opening artery. At the point when the person listening with the stethoscope first hears the sounds of the pulse beats, the reading on the device attached to the cuff shows the higher, systolic, blood pressure (pressure in the artery when the ventricles are contracting).

As air continues to escape, the sounds become progressively louder. Finally, when a change in sound from loud to soft occurs, the observer makes note of the pressure on the recording device. This is called the diastolic blood pressure (pressure in the artery when the ventricles are relaxing).

Blood pressure is usually expressed as a fraction: for example, 120/80, in which 120 represents the systolic pressure and 80 the diastolic pressure.

VII. COMBINING FORMS AND TERMINOLOGY

Combining Form	Meaning	Terminology	Meaning
cardi/o	heart	bradycardia	_____
		tachycardia	_____
		cardiomegaly	_____
coron/o	heart	coronary arteries	_____
aort/o	aorta	aortic stenosis	_____
angi/o	vessel	angionecrosis	_____
		angiogram	_____
		angiorrhaphy	_____
		angiostenosis	_____
		hemangioma	_____
vas/o	vessel	vasoconstriction	_____
		vasodilation	_____
arteri/o	artery	arteriosclerosis	_____
		arterial anastomosis	_____
		arteritis	_____
arteriol/o	arteriole, small artery	arteriolitis	_____
phleb/o	vein	phlebitis	_____
		phlebotomy	_____
		phlebolith	_____
ven/o	vein	venotomy	_____
		venospasm	_____

venul/o	venule, small vein	<u>venul</u>itis _____
atri/o	atrium	<u>atri</u>oventricular _____
ventricul/o	ventricle	<u>ventricul</u>otomy _____
		<u>ventricul</u>ar _____
valv/o	valve	<u>valv</u>otomy _____
steth/o	chest	<u>steth</u>oscope _____
		A misnomer since the examination is by ear, not by eye.
sphygm/o	pulse	<u>sphygm</u>omanometer _____
ox/o	oxygen	hyp<u>ox</u>ia _____
ather/o	yellowish plaque, fatty substance	<u>ather</u>osclerosis _____
		<u>ather</u>oma _____
aneurysm/o	aneurysm	<u>aneurysm</u>ectomy _____
de	lack of	<u>de</u>oxygenation _____

VIII. PATHOLOGICAL CONDITIONS OF THE HEART

coronary artery disease   Disease of the arteries surrounding the heart.

The coronary arteries are two large vessels which arise from the aorta and supply oxygenated blood to the heart. It is interesting that the blood which constantly flows through the four hollow chambers of the heart does not itself nourish the myocardial tissue. Instead, after blood leaves the heart via the aorta, a portion is at once led back over the surface of the heart through the coronary arteries so that the heart feeds itself before any other organ. This seems logical since the energy requirements of the heart are greater than those of any other organ. Figure 12–10 shows the right and left coronary arteries as they branch from the aorta.

Coronary artery disease is usually the result of **atherosclerosis** (ather/o = paste, porridge). This is the deposition of fatty compounds on the inner lining of the arteries (any other artery in the body can be similarly affected). The ordinarily smooth lining of the artery becomes roughened and seems to look like grains of porridge. Atherosclerosis is a

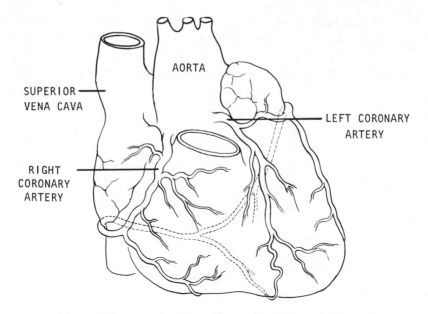

Figure 12–10 Coronary arteries supplying the heart.

form of **arteriosclerosis**, which generally means the deposition of any hard material in the walls of arteries, resulting in inflexibility.

Atherosclerosis is dangerous for two important reasons. First, the roughened lining of the artery can cause abnormal clotting of blood in the coronary arteries leading to a thrombotic occlusion (blocking of the artery by a clot). Second, narrowing of the vessel due to atherosclerotic deposits may itself lead to inflexibility and plugging up of the vessel. In both cases, blood flow is decreased or stopped entirely, leading to death of the myocardium. The area of dead myocardial tissue is known as an **infarction**. The infarcted area is eventually replaced by scar tissue.

The severity of a myocardial infarction (also known as a **heart attack**) depends on the size of the artery which is blocked and the extent of the blockage. If the blocked artery is small enough the result may be death of only a small portion of the heart immediately fed by the artery. After scar tissue forms, the patient may be able to resume completely normal activity.

An enzyme, **transaminase**, is liberated from the myocardium during a myocardial infarction and passes into the blood. The blood levels of transaminase may rise 20 times normal within 24 hours after an infarction. Measurement of this enzyme, as well as other enzymes, is useful in determining proof of an infarction.

arrhythmias	Abnormal heart rhythms.

Some examples of cardiac arrhythmias are:

1. **heart block** (**atrioventricular block**)	Failure of proper conduction of impulses through the A-V node to the bundle of His.

If conduction of the electrical impulse down the bundle of His is prevented by a disease process, the result is known as heart block. The heart then has a much slower rate of contraction. The implantation of an electric pacemaker can overcome heart block and establish a new rate for the heart by serving as an artificial source of excitation for the heart.

2. **flutter**   Rapid but regular contractions of the heart.

This condition occurs mainly in patients with heart disease. The heart rhythm can reach up to 240 to 260 beats per minute.

3. **fibrillation**   Rapid random and irregular contractions of the heart.

In atrial fibrillation the wave of excitation passes through the atrial myocardium even more quickly than in atrial flutter. An electrical defibrillator is a device used to reverse fibrillation. The device applies shocks to the heart using electrodes on the chest wall.

rheumatic heart disease   Heart disease caused by rheumatic fever.

Rheumatic fever is caused by a streptococcal infection which indirectly affects all parts of the heart—endocardium, myocardium, and pericardium (**pancarditis**)—particularly the heart valves. The valves, especially the mitral valve, become inflamed (**endocarditis**). As the cusps become thickened, they adhere and the valvular opening becomes narrowed, leading to **mitral stenosis**. This means that not enough blood can flow from the left atrium to the left ventricle, and the blood is held back, first in the lungs and then in the right side of the heart, and finally in the veins. The condition called atrial fibrillation is apt to develop in which the atria no longer contract in a regular manner. The pulse becomes irregular and the ventricles of the heart are exhausted because of a shortened period of diastole (relaxation). **Digitalis** is one drug which prevents the irregular impulses from the atria from reaching the ventricles, and the patient experiences relief as the heart begins to beat in a slower and more regular manner.

bacterial endocarditis   Inflammation of the inner lining of the heart.

This condition is caused by bacteria which infect the heart valves. There is great damage to the heart valves producing large lesions, called vegetations, which may break off into the bloodstream as **emboli** (floating clots). The emboli may lodge in the arteries of the brain and cause ischemia and paralysis, may appear in the kidney and cause hematuria, or may lodge in the small vessels of the skin to form multiple pinpoint hemorrhages known as **petechiae**. Antibiotics are effective in curing this disease.

heart murmur   Abnormal sounds in the heartbeat.

This abnormal heart sound is heard with the aid of a stethoscope, and is usually caused by a valvular defect or disease which disrupts the smooth flow of blood in the heart. Murmurs can also be heard in cases of interseptal defects where blood is abnormally flowing between chambers through holes in the septa. A functional murmur is one that is not caused by a valve or septal defect and is not a serious danger to the patient's health.

hypertensive heart disease   High blood pressure affecting the heart.

This disease is caused by the contracting of the arterioles of the body leading to increased pressure in arteries. The increased pressure may result in the bursting of a blood vessel in the brain (**cerebral hemorrhage**), or atrophy of an organ like the kidney, which could lead to **renal failure**. The heart itself is affected because it has to pump more vigorously to overcome the increased resistance in the arteries. The vessels lose their elasticity, become like solid pipes, and place increased burden on the heart to pump blood through the body.

congenital heart disease   Abnormalities in the heart at birth.

The following conditions are congenital anomalies resulting from some failure in the development of the fetus. A diagnostic method called **cardiac catheterization** may be used to provide a precise description of any anatomic abnormality in the heart, including congenital anomalies. In this procedure, a catheter (tube) is introduced into the heart via a vein. The catheter is used to sample pressures and oxygen content in the heart chambers, to introduce dye which can be seen on x-ray, and to provide information about structural abnormalities of the heart.

1. **septal defects**   Small holes in the septa between the atria or ventricles.

Septal defects can be closed while maintaining a general circulation by means of a heart-lung machine.

2. **tetralogy of Fallot**   A combination of four congenital defects in the heart which results in most of the blood failing to go to the pulmonary circulation to pick up needed oxygen.

Figure 12–11 illustrates the defects in tetralogy of Fallot:

(1) Pulmonary stenosis: Narrowing of the pulmonary artery and its valve so that blood is not adequately passed to the lungs and less blood is oxygenated.

(2) A gap is present in the septum and deoxygenated blood passes to the aorta and travels all over the body.

(3) The septum which separates the right and left sides of the heart is shifted to the right, which further narrows the pulmonary opening.

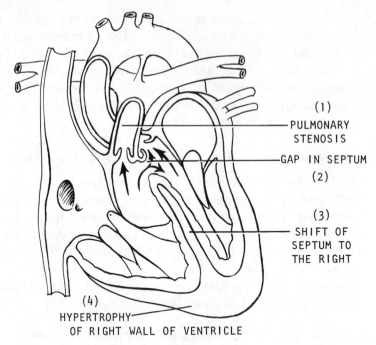

(1)
PULMONARY
STENOSIS

GAP IN SEPTUM
(2)

(3)
SHIFT OF
SEPTUM TO
THE RIGHT

(4)
HYPERTROPHY
OF RIGHT WALL OF VENTRICLE

Figure 12–11 Tetralogy of Fallot.

(4) The wall of the right ventricle is hypertrophied and thus increases the need of the myocardium for oxygen and nourishment.

An infant with this condition is known as a "blue baby" because of the extreme degree of **cyanosis** (cyan/o = blue) present upon birth. Several operations may be performed to alleviate this condition: repair of the septal defect using a synthetic patch; anastomosis of the pulmonary artery to an aortic branch so that poorly oxygenated aortic blood can flow back to the lungs; and enlargement of the outflow tract of the right ventricle.

3. **patent ductus arteriosus**   Failure of a vessel in the fetal heart to close after birth.

The ductus arteriosus is a short vessel which connects the pulmonary artery and the aorta during fetal life. Hence, *in utero* while the lungs are not used, much blood can pass from the right side of the heart into the aorta without passing through the lungs. After birth, the ductus normally closes. However, it may remain **patent** (open) in this condition. The blood then flows from the aorta to the pulmonary artery since the pressure is higher in the former. This results in dilation of the pulmonary artery and overload of the right side of the heart. The treatment is a surgical operation to close the ductus. Figure 12–12 shows the ductus arteriosus connecting the aorta to the pulmonary artery.

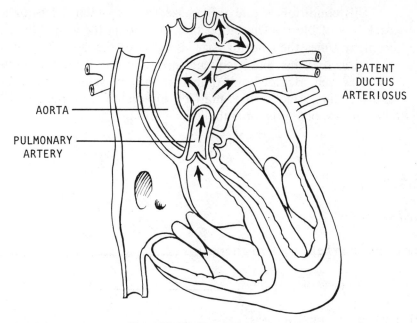

AORTA

PULMONARY
ARTERY

PATENT
DUCTUS
ARTERIOSUS

Figure 12-12   Patent ductus arteriosus.

IX. BLOOD VESSEL DISORDERS

arterial hypertension High blood pressure in arteries.

There are two kinds of high blood pressure, or hypertension: **essential** and **secondary**. In essential hypertension, the cause of the increased pressure is **idiopathic** (unknown). In secondary hypertension, there is always some associated lesion, such as glomerulonephritis, pyelonephritis, or adenoma of the adrenal cortex, which is responsible for the elevated blood pressure.

aneurysm Local widening of an artery.

Aneurysms may be due to a weakness in the arterial wall or breakdown of the wall due to atherosclerosis. The weak part of the wall bellies out with each beat of the heart. An **aneurysmectomy** is a surgical procedure which removes an aneurysm. After removal, a bypass arterial segment is necessary.

varicose veins Dilated, twisted veins.

This condition is due to damaged valves which fail to prevent the backflow of blood. The blood then collects in the veins, which distend to many times their normal size. Because of the slow flow of blood in the varicose veins and frequent injury to the vein, thrombosis may occur as well. Hemorrhoids (piles) are varicose veins at the distal end of the intestinal tract. They may be internal or external, and lead to thrombosis, phlebitis, or embolism.

X. EXERCISES

A. *Build medical words:*

1. New connection between two arteries _____

2. Instrument to measure the pulse _____

3. Inflammation of small arteries _____

4. Suture of a vein _____

5. Tumor of yellowish plaque _____

6. Pertaining to the atria and ventricles _____

7. Slow heartbeat _____

8. Dilation of a lymph vessel _____

9. Enlargement of the heart _____

10. Removal of an aneurysm _____

11. High blood pressure _____

12. Narrowing of the mitral valve _____

13. Heart muscle _____

14. Floating clot _____

15. Inflammation of a vein _____

16. Rapid heartbeat _____

17. Hardening of arteries _____

B. *Give the meaning of the following:*

1. atherosclerosis _____

_____

2. bundle of His _____

3. endocardium _____

4. vasoconstriction _____

5. pacemaker _____

6. deoxygenation _____

7. cardiac murmur _____

8. angiocardiography _____

9. systole _____

10. diastole _____

11. cardiac catheterization _____

_____

12. transaminase _____

13. aneurysm _____

14. angina pectoris _____

15. ischemia _____

16. nitroglycerin _____

17. digitalis _____

18. varicose veins _____

19. infarction _____

20. petechiae _____

C. *Trace the path of blood through the heart.* Begin as the blood enters the right atrium from the venae cavae (include the valves between the heart chambers):

1. _____*right atrium*_____   6. _____

2. _____   7. _____

3. _____   8. _____

4. _____   9. _____

5. _____   10. _____

D. *Match the term for the cardiovascular structure in Column I with an appropriate meaning in Column II:*

Column I	Column II
1. arteriole	_____ Small vein.
2. capillary	_____ Only artery which carries deoxygenated blood.
3. atrium	
	_____ Largest vein in the body.
4. aorta	
	_____ Lies between the left atrium and left
5. venule	ventricle.
6. mitral valve	_____ Upper chamber of the heart.
7. vena cava	_____ Smallest of the blood vessels.
8. tricuspid valve	_____ Only vein which carries oxygenated blood.
9. pulmonary artery	_____ Small artery.
10. pulmonary vein	_____ Lies between the right atrium and right ventricle.
	_____ Largest artery in the body.

E. *Match the blood vessel or heart condition in Column I with its description in Column II:*

<table>
<tr><td>*Column I*</td><td>*Column II*</td></tr>
<tr><td>1. heart block</td><td>_____ Small holes within the walls between the right and left sides of the heart.</td></tr>
<tr><td>2. rheumatic heart disease</td><td>_____ A fetal vessel connecting the aorta and pulmonary artery; remains open long after birth.</td></tr>
<tr><td>3. atrial fibrillation</td><td></td></tr>
<tr><td>4. patent ductus arteriosus</td><td>_____ High blood pressure of idiopathic origin.</td></tr>
<tr><td>5. tetralogy of Fallot</td><td>_____ Blockage of the two major arteries which circle the heart and supply blood to the myocardium.</td></tr>
<tr><td>6. septal defects</td><td></td></tr>
<tr><td>7. coronary artery disease</td><td>_____ Bradycardia or tachycardia.</td></tr>
<tr><td></td><td>_____ Streptococcal infection which indirectly leads to pancarditis.</td></tr>
<tr><td>8. bacterial endocarditis</td><td></td></tr>
<tr><td>9. arrhythmias</td><td>_____ Failure of electrical impulse to travel from the A-V node to the bundle of His.</td></tr>
<tr><td>10. essential hypertension</td><td>_____ Random and irregular contraction of the upper chambers of the heart.</td></tr>
<tr><td></td><td>_____ Inflammation of the inner lining of the heart, especially heart valves.</td></tr>
<tr><td></td><td>_____ "Blue baby"—a combination of four congenital heart defects resulting in failure of enough blood reaching the lungs.</td></tr>
</table>

ANSWERS

A.
1. arterial anastomosis
2. sphygmomanometer
3. arteriolitis
4. phleborrhaphy
5. atheroma
6. atrioventricular
7. bradycardia
8. lymphangiectasis
9. cardiomegaly

10. aneurysmectomy
11. hypertension
12. mitral stenosis
13. myocardium
14. embolus
15. phlebitis
16. tachycardia
17. arteriosclerosis

B.
1. Collection of fatty, yellowish plaques in arteries, leading to hardening and inflexibility.
2. Specialized conductive tissue in the ventricle wall.
3. Inner lining of the heart.
4. Tightening of a vessel.
5. S-A node; specialized muscle tissue in the wall of the right atrium.
6. Lack of oxygen in blood.
7. Abnormal sound in the heart.
8. Process of recording (x-ray) the heart and major vessels.
9. Active, contracting phase of heartbeat; heart pumps blood out to lungs and body.
10. Heart fills with blood; relaxation phase of heartbeat.
11. Inserting a catheter (tube) into the heart via a vein; measurements of pressure are made, and dye is injected for x-ray.
12. Enzyme released by myocardium during a myocardial infarction (heart attack).
13. Local widening of an artery.
14. Chest pain.
15. Holding back of blood due to blockage of a vessel.
16. Drug given for the relief of angina pectoris; arteries become more relaxed and more blood flows to the myocardium.
17. Drug used to overcome fibrillation of the heart.
18. Twisted, dilated veins.
19. Area of dead tissue.
20. Small pinpoint hemorrhages.

C.
1. right atrium	6. pulmonary veins
2. tricuspid valve	7. left atrium
3. right ventricle	8. mitral valve
4. pulmonary artery	9. left ventricle
5. lung capillaries	10. aorta

D.
5
9
7
6
3
2
10
1
8
4

E.
6
4
10
7
9
2
1
3
8
5

REVIEW SHEET 12

Combining Forms

aneurysm/o	_____	lith/o	_____
angi/o	_____	necr/o	_____
aort/o	_____	ox/o	_____
arteri/o	_____	phleb/o	_____
arteriol/o	_____	pulmon/o	_____
ather/o	_____	sphygm/o	_____
atri/o	_____	steth/o	_____
axill/o	_____	thromb/o	_____
brachi/o	_____	valv/o	_____
cardi/o	_____	vas/o	_____
coron/o	_____	ven/o	_____
idi/o	_____	ventricul/o	_____
isch/o	_____	venul/o	_____
lip/o	_____		

Suffixes

-emia	_____	-sclerosis	_____
-orrhaphy	_____	-spasm	_____
-megaly	_____	-stasis	_____
-meter	_____	-stenosis	_____

Prefixes

brady	_____	inter	_____
de	_____	peri	_____
endo	_____	tachy	_____
hyper	_____	tetra	_____
hypo	_____	tri	_____

Additional Terms

aneurysm _____

angina pectoris _____

aorta _____

arrhythmia _____

arteriosclerosis _____

atherosclerosis _____

atria _____

atrioventricular node (A-V node) _____

bacterial endocarditis _____

bundle of His _____

capillary _____

cardiac catheterization _____

coronary arteries _____

deoxygenated _____

diastole _____

digitalis _____

dilatation (dilation) _____

emboli _____

fibrillation _____

flutter _____

heart block _____

heart murmur _____

hemorrhoids _____

hypertension _____

idiopathic _____

infarction _____

mitral valve _____

nitroglycerin _____

occlusion _____

pacemaker _____

patent ductus arteriosus _____

petechiae _____

pulmonary artery _____

pulmonary circulation _____

pulmonary vein _____

septum _____

sinoatrial node (S-A node) _____

sphygmomanometer _____

systemic circulation _____

systole _____

tetralogy of Fallot _____

_____

transaminase _____

tricuspid valve _____

varicose veins _____

vegetations _____

venae cavae _____

ventricle _____

CHAPTER 13

RESPIRATORY SYSTEM

In this chapter you will:

Learn the terms which describe the anatomic structures and pathological conditions of the respiratory system; and

Recognize and use the combining forms, prefixes, and suffixes which apply to respiration and respiratory diseases.

This chapter is divided into the following sections:

I. INTRODUCTION

We usually think of **respiration** as the mechanical process of breathing, that is, the repetitive and, for the most part, unconscious exchange of air between the lungs and the external environment. This exchange of air at the lungs is also called **external respiration**. In external respiration, oxygen is inhaled (air inhaled contains about 21 per cent oxygen) into the air spaces (sacs) of the lungs and immediately passes into tiny capillary blood vessels surrounding the air spaces. Simultaneously, carbon dioxide, a waste product of the chemical combination of oxygen and food in cells, passes from the capillary blood vessels into the air spaces of the lungs to be exhaled (exhaled air contains about 16 per cent carbon dioxide).

While external respiration occurs between the outside environment and the capillary bloodstream of the lungs, another form of respiration is occurring simultaneously between the individual body cells and the tiny capillary blood vessels which surround them. This process is called **internal** (cellular) **respiration**. Internal respiration is the exchange of gases not at the lungs but at the cells within all the organs of the body. In this process, oxygen carried in the blood from the capillaries of the lung to the capillaries surrounding body cells passes out of the bloodstream and into the cells. At the same time, carbon dioxide, the waste produced in cells as oxygen chemically combines with food, passes from the tissue cells into the bloodstream and is carried by the blood back to the lungs to be exhaled.

Figure 13–1 summarizes the events which occur simultaneously during both external and internal respiration.

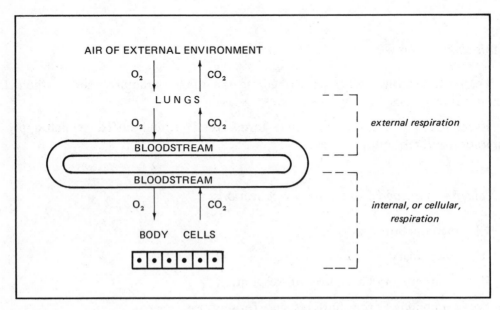

Figure 13–1   Events which occur simultaneously during external and internal respiration.

II. VOCABULARY

abscess	Local area of pus formation.
adenoids	Collections of lymph tissue in the throat. Also called pharyngeal tonsils.
alveolus (plural: alveoli)	Air sac in the lung. (Also used to describe the sockets of the jaws in which the roots of teeth are embedded.)
bacillus (plural: bacilli)	Rod-shaped bacterium.
bronchus (plural: bronchi)	Branch of the trachea (windpipe) which acts as a passageway into the air spaces of the lung.

bronchioles	Smallest branches of the bronchi.
carbon dioxide (CO_2)	A gaseous waste produced by body cells when oxygen and food combine.
cilia	Thin hairs attached to the mucous membrane epithelium lining the respiratory tract.
edema	Swelling; fluid in the tissues.
effusion	Pouring out of fluid into a part or tissue.
embolus	"To throw in"—a floating clot or other material in circulation.
epiglottis	Fold of cartilage which covers the larynx (voice box).
external respiration	Exchange of gases in the lungs.
glottis	Mouth of, or entrance to, the larynx and trachea.
internal respiration	Exchange of gases at the tissue cells.
larynx	Voice box.
lobes	Divisions of the lungs.
mediastinum	Region between the lungs in the chest cavity. It contains the heart, aorta, esophagus, and bronchial tubes.
oxygen (O_2)	Gas which passes into the bloodstream at the lungs, and travels to all body cells.
parietal pleura	The outer fold of pleura lying closest to the ribs and wall of the thoracic cavity.
paroxysmal	Pertaining to a sudden, violent event.
pharynx	Throat.
pleura	Double-folded membrane surrounding each lung.
pleural cavity	Space between the folds of the pleura.
pulmonary parenchyma	The working, active cells of the lung; the air sacs and small bronchioles.

stridor	Harsh, high-pitched respiratory sound.
tonsils	Two rounded masses of lymph tissue in the throat.
trachea	Windpipe.
visceral pleura	The inner fold of pleura lying closest to the lung tissue.

III. ANATOMY AND PHYSIOLOGY OF RESPIRATION

Label Figure 13–2 as you read the following paragraphs.

Air enters the body through the **nose** (1) and passes through the **nasal cavities** (2) which are lined with a mucous membrane and fine hairs (cilia) to help filter out foreign bodies, as well as to warm and moisten the air. **Paranasal sinuses** (3) are hollow, air-containing cavities within the cranium. They, too, have a mucous membrane lining and function to provide the lubricating fluid mucus, as well as to lighten the bones of the skull and help produce sound.

After passing through the nasal cavities, the air next reaches the **pharynx** (throat). There are three divisions of the pharynx. The **nasopharynx** (4) is the first division, and is nearest to the nasal cavities. It contains the **adenoids** (5), which are masses of lymphatic tissue. The adenoids are more prominent in children, and if enlarged can obstruct air passageways. Below the nasopharynx and closer to the mouth is the second division of the pharynx, the **oropharynx** (6). The **tonsils** (7), two rounded masses of lymphatic tissue, are located in the oropharynx. The third division of the pharynx is the **hypopharynx** (also called the **laryngopharynx**) (8). It is in the hypopharyngeal region that the pharynx, serving as a common passageway for food from the mouth and air from the nose, divides into two branches, the **larynx** (voice box) (9), and the **esophagus** (10).

The esophagus leads into the stomach and carries food to be digested. The larynx contains the vocal cords and is surrounded by pieces of cartilage for support. Sounds are produced as air is expelled past the vocal cords and the cords vibrate. The tension of the vocal cords determines the high or low pitch of the voice.

Since food entering from the mouth and air entering from the nose mix in the pharynx, what prevents the passing of food or drink into the larynx and respiratory system after it has been swallowed? Even with a small quantity of solid or liquid matter finding its way into the air passages, breathing could be seriously blocked. A special deterrent to this event is provided for by a flap of cartilage attached to the root of the tongue which acts like a lid over the larynx. This flap of cartilage is called the **epiglottis** (11). The epiglottis lies over the mouth of the larynx (also called the glottis). In the act of swallowing, when food and water move through the throat, the glottis automatically moves under the epiglottis, closing off the larynx so that food cannot enter.

On its way to the lungs, air passes from the larynx to the **trachea** (windpipe) (12), a vertical tube about 4½ inches long and an inch in diameter. The trachea is kept open by 16 to 20 C-shaped rings of cartilage separated by fibrous connective tissue which stiffen the front and sides of the tube.

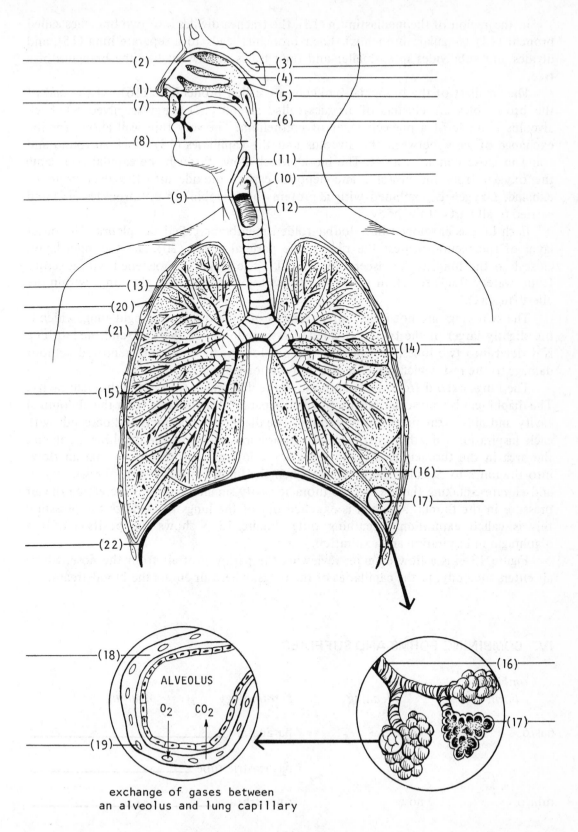

exchange of gases between
an alveolus and lung capillary

Figure 13-2 Organs of the respiratory system.

In the region of the **mediastinum** (13), the trachea divides into two branches called **bronchi** (14) (singular: bronchus). Each bronchus leads to a separate **lung** (15), and divides and subdivides into smaller and finer tubes, somewhat like the branches of a tree.

The smallest of the bronchial branches are called **bronchioles** (16). At the end of the bronchioles are clusters of air sacs called **alveoli** (17) (singular: alveolus). Each alveolus is made of a one-cell layer of epithelium. The very thin wall allows for the exchange of gases between the alveolus and the **capillaries** (18) which surround and come in close contact with it. The blood which flows through the capillaries accepts the oxygen from the alveolus and deposits carbon dioxide into the alveolus to be exhaled. Oxygen is combined with a protein (hemoglobin) in **erythrocytes** (19) and carried to all parts of the body.

Each lung is enveloped in a double-folded membrane called the **pleura**. The outer layer of the pleura, nearest the ribs, is the **parietal pleura** (20), and the inner layer, closest to the lung, is the **visceral pleura** (21). The pleura is moistened with a serous (thin, watery fluid) secretion which facilitates the movements of the lungs within the chest (thorax).

The two lungs are not quite mirror images of each other. The right lung, which is the slightly larger of the two, is divided into three **lobes**, or divisions, and the left lung is divided into two lobes. It is possible for one lobe of the lung to be removed without damage to the rest, which can continue to function normally.

The lungs extend from the collarbone to the **diaphragm** (22) in the thoracic cavity. The diaphragm is a muscular partition which separates the thoracic from the abdominal cavity and aids in the process of breathing. The diaphragm contracts and descends with each **inspiration** (breathing in). The downward movement of the diaphragm enlarges the area in the thoracic cavity and reduces the internal air pressure so that air flows into the lungs to equalize the pressure. When the lungs are full, the diaphragm relaxes and elevates, making the area in the thoracic cavity smaller, and thus increasing the air pressure in the thorax. Air then is expelled out of the lungs to equalize the pressure; this is called **expiration** (breathing out). Figure 13–3 shows the position of the diaphragm in inspiration and expiration.

Figure 13–4 is a flow diagram reviewing the pathway of air from the nose, where air enters the body, to the capillaries of the lungs, where air enters the bloodstream.

IV. COMBINING FORMS AND SUFFIXES

Combining Form	Meaning	Terminology	Meaning
nas/o	nose	paranasal	_____
		nasogastric tube	_____
rhin/o	nose	rhinorrhea	_____
		rhinoplasty	_____

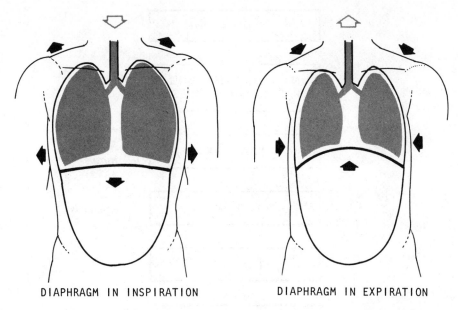

DIAPHRAGM IN INSPIRATION   DIAPHRAGM IN EXPIRATION

Figure 13-3 Position of the diaphragm during inspiration and expiration.

		rhinostenosis _____
adenoid/o	adenoids	adenoid hypertrophy _____
		adenoidectomy _____
tonsill/o	tonsils	tonsillectomy _____
pharyng/o	throat	pharyngeal _____
		nasopharyngitis _____
laryng/o	voice box, larynx	laryngotracheobronchitis _____
		_____
		laryngostomy _____
		laryngoplasty _____
		laryngoscopy _____
epiglott/o	epiglottis	epiglottitis _____
trache/o	windpipe, trachea	tracheotomy _____

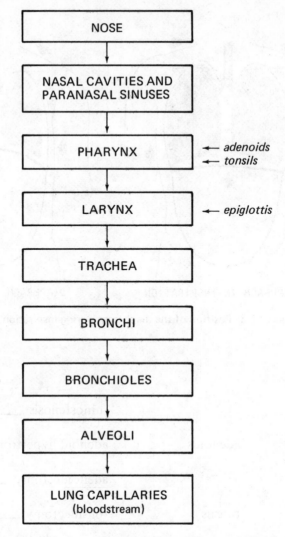

Figure 13-4 Pathway of air from the nose to the capillaries of the lungs.

tracheoesophageal _____

endotracheal _____

bronch/o   bronchial tube   bronchitis _____
bronchi/o
                                     bronchorrhagia _____

                                     bronchostenosis _____

                                     bronchiectasis _____

bronchiol/o	bronchiole, small bronchus	bronchiolitis _____
pulmon/o	lung	pulmonary _____
		pulmono-aortic _____
pneumon/o pneum/o	lung, air	pneumonectomy _____
		pneumonitis _____
		pneumoencephalography _____
lob/o	lobe of the lung	lobectomy _____
phren/o	diaphragm	phrenic _____
	(also can mean the "mind" in some medical terms)	schizophrenia _____
		("Split mind," an altered sense of reality.)
		phrenodynia _____
pector/o	chest	expectoration _____
pleur/o	pleura	pleuritis _____
		pleurocentesis _____
spir/o	to breathe	inspiration _____
		expiration _____
		Note that the "s" is omitted.
		respiration _____
sinus/o	sinus, cavity	sinusitis _____
		sinusoid _____
coni/o	dust	pneumoconiosis _____
anthrac/o	coal dust	anthracosis _____
alveol/o	alveolus; air sac; small hollow or cavity	alveolar _____
		alveolitis _____
ox/o	oxygen	anoxia _____

		hypoxia _____
		hypoxemia _____
cyan/o	blue	cyanosis _____
-osmia	smell	anosmia _____
-capnia	carbon dioxide	hypercapnia _____
-phonia	voice	dysphonia _____
-ptysis	spitting	hemoptysis _____
-pnea	breathing	dyspnea _____
orth/o	straight	orthopnea _____
-thorax	pleural cavity, chest	hemothorax _____
em	in	empyema _____

V. DIAGNOSTIC AND PATHOLOGICAL TERMS

Diagnostic Terms

auscultation

Listening to sounds within the body.

This procedure, using a stethoscope, is used chiefly for discerning the condition of the lungs, pleura, heart, and abdomen, as well as the condition of the fetus during pregnancy.

percussion

Sharp, short blows to the surface of the body with a finger or instrument.

This technique is used to diagnose a condition by determining the density of structure from the sounds obtained.

rales

Abnormal rattling sounds heard on auscultation.

Rales may be produced by secretions within the bronchi and lungs, as well as by spasm or stenosis of the bronchial walls.

sputum

Material expelled from the chest by coughing or clearing the throat.

Sputum often contains mucus, pus, and microorganisms, and its contents may indicate the type of disease process which is going on in the lower respiratory airways.

Pathological Terms

Upper Respiratory Disorders

diphtheria

An acute infectious disease of the throat and upper respiratory tract caused by the presence of diphtheria bacteria.

This disease is characterized by the appearance of inflammation and the formation of a leathery, opaque membrane in the pharynx and respiratory tract. Swelling of the larynx and pharynx lead to dyspnea, aphonia, and dysphagia. Fever, heart weakness, and anemia are other symptoms. This condition can be fatal if not treated promptly with diphtheria antitoxin.

pertussis

Whooping cough.

This is a contagious bacterial infection of the upper respiratory tract (pharynx, larynx, and trachea). It is characterized by a **paroxysmal** (sharp, painful) cough.

croup

Acute respiratory syndrome in children and infants; characterized by obstruction of the larynx, hoarseness, barking cough, and a croaking sound called **stridor** heard during inspiration.

Croup itself is not a disease condition but a group of symptoms which may result from a variety of pathological conditions. Some of these are infection, allergy, foreign body, or new growth in the laryngeal region of the respiratory tract.

epistaxis

Nosebleed.

Bronchial Tube Disorders

asthma

A disease characterized by recurrent attacks of paroxysmal dyspnea, wheezing, gasps, and cough.

Episodes (attacks) of asthma are chiefly due to an allergic reaction in the bronchial and bronchiolar tubes (bronchial asthma) caused by the absorption of something to which the patient is hypersensitive. Some cases of asthma appear to be chiefly due to nervous tension and emotional problems. In this sense, asthma would be classified as a psychosomatic (pertaining to the mind and body) condition.

bronchogenic carcinoma

Cancerous tumor arising from a bronchus.

This malignant tumor may be either **epidermoid** (derived from the lining of the bronchus) or **oat cell** (a small cell of uncertain origin). Metastases spread readily to the brain, liver, and other organs. These types of tumors are commonly known as lung cancers.

alveolar cell carcinoma   Carcinoma arising from an alveolus.

Lung Disorders

atelectasis (a/tel/ectasis)   Imperfect expansion of the air sacs; functionless, airless lung or portion of a lung.

In this condition, the pulmonary parenchymal tissue (bronchioles and air sacs) may be partially or totally collapsed, like a collapsed balloon. This may be caused by obstruction of the bronchus by foreign bodies, tumors, enlarged lymph nodes, or excessive secretions (mucus).

emphysema   Abnormal swelling or inflation of the lung tissue.

In this condition, the alveoli lose their elasticity, become distended and overexpanded, and often are covered with fibrous scar tissue. The lungs lose their ability to contract, and the patient has shortness of breath with a chronic cough. Emphysema may arise from a condition of chronic bronchitis. The inflammatory bronchiolar changes, mucorrhea, and edema produced by chronic bronchitis lead to airway obstruction. This, in turn, by disturbing the blood-gas exchange, promotes hypoxemia, and may lead to ventricular hypertrophy and right-sided heart failure. **Cor pulmonale** is right-sided heart failure due to progressive pulmonary disease such as emphysema or bronchitis.

Figure 13–5 illustrates the structural differences in alveoli in normal lung tissue, atelectasis, and emphysema.

pneumoconiosis   Abnormal condition of dust in the lungs.

There are several forms of pneumoconiosis (coni/o = dust), named according to the type of dust particle which is inhaled. **Silicosis** is an occupational disease (grinder's disease) caused by inhalation of silica dust (sand, stone, or flint) over a period of years. **Anthracosis** (black lung disease) is a disease of the lungs caused by a prolonged inhalation of coal dust. **Asbestosis** is an occupational disease due to prolonged inhalation of asbestos particles, as in the construction and shipbuilding trades.

pulmonary abscess   Localized area of pus formation in the lungs.

pulmonary edema   Swelling and fluid in the air sacs and bronchioles.

This condition may be caused by failure of the left ventricle to pump blood out the aorta. Backed-up blood and fluid in the lungs seep out into the alveoli and disturb the exchange of gases between the capillaries and alveoli.

pulmonary embolism   Floating clot or other material blocking the blood vessels of the lung.

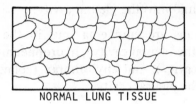

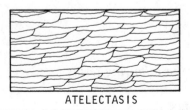

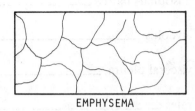

Figure 13–5 Alveoli in normal lung tissue, atelectasis, and emphysema.

pneumonia	Inflammation of the lungs.

Pneumonia is an infectious condition usually caused by pneumococci and less frequently by staphylococcal, fungal, or viral agents. The infection damages the alveolar membranes and they become porous, allowing fluid and sometimes blood cells to escape from the blood into the alveoli. Oxygenation of the blood is diminished because of inflammatory material in the damaged alveoli. **Lobar pneumonia** is an acute inflammation of one or more lobes of the lung.

tuberculosis	A pulmonary infection leading to the formation of small tubercles (nodes) in the lung.

Tuberculosis is caused by a bacterium called the tubercle **bacillus** (rod-shaped bacterium). Small tubercles composed of inflammatory cells, such as lymphocytes and monocytes, and bacteria form in the lung tissue. These diseased tubercles can spread not only in the lung but throughout the lymph and blood vessels to other parts of the body.

Disorders of the Pleura

pleurisy	Inflammation of the pleura.

This condition, also called pleuritis, causes pain and dyspnea and, in chronic cases, escape of fluid into the pleural cavity (space between the pleura surrounding the lungs).

pleural effusion   Escape of fluid into the pleural cavity.

Examples of pleural effusions are **empyema** (pus in the pleural cavity), **hemothorax** (blood in the pleural cavity), **hydropneumothorax** (water and air in the pleural cavity), and **chylothorax** (collection of lymphatic fluid called chyle in the pleural cavity).

VI. EXERCISES

A. *Give the meaning of the following terms:*

1. pneumopyothorax _____

2. nasopharyngitis _____

3. alveolus _____

4. visceral pleura _____

5. rales _____

6. bronchiolar _____

7. empyema _____

8. pulmonary embolism _____

9. hemothorax _____

10. pneumonia _____

11. bronchiectasis _____

12. pleurisy _____

13. paroxysmal _____

14. internal respiration _____

_____

15. auscultation _____

16. percussion _____

17. eupnea _____

18. hypercapnia _____

B. *Build medical terms:*

1. Pertaining to bronchi and lungs _____

2. Instrument to visually examine the bronchi _____

3. Removal of a lung (right or left) _____

4. Imperfect or incomplete expansion _____

5. Nosebleed _____

6. Pleural pain _____

7. Difficult (hoarse) voice _____

8. Increased (excessive) breathing _____

9. Inflammation of the voice box _____

10. Surgical repair of the windpipe _____

11. Collection of pus in the lungs _____

12. Abnormal condition of dust in the lungs _____

C. *Give the meaning of the following medical terms:*

1. pulmonary edema _____

2. pleural effusion _____

3. anosmia _____

4. anoxia _____

5. dysphasia _____

6. dysphagia _____

7. dysplasia _____

8. hemoptysis _____

9. bronchiolitis _____

10. glottis _____

11. cilia _____

12. bacillus _____

13. adenoids _____

14. pulmonary parenchyma _____

15. stridor _____

D. *Identify the respiratory condition which is described by the following:*

1. Infectious disease of upper respiratory tract marked by inflammation and formation of a leathery membrane in the pharynx and respiratory passages

   _____

2. Abnormal condition from coal dust _____

3. Allergic disorder marked by wheezing, coughing, and dyspnea _____

   _____

4. Whooping cough _____

5. Infectious condition caused by a bacillus and leading to the formation of

   diseased nodes or tubercles in the lung _____

   _____

6. Cancerous tumor arising from a bronchus _____

7. Collapsed lung (imperfect expansion of lung tissue) _____

   _____

8. Chronic bronchitis may lead to this condition of swelling and distention and

   loss of elasticity of alveoli _____

9. Inflammation of pleura _____

10. Infectious condition caused by pneumococci and leading to inflammation of

    lungs _____

11. Syndrome consisting of laryngeal obstruction, hoarseness, barking cough, and

    stridor _____

ANSWERS

A. 1. Air and pus in the chest (pleural cavity—area between the pleura).
  2. Inflammation of the nose and throat.
  3. Air sac.
  4. Part of pleural membrane lying closest to the lungs.
  5. Rattling sounds heard on auscultation, usually abnormal.
  6. Pertaining to the small branches of bronchi.
  7. Pus in the pleural cavity; pyothorax.
  8. Floating clot trapped in a blood vessel of the lung.
  9. Blood in the chest (pleural cavity).
  10. Inflammation of the lung caused by a virus or bacterium.
  11. Dilation of the bronchial tube.
  12. Inflammation of the pleura; pleuritis.
  13. Abnormally sharp, sudden event.
  14. Cellular respiration; the exchange of oxygen and carbon dioxide between the bloodstream and tissue cells.
  15. Listening to sounds in the body.
  16. Striking short, sharp blows to the body surface with finger or instrument to diagnose a condition by the kind of sound that is heard.
  17. Good, normal breathing.
  18. Excessive carbon dioxide in the blood.

B. 1. bronchopulmonary
  2. bronchoscope
  3. pneumonectomy
  4. atelectasis (collapsed lung)
  5. epistaxis
  6. pleurodynia
  7. dysphonia
  8. hyperpnea
  9. laryngitis
  10. tracheoplasty
  11. pulmonary abscess
  12. pneumoconiosis

C. 1. Swelling; collection of fluid in tissue spaces.
  2. Pouring out of fluid into pleural cavity.
  3. Lack of sense of smell.
  4. Deficient oxygen in blood; hypoxia.
  5. Difficult speech.
  6. Difficult swallowing.
  7. Difficult (poor) formation, development.
  8. Spitting blood.
  9. Inflammation of small branches of bronchi.
  10. Mouth of the windpipe (trachea) and voice box (larynx).
  11. Thin hairs attached to the mucous membrane epithelium lining the respiratory tract.
  12. Rod-shaped bacterium.
  13. Masses of lymph tissue in the nasopharynx.
  14. Air sacs and bronchioles; active, essential cells of the lung.
  15. Croaking harsh sounds heard during respiration.

D. 1. diphtheria
  2. anthracosis
  3. asthma
  4. pertussis
  5. tuberculosis
  6. bronchogenic carcinoma
  7. atelectasis
  8. emphysema
  9. pleurisy; pleuritis
  10. pneumonia
  11. croup

REVIEW SHEET 13

Combining Forms

adenoid/o	_____	ox/o	_____
alveol/o	_____	pector/o	_____
anthrac/o	_____	pharyng/o	_____
asbest/o	_____	phren/o	_____
atel/o	_____	pleur/o	_____
auscult/o	_____	pneum/o	_____
bronch/o	_____	pneumon/o	_____
bronchi/o	_____	pulmon/o	_____
bronchiol/o	_____	py/o	_____
coni/o	_____	rhin/o	_____
epiglott/o	_____	silic/o	_____
hydr/o	_____	sinus/o	_____
laryng/o	_____	spir/o	_____
lob/o	_____	steth/o	_____
nas/o	_____	thorac/o	_____
or/o	_____	tonsill/o	_____
orth/o	_____	trache/o	_____

Suffixes

-algia	_____	-centesis	_____
-capnia	_____	-ectasis	_____

-ectomy	_____	-oxia	_____
-lysis	_____	-phonia	_____
-odynia	_____	-plasty	_____
-orrhagia	_____	-pnea	_____
-orrhea	_____	-ptysis	_____
-osmia	_____	-stenosis	_____
-ostomy	_____	-thorax	_____
-otomy	_____	-trophy	_____

Prefixes

brady	_____	hypo	_____
dys	_____	para	_____
em	_____	per	_____
eu	_____	re	_____
ex	_____	tachy	_____
hyper	_____		

Additional Terms

abscess _____

adenoids _____

alveoli _____

anthracosis _____

asbestosis _____

asthma _____

atelectasis _____

auscultation _____

bacillus _____

bronchus _____

carbon dioxide _____

cilia _____

croup _____

diaphragm _____

diphtheria _____

edema _____

embolism _____

emphysema _____

empyema _____

epiglottis _____

epistaxis _____

external respiration _____

glottis _____

hypopharynx _____

internal respiration _____

larynx _____

lobe _____

mediastinum _____

oxygen _____

parietal pleura _____

paroxysmal _____

percussion _____

pertussis _____

pharynx _____

pleura _____

pleural cavity _____

pleural effusion _____

pleurisy _____

pneumoconiosis _____

pulmonary parenchyma _____

rales _____

silicosis _____

sputum _____

stethoscope _____

stridor _____

tonsils _____

trachea _____

tuberculosis _____

visceral pleura _____

CHAPTER 14

BLOOD AND LYMPHATIC SYSTEMS

In this chapter you will:

Learn the terms relating to the composition, formation, and function of blood and lymph;

Learn the terminology of blood grouping;

Build words and recognize combining forms used in the blood and lymphatic systems; and

Become acquainted with the names for and descriptions of various pathological conditions affecting blood and lymph.

This chapter is divided into the following sections:

I. INTRODUCTION

Blood and lymph are the liquid tissues of the body; each is composed of cells suspended and carried within a watery fluid.

Blood contains cells called **leukocytes, erythrocytes,** and **platelets (thrombocytes)** within a fluid portion called **plasma.** Plasma and cells circulate throughout the body in blood vessels called arteries, capillaries, and veins.

Lymph does not contain erythrocytes or platelets, but is rich in two types of white blood cells called **lymphocytes** and **monocytes.** The liquid medium of lymph is similar to blood plasma but contains much less protein. Lymph actually originates from the blood as fluid is squeezed out of tiny blood capillaries into the spaces between cells. This fluid is called **interstitial fluid.** The interstitial fluid passes continuously into special thin-walled vessels called lymph capillaries, which begin at the tissue spaces. The fluid, now called lymph, passes through larger lymphatic vessels and glands (nodes), finally to reach large veins in the thoracic region of the body. Lymph enters the veins and thus empties back into the bloodstream. Figure 14–1 illustrates the close relationship between the blood and lymph circulation in the body.

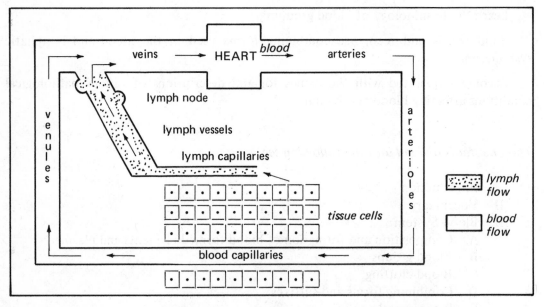

Figure 14–1 Relationship between the circulatory systems of blood and lymph.

The blood and lymphatic systems have many functions. Blood carries vital materials such as oxygen, nutrients, and hormones to tissue cells and transports waste materials, such as carbon dioxide and urea, away from tissue cells to be excreted from the body. Lymph transports needed proteins which have leaked out of the blood capillaries back to the bloodstream via the veins. Both blood and lymph protect the body by carrying disease-fighting cells (phagocytes) and protein substances called **antibodies** which combat infection. Also, plasma proteins and blood-clotting cells (platelets) contribute in the important **coagulation** (clotting) function of blood.

II. VOCABULARY

agglutinins	Protein substances (antibodies) formed in the body or present at birth. Agglutinins are formed in response to the presence of antigens, such as foreign substances (bacteria and viruses), in the blood or to proteins on the red blood cells of some individuals. Anti-A agglutinin and anti-B agglutinin are antibodies present in the different blood groups.
agglutinogens	Proteins in the red blood cells of some individuals. Blood groups are differentiated on the basis of the presence or absence of agglutinogens called A and B. Agglutinogens are also called antigens.
albumin	Protein found in blood plasma.
antibodies	Protein substances whose formation is stimulated by the presence of antigens in the body. An antibody then neutralizes or inactivates the antigen which stimulated its formation.
antigens	Foreign material which causes the production of an antibody. Naturally occurring antigens called iso-antigens (agglutinogens) are present at birth in some individuals.
B-cells	Lymphocytes formed in the bone marrow that are capable of producing antibodies.
basophil	White blood cell with large, dark-staining granules which have an affinity for basic dyes.
biconcave disk	A platelike structure having a depressed hollow surface on two sides; shape of a mature red blood cell.
bilirubin	Orange-yellowish pigment produced from hemoglobin when red blood cells are destroyed. Bilirubin is concentrated in bile by the liver and excreted in the feces.
bleeding time	Time it takes a small puncture wound in skin to be plugged up by platelets and clot.
blood dyscrasia	Any abnormal or pathological condition of the blood.

chyle	Lymph fluid flowing from the villi of the small intestine; it contains absorbed fats.
coagulation time	Time it takes a clot to form in the bloodstream.
corpuscle	"Little body"—refers to blood cells.
differentiation	Change in structure and function of a cell as it matures; specialization.
electrophoresis	Method of separating out plasma proteins by exposure to an electric force.
eosinophil	White blood cell with dense, reddish granules having an affinity for acid dyes.
erythroblast	Immature red blood cell found in the bone marrow; it has a nucleus and no hemoglobin.
fibrin	Protein threads which form the basis of a blood clot.
fibrinogen	Plasma protein which takes part in the clotting process.
formed elements	The cellular elements in blood.
globulin	Plasma protein; separates into alpha, beta, and gamma types by electrophoresis.
granulocytes	White blood cells with granules, eosinophils, neutrophils, and basophils.
hemoglobin	Blood protein found in red blood cells; enables the red blood cell to carry oxygen and carbon dioxide.
heparin	A substance found in the blood and tissues which prevents formation of new blood clots.
histiocyte	Cell found in lymph nodes and tissue spaces which engulfs foreign substances.
immune reaction	Reaction between an antigen and an antibody in which the antigen is neutralized or inactivated by the antibody.
interstitial fluid	Fluid which is squeezed out of tiny blood capillaries into tissue spaces. This fluid enters lymph capillaries and is called lymph.

isoantigen	An antigen that occurs naturally in some individuals, such as the blood group isoantigens (A and B) in man. An isoantigen is also called an agglutinogen.
lacteals	Lymph vessels in villi. Lacteals absorb fats from the intestine. Chyle flows in lacteals.
lymphocyte	White blood cell found in lymph tissue, e.g., in the spleen, lymph nodes, thymus, and sometimes bone marrow.
megakaryocyte	Immature platelet precursor (forerunner) formed in the bone marrow.
monocyte	White blood cell formed in lymph tissue. It has one large nucleus and no cytoplasmic granules.
neutrophil	White blood cell formed in bone marrow which has neutral-staining granules; also called a polymorphonuclear leukocyte because of its many-lobed nucleus.
plasma	Liquid portion of blood; contains water, proteins, salts, nutrients, hormones, and vitamins.
plasmapheresis	Process of using a centrifuge (machine which quickly spins blood so that the elements in blood separate out according to their different weights) to separate the formed elements from the blood plasma.
prothrombin	Plasma protein; important in clotting.
reticulocytes	Immature red blood cells found in the bone marrow, nucleated and possessing a granular network structure (reticulum) in cytoplasm.
reticuloendothelial cells	Special phagocytic cells found all over the body, in liver, spleen, lymph nodes, bone marrow, nervous system, and other locations. As phagocytes they eliminate aging erythrocytes, ingest foreign antigens, and help to repair injured tissue. Lymph node histiocytes are an example.
Rh factor	An isoantigen on red blood cells of Rh-positive individuals.

serum	Plasma minus the clotting proteins and clotting cells.
spleen	A vascular organ which forms blood cells in the fetus; stores blood cells in the adult for use when needed; and destroys bacteria, germs, and worn-out red blood cells (reticuloendothelial function).
stem cell	A cell in bone marrow which gives rise to different types of blood cells; also called a hemocytoblast.
T-cells	Special lymphocytes made in the thymus gland. T-cells fight disease by attaching to and destroying foreign materials.
thrombin	An enzyme which helps to convert fibrinogen to fibrin during coagulation (clotting).
thromboplastin	A clotting factor found in blood and tissues which aids in coagulation.
thymus gland	Organ composed of lymphocytes and found in the chest; it produces T-cell lymphocytes which fight infection.
type A blood group	Persons who possess type A isoantigen on red blood cells and anti-B agglutinin in plasma.
type B blood group	Persons who possess type B isoantigen on red blood cells and anti-A agglutinin in plasma.
type AB blood group	Persons who possess types A and B isoantigens on red blood cells and no agglutinin in plasma.
type O blood group	Persons who possess no isoantigens on red blood cells but whose plasma contains anti-A and anti-B agglutinins.

III. BLOOD SYSTEM

A. Composition and Formation of Blood

Whole blood is composed of **formed elements** (blood cells) and a clear, straw-colored liquid called **plasma**.

Formed Elements

The formed elements of the blood are the **erythrocytes** (red blood cells), **leukocytes** (white blood cells), and **thrombocytes**, or **platelets** (clotting cells). All blood cells originate from immature cells called **stem cells (hemocytoblasts)**. These stem cells mature in the red bone marrow tissue of adults and in the liver and spleen of the growing fetus. In an adult, the skull, vertebrae, ribs, breastbone, pelvis, thigh bone, and upper arm bone are the sites of active red bone marrow and blood cell formation. During the development of blood cells in the bone marrow tissue, the primitive, immature stem cells change shape and structure several times as the mature, **differentiated** (specialized) blood cell is formed.

Erythrocytes. An erythrocyte gets its name from the red color of one form of **hemoglobin** (oxygen-carrying pigment) which is contained within it. When hemoglobin combines with oxygen, oxyhemoglobin is formed. It is the oxyhemoglobin that is the bright red we actually think of as the color of blood. The blood in veins, however, is deoxygenated and appears bluish purple through the skin because oxyhemoglobin is not present.

There are striking differences in content and structure between mature erythrocytes (sometimes called red blood **corpuscles**, meaning small bodies) and the immature red cells from which they develop. The immature cells, formed in bone marrow, possess nuclei and do not contain hemoglobin at their youngest stage. Mature erythrocytes, however, lack nuclei, and are hemoglobin-filled, and thus can carry oxygen as they circulate through the bloodstream. The gradual development of an immature red cell to maturity is accomplished in various stages.

The most immature red blood cells, which develop from stem cells in the bone marrow, are called **erythroblasts**. They are large, **nucleated** cells which do not contain hemoglobin. Erythroblasts divide within the bone marrow and their offspring develop into other immature cells called **normoblasts**. Normoblasts are smaller cells (more the size of a normal erythrocyte) filled with hemoglobin but still containing a nucleus.

The normoblast then divides and the cells it produces develop into cells called **reticulocytes**. Reticulocytes also contain hemoglobin and, when stained with a dye, their cytoplasm reveals a dense network (reticulum) of granules. The reticulocytes still possess a nucleus, as do erythroblasts and normoblasts.

The last stage in red blood cell development is the progression from reticulocyte to erythrocyte. During this change the hemoglobin-filled reticulocyte loses its nucleus. The mature, developed erythrocyte then lacks a nucleus and contains hemoglobin as its major protein. In addition, the mature erythrocyte possesses the characteristic shape of a **biconcave disk**. This shape (a depressed or hollow surface on each side of the cell) allows for a large surface area on the erythrocyte so that absorption and release of gases can take place.

Figure 14–2 recapitulates the development of the mature red blood cell from stem cell to erythrocyte.

Just as the bone marrow is continually producing erythrocytes, special liver and spleen cells are continually destroying worn-out erythrocytes. These special cells are called **reticuloendothelial cells**. The hemoglobin in the destroyed erythrocyte is released and broken down in the liver and spleen. Bile pigments are formed from the destroyed hemoglobin (**bilirubin** is one such pigment), and these pigments are excreted with bile from the liver into the intestines and out of the body in solid wastes (feces).

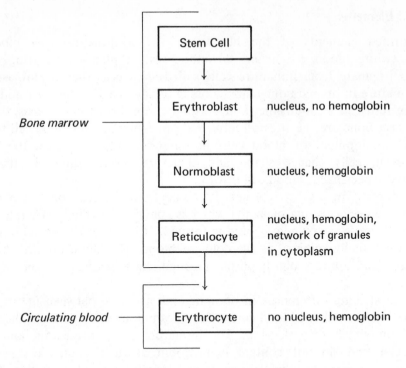

Figure 14-2 Development of the mature red blood cell from stem cell to erythrocyte.

Leukocytes. While mature erythrocytes lack nuclei and contain hemoglobin, other blood cells are devoid of pigmentation and contain large nuclei. These are the leukocytes, also called white blood corpuscles. Although there is only one type of mature erythrocyte, there are several types of mature leukocytes. The characteristics of leukocytes were discussed in Chapter 4 (see Figure 4–1), and will be reviewed in the following paragraphs.

Leukocytes are divided into two major types: **granulocytes**, containing large granules in their cytoplasm; and **agranulocytes**, lacking granules in their cytoplasm.

Granulocytes are divided into three types of cells, determined by the staining of the granules in their cytoplasm. The granules in **eosinophils** turn red, or a rosy color, with the addition of an acid dye. Eosinophils make up 3 per cent of all leukocytes and are increased in allergic conditions.

The granules in **basophils** turn blue with the addition of a basic dye. These leukocytes account for less than 1 per cent of all white blood cells. Their exact function is not known, but they appear to increase in number in inflammatory reactions.

The granules in **neutrophils** stain purple with the addition of acid or basic dye. Neutrophils compose about 60 per cent of all leukocytes, and they are phagocytes (fight disease by engulfing or swallowing up germs). Neutrophils increase in number in **pyrogenic** (fever-producing) infections and in certain forms of leukemia.

All granulocytes are polymorphonuclear; that is, they have multilobed nuclei. The term **polymorphonuclear leukocyte** is used most often to describe the most numerous of the granulocytes, the neutrophil.

Agranulocytes are the other major category of white blood cells. They are divided into two types. **Monocytes**, which make up 6 per cent of leukocytes, lack granules in their cytoplasm and are large cells with kidney-shaped nuclei. They are phagocytic and, like scavengers, dispose of dead and dying cells or other debris.

The other type of agranulocyte is the **lymphocyte**, which composes about 30 per cent of all leukocytes. Lymphocytes are smaller cells with less cytoplasm than monocytes but are also lacking in cytoplasmic granules. They are made in lymphatic tissue, such as lymph nodes, the spleen, and the thymus gland, as well as in the bone marrow. Lymphocytes are not phagocytic, but they play an important role in fighting disease. Lymphocytes are a source of **antibodies** which can neutralize and destroy **antigens** (bacteria, viruses) that may enter the body. The reaction between an antibody and antigen is called an **immune reaction** (immun/o = protection, safe).

Most leukocytes, like erythrocytes, develop in the red bone marrow from undifferentiated, immature stem cells. An understanding of the terminology used to describe the different stages in leukocyte growth and development is important because the presence or absence of these different types of cells in the marrow and circulating blood is a valuable diagnostic clue to the nature of various pathological conditions.

Figure 14–3 is a chart depicting the various stages in the development of leukocytes from stem cell to mature leukocyte.

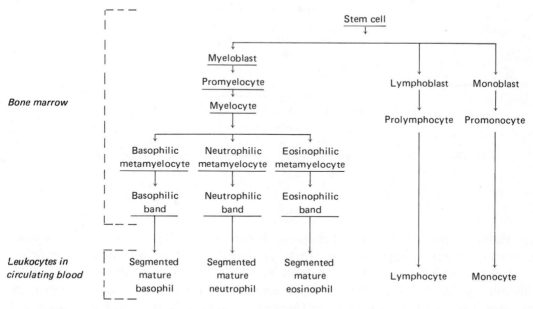

KEY

Myel/o = bone marrow; -blast = immature; pro = before.
Meta = change, transformation.
Bands are identical to mature polymorphonuclear leukocytes, except that the nucleus is U-shaped and its lobes are connected by a band rather than a thin thread as in segmented cell forms.

Figure 14–3 Stages in the development of leukocytes from stem cell to mature leukocyte.

Platelets. The third type of formed element in the blood, smaller than an erythrocyte and with a platelike flatness to its shape, is called a platelet (thrombocyte). Platelets are formed in the bone marrow, and are actually fragments which have broken away from giant multinucleated cells called **megakaryocytes**. A week after its formation in bone marrow, a megakaryocyte will fall apart into the small pieces known as platelets.

Megakaryocytes and platelets develop from bone marrow stem cells as do erythrocytes and leukocytes. Study Figure 14–4, which is a chart tracing the development of a platelet from an immature stem cell in the bone marrow.

Although platelets are cell fragments, they contain the important cytoplasmic structures common to all cells. Their primary function is **hemostasis** (stoppage of blood flow). The terminology of blood clotting will be explained in a later section of this chapter.

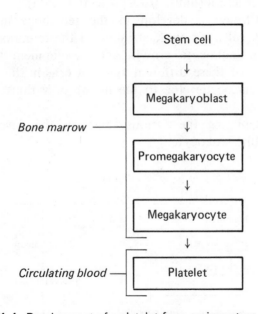

Figure 14–4 Development of a platelet from an immature stem cell in the bone marrow.

Plasma

Plasma is the liquid part of the blood. It consists of 91 per cent water and 9 per cent solid materials. These solid materials are largely proteins, with lesser amounts of salts, sugar, hormones, wastes, and food substances. Four major plasma proteins are **albumin**, **globulin**, **fibrinogen**, and **prothrombin**. Fibrinogen and prothrombin are proteins which participate in the clotting process and will be discussed in a subsequent section.

The plasma concentrations of albumin and globulin serve to maintain the proper water content of the blood. These proteins by their presence hold water in the blood, opposing its tendency to leak out into the tissue spaces. When these proteins are lacking in the blood, water tends to leave the blood and fill the tissue spaces, causing **edema** (swelling).

The globulin fraction of plasma has added importance because it contains antibodies which can fight foreign antigens in the body. There are three different kinds of globulins in plasma; they are called **alpha**, **beta**, and **gamma**, and they can be distinguished by **electrophoresis**. The technique of electrophoresis involves placing the plasma in a special solution and passing an electric current through the solution. The different protein molecules in the plasma separate out as they migrate at different speeds to the source of electricity.

Plasmapheresis is the process of separating out the plasma from the formed elements in the blood. This separation is mechanical, not electrical, in nature. The blood is spun down using a centrifuge, and the plasma, being lighter in weight than red cells, collects above as a clear liquid.

Figure 14—5 reviews the composition of blood.

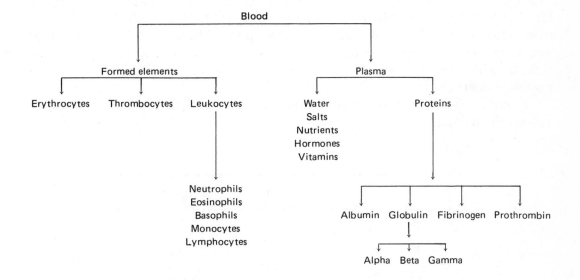

Figure 14–5 Composition of blood.

B. Blood Groups

Although blood cells and plasma are formed continuously in the bone marrow, if large amounts of blood are lost from the body, the body's machinery may be incapable of bringing about a reasonable recovery quickly enough for its needs. It would be advisable then to transfer blood directly into the patient's bloodstream. This process is called a **transfusion** (meaning to pour across).

A transfusion, however, cannot be made between any two people at random. Human blood falls into four main groups called O, A, B, and AB, and there are widely recognized harmful effects of transfusing blood from a donor of one blood group into a recipient who is of another blood group.

Blood groups are named for the presence of a specific substance (called an **isoantigen**, or **agglutinogen**) which is found on the red blood cells of an individual of that particular group. For example, group A individuals have A-type isoantigens on their red blood cells; group B individuals have B-type isoantigens on their red blood cells; group AB individuals have both A- and B-type isoantigens; and group O individuals are lacking both A- and B-type isoantigens.

In addition to isoantigens (agglutinogens) on their red blood cells, the individuals in the different blood groups have certain compounds in their blood plasma which are capable of reacting with A- and B-type isoantigens to clump together, or **agglutinate**, red blood cells. These compounds are called **agglutinins**. Agglutinins are special types of antibodies.

There are two major types of agglutinins. The agglutinin which reacts with A-type isoantigen and causes the clumping together of those red blood cells which contain A-type isoantigen is called **anti-A**. The agglutinin which reacts with B-type isoantigen and causes the clumping together of B-type red blood cells is called **anti-B**.

It is obvious that a person of blood group A, with A-type isoantigens, would have anti-B in her plasma (if she had anti-A isoantigen it would agglutinate her own red blood cells and be fatal). Similarly, a person of blood group B would be expected to have anti-A in her plasma. A person of blood group AB, with both A- and B-type isoantigens, would have neither anti-A nor anti-B in her plasma, and a person of blood type O, with neither A- nor B-type isoantigen, would have both anti-A and anti-B agglutinin in her plasma.

Figure 14–6 is a chart summarizing the types of isoantigens and agglutinins in the various blood groups.

Blood Groups	Isoantigen	Agglutinin
A	A	Anti-B
B	B	Anti-A
AB	AB	no agglutinins
O	no isoantigens	Anti-A and Anti-B

Figure 14–6 Types of isoantigens and agglutinins in the various blood groups.

When making a transfusion, it is ideal to have both donor and recipient of the same blood group. But what would happen if by mistake the donor and recipient were not of the same blood group? Suppose blood from an A-group donor is given to a B-group patient. Remember, there is anti-A agglutinin in the plasma of the patient. The A-type isoantigens on the red blood cells of the donor will then react with the patient's anti-A agglutinins and cause clumping together of the red blood cells as they enter the patient's bloodstream. These agglutinated red blood cells block the blood vessels of the patient, with fatal results.

The A-group donor does have anti-B agglutinins which you might think would react with the B-type isoantigens on the patient's red blood cells. This does not happen, however, because the quantity of agglutinins in the plasma being transfused is small and the agglutinins which are present are diluted by the larger quantity of opposite agglutinins in the patient's blood. The important precaution, then, is to prevent the donation of A- and B-type isoantigens on red blood cells which might be agglutinated by the agglutinins in the recipient's plasma.

For example, a patient of blood group A has anti-B agglutinins in his plasma. He cannot receive blood from a B- or AB-group person because his anti-B agglutinins will clump together the donor's red cells which contain B-type isoantigens. He can receive blood from another A-group individual or an O-group individual, both of whom do not have B-type isoantigens.

Similarly, a patient of blood group B with anti-A agglutinins cannot receive blood from an A or AB person because his anti-A agglutinins will clump together the donor's red blood cells which contain A-type isoantigens. B-group patients can thus receive blood from other B-group individuals or from O-group individuals.

An AB-group patient contains no anti-A or anti-B agglutinins in his plasma, so he can receive blood from not only another AB person but from O-, A-, and B-group individuals as well. An O-group patient, who has no isoantigens but only anti-A and anti-B agglutinins in his plasma, can receive blood only from another O-type person because groups A, B, and AB contain isoantigens which would cause agglutination of red blood cells upon transfusion.

Figure 14–7 summarizes the possible donors which can be used in transfusions between the various blood groups.

Recipient/Patient	Donor
O	O
A	A, O
B	B, O
AB	AB, A, B, O

Figure 14–7 Possible donors which can be used in transfusions between the blood groups.

Besides A- and B-type isoantigens, there are many other isoantigens on red blood cells. One of these is called the **Rh factor** (named because it was first found in the blood of a rhesus monkey). The term **Rh-positive** refers to the presence of the Rh isoantigen on an individual's red blood cells. An **Rh-negative** person does not possess the Rh isoantigen. There are no anti-Rh agglutinins (antibodies) normally present in the blood of an Rh-positive or Rh-negative person.

If, however, Rh-positive blood (with Rh isoantigens) is transfused into an Rh-negative person, the recipient will begin to develop agglutinins which would clump together any Rh-positive blood if another transfusion were to occur subsequently.

The same reactions occur during pregnancy if the fetus of an Rh-negative mother happens to be Rh-positive. This situation is discussed in Chapter 5 as an example of an antigen-antibody reaction.

C. Blood Clotting

Blood clotting, or hemostasis, is a complicated process involving several different substances and chemical reactions. Study Figure 14–8 as you read the following.

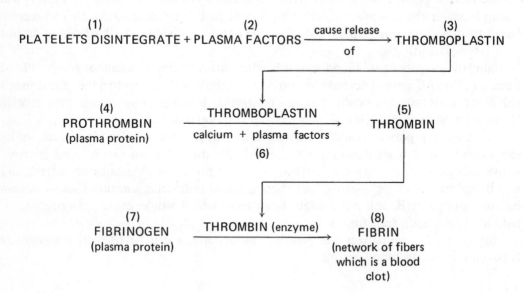

Figure 14–8   Sequence of blood clotting.

When platelets (thrombocytes) come in contact with the roughened or injured lining of a blood vessel, the platelet cells disintegrate (1) and, combined with factors present in the blood plasma (2), cause the release of a substance called **thromboplastin** (3). Thromboplastin is necessary to allow a plasm protein called **prothrombin** (4) to be converted to a substance called **thrombin** (5). This important conversion takes place with the help of **calcium** (6) and other plasma factors.

As thrombin is formed, it acts as an enzyme to change another blood protein called **fibrinogen** (7) to a network of threads called **fibrin** (8). It is this network of fibrin threads that forms the substance of a blood clot.

After the fibrin threads of the clot form, most of the plasma leaves the clot, and this fluid (plasma minus the clotting proteins and clotting factors) is called **serum**. The period of time it takes for the fibrin-threaded clot to form in the blood is known as the **coagulation** (clotting) **time** (normally 3 minutes). **Bleeding time** (normally 2 minutes) refers to the time it takes for platelets to plug up a small puncture of the skin.

A clot which forms within a blood vessel is called a **thrombus**, and the actual stopping up of the vessel by the thrombus is called **thrombosis**. If a thrombus should be dislodged from its place in a vessel and travel through the bloodstream, it is called an **embolus**. Traveling air bubbles, fragments of tissue, and other substances may be called emboli as well. The obvious danger of emboli is the closing up of blood vessels and stoppage of the flow of blood to a vital vessel or organ. This is particularly dangerous in the lungs, where a pulmonary embolus may be fatal.

Anticoagulant substances within the body prevent the spontaneous clotting of blood as it flows through the blood vessels. These substances are called **fibrolytic** enzymes. **Heparin** is such an anticlotting chemical which is found in several tissues. Heparin blocks the change of prothrombin to thrombin.

D. Combining Forms and Suffixes

Combining Form	Definition	Terminology	Meaning
hem/o hemat/o	blood	hemocytoblast _____	
		hemorrhage _____	
		hematocrit _____	
		hemolysis _____	
erythr/o	red	erythropoiesis _____	
		erythropenia _____	
is/o	same, equal	anisocytosis _____	
		isoantigen _____	
chrom/o	color	hypochromia _____	
		Reduction in hemoglobin in red cells.	
poikil/o	varied, irregular	poikilocytosis _____	
		_____	
		Variation in shape of erythrocyte.	
spher/o	globe, round	spherocytosis _____	
		One type of poikilocytosis found in hemolytic anemias.	
leuk/o	white	leukotoxic _____	
		leukopenia _____	
eosin/o	red, dawn, rosy	eosinophil _____	
		eosinopenia _____	

bas/o	base, opposite of acid	basophil _____
neutr/o	neither, neutral *(neither base nor acid)*	neutropenia _____ neutrophil _____
granul/o	granules	granulocytosis _____ granulocytopoiesis _____ _____ agranulocytopenia _____ _____
myel/o	bone marrow	metamyelocyte _____ myeloblast _____ myeloid _____
phag/o	eat, swallow	phagocytosis _____ macrophage _____
mon/o	one, single	monoblast _____ promonocyte _____ monocytosis _____
thromb/o	clot	thrombocytopenia _____ _____ thrombocytopathy _____ _____ prothrombin _____ thromboplastin _____ thrombin _____
fibrin/o	fibrin, threads of a clot	fibrinolysis _____

nucle/o	nucleus	nucleated _____
kary/o	nucleus	mega<u>kary</u>ocyte _____
		mega<u>kary</u>oblast _____
morph/o	shape, form	poly<u>morph</u>onuclear _____
		_____
reticul/o	network	<u>reticul</u>ocyte _____
norm/o	normal, rule	<u>norm</u>oblast _____

Resembles the normal shape of mature erythrocytes.

agglutin/o	clumping, sticking together	<u>agglutin</u>ation _____
		<u>agglutin</u>in _____
immun/o	safe, protection	<u>immun</u>ogenic _____
		<u>immun</u>ology _____
sider/o	iron	<u>sider</u>openia _____
-globin	protein	hemo<u>globin</u> _____
-globulin	protein	gamma <u>globulin</u> _____
-blast	embryonic, immature	erythro<u>blast</u> _____
		megalo<u>blast</u>ic _____
-emia	blood condition *(usually large increase in cell numbers)*	leuk<u>emia</u> _____
-cytosis	condition of cells *(slight increase in cell numbers)*	leuko<u>cytosis</u> _____
		mono<u>cytosis</u> _____
-philia	attraction for *(usually increase in numbers)*	neutro<u>philia</u> _____
		_____

		eosinophilia _____
		_____
-poiesis	formation	myelopoietic _____
-stasis	stop, control	hemostasis _____
-pheresis	removal	plasmapheresis _____
	(use of a centrifuge to spin down blood to separate out elements)	leukapheresis _____
		plateletpheresis _____
-phoresis	carrying, transmission	electrophoresis _____

E. Pathological Conditions

Any abnormal or pathological condition of the blood is generally referred to as a blood **dyscrasia**. The blood dyscrasias discussed in this section are organized in the following manner: diseases of red blood cells, diseases of blood clotting, and diseases of white blood cells.

Diseases of Red Blood Cells

anemia   Deficiency in erythrocytes or hemoglobin.

Anemia implies a reduction in red blood cells. This can be exhibited by a decrease in number of red cells or decrease in the amount of hemoglobin in red cells. The most common type is iron-deficiency anemia caused by a lack of iron, which is required for hemoglobin production. Other types of anemia include:

pernicious anemia   Lack of mature erythrocytes due to inability to absorb vitamin B_{12} into the body.

Vitamin B_{12} is necessary for the proper development and maturation of nucleated erythroblasts to normoblasts, to reticulocytes, and finally to mature, non-nucleated erythrocytes. While vitamin B_{12} is a common constituent of food matter, it cannot be absorbed into the bloodstream without the aid of a special factor in the gastric juice. This factor facilitates the passage of vitamin B_{12} through the lining of the small intestine into the bloodstream. Individuals with pernicious anemia lack this factor in their gastric juice, and the result is unsuccessful maturation of red cells and an excess of large, immature, nucleated, and poorly functioning red cells in the circulation.

aplastic anemia   Failure of blood cell production due to aplasia (absence of development, formation) of bone marrow cells.

The bone marrow stem cells fail to produce leukocytes and platelets as well as erythrocytes. The cause of aplastic anemia is unknown.

hemolytic anemia   Reduction in red cells due to excessive destruction.

This is anemia due to excessive breakdown of red cells. One example of hemolytic anemia is congenital spherocytic anemia. Instead of their normal biconcave shape, erythrocytes are spheroidal in shape in this blood disorder. This spheroidal shape makes them very fragile and they are easily destroyed, or hemolyzed, leading to anemia. The spherocytosis causes increased numbers of reticulocytes in the circulating blood as the bone marrow attempts to compensate for the hemolysis of mature erythrocytes. The excessive hemolysis leads to jaundice because of accumulation of bilirubin (product of hemolysis) in the circulating bloodstream. Since the spleen is an organ where red cells are destroyed, it may be removed in this condition with helpful results.

sickle-cell anemia   Hereditary condition characterized by abnormal shape of erythrocytes and by hemolysis.

This is a congenital anomaly in the structure of erythrocytes. Sickling is an abnormal change in the shape of erythrocytes when they are exposed to low oxygen content in the bloodstream. The hemoglobin in the erythrocyte comes out of solution and the red cell assumes a sickle, or crescent, shape. This change in shape impairs the oxygen-carrying capacity of the red blood cell. The genetic defect of sickling is found predominantly in blacks, and the defect appears with different degrees of severity, depending on the presence of one or two inherited genes for the trait. Reticulocytosis is a prominent feature, as well as bilirubinemia, which is due to the hemolysis of the sickled cells.

thalassemia   An inherited defect in the ability to produce hemoglobin, usually seen in persons of Mediterranean (thalass = sea) background.

This condition, consisting of various forms and degrees of severity, usually leads to hypochromic anemia (diminished hemoglobin content in red cells). Treatment may involve splenectomy (the spleen is a site of red cell destruction) and blood transfusions.

polycythemia vera   Excessive increase in red blood cells.

Erythremia is another name for this pathological condition. Red cell volume is increased and the blood consistency is viscous (sticky) because of greatly increased numbers of erythrocytes. The bone marrow is hyperplastic, and leukocytosis and thrombocytosis accompany the increase in red blood cells. Treatment consists of reduction of red cell volume to normal levels with phlebotomy (removal of blood from a vein) and myelosuppressive drugs.

Disorders of Blood Clotting

hemophilia

Excessive bleeding caused by a congenital lack of a substance necessary for blood clotting.

In this hereditary disorder, **bleeding time** is normal, whereas **coagulation time** is greatly prolonged. Thus, while the platelet count of a hemophiliac is normal (as evidenced by the normal bleeding time), there is a marked deficiency in a plasma clotting factor, which results in a very prolonged coagulation, or clotting, time. Treatment consists of administration of the deficient factor.

purpura

Multiple pinpoint hemorrhages and accumulation of blood, under the skin.

Purpura means purple, and in this bleeding condition, hemorrhages into the skin and mucous membranes produce red-purple discoloration of the skin. The bleeding is caused by a fall in the number of blood platelets (thrombocytopenia) so that, while the clotting time is normal (all the plasma factors are present), bleeding time is prolonged. The etiology of the disorder may be immunologic, meaning that the body produces an antiplatelet factor which harms its own platelets. Splenectomy (spleen is the site of platelet destruction) and drug therapy to discourage antibody synthesis are methods of treatment. Purpura is also seen in any other condition associated with a low platelet count, such as leukemia and drug reactions.

Diseases of White Blood Cells

leukemia

Excessive increase in white blood cells.

This disease is characterized by proliferation of malignant leukocytes in the bone marrow. There are several varieties of leukemia, depending upon the particular leukocyte that is involved. In **acute myelogenous leukemia**, also known as **acute myelocytic leukemia** and **acute granulocytic leukemia**, there is a proliferation of immature granulocytes called myeloblasts. Since leukemia is essentially a bone marrow disease, other blood cell abnormalities are evident as well. In acute myelogenous leukemia, platelets and erythrocytes are diminished because of infiltration and replacement of the bone marrow by large numbers of myeloblasts.

In **acute lymphocytic leukemia**, immature lymphocytes called lymphoblasts are increased, while in **acute monocytic leukemia** there is monocytic proliferation.

There are also chronic, or more slowly progressive, forms of myelogenous and lymphocytic leukemias in which patients live many years before encountering life-threatening problems.

All forms of leukemia are treated with chemical therapy (chemotherapy), using drugs which prevent cell division and selectively injure rapidly dividing cells. Effective treatment leads to a **remission**, or disappearance of evidence, of leukemia in the bone marrow and blood. **Relapse** occurs when leukemia cells reappear in blood or bone marrow, necessitating further treatment.

granulocytosis   Abnormal increase in granulocytes in the blood.

An increase in granulocytes in the blood may occur in response to infection or inflammation of any type. **Eosinophilia** is an increase in eosinophilic granulocytes, which is seen in certain allergic conditions, such as asthma, or in parasitic infections (tapeworm, pinworm). **Basophilia** is an increase in basophilic granulocytes seen in certain types of leukemia.

infectious mononucleosis   Acute infectious disease with enlarged lymph nodes and spleen, and increased number of lymphocytes and monocytes.

This disease is caused by a virus and is characterized by a greatly increased number of large lymphocytes in the blood (monocytosis). Lymphadenopathy is present, with sore throat and enlarged, tender lymph nodes in the cervical and sometimes axillary and inguinal regions.

IV. LYMPHATIC SYSTEM

A. Composition, Anatomy, and Function

Composition

Lymph is interstitial tissue fluid which is found in special lymphatic vessels all over the body. Lymph is clear and colorless and contains less protein than blood plasma. Other noncellular constituents of lymph are water, salts, sugar, and wastes of metabolism, such as urea and creatinine. Lymph passing from the villi of the small intestine is called **chyle**, and it is milky in appearance from fats absorbed through the villi into the lymph vessels which are called **lacteals**. The cellular composition of lymph includes lymphocytes, monocytes, and a few platelets and erythrocytes.

Label Figure 14–9 as you read the following paragraphs.

Anatomy

Lymph capillaries (1) begin at the tissue spaces from microscopic blind ends. They, like blood capillaries, are thin-walled tubes. Lymph capillaries carry lymph from the tissue spaces to larger **lymphatic vessels** (2). Lymphatic vessels are thicker than lymph capillaries and, like veins, contain valves so that lymph fluid flows only in one direction, toward the thoracic cavity. Two ducts in the thoracic cavity receive the

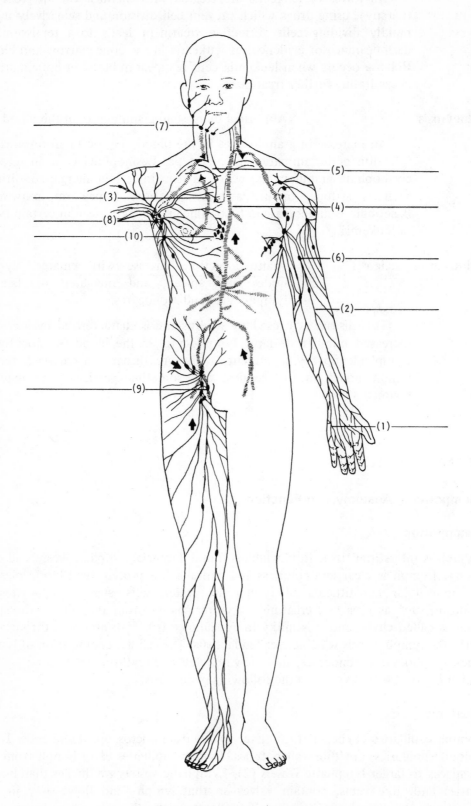

Figure 14-9 Lymphatic system.

lymph from the lymph vessels. These ducts are the **right lymphatic duct** (3) and the **thoracic duct** (4). They empty lymph into veins (5) in the upper thoracic region.

Function

By serving as a channel for the flow of substances from tissue spaces to the bloodstream, lymph has an important function in the body. Valuable proteins which may have leaked out of blood capillaries at the tissue spaces can be returned to the bloodstream by flowing through the lymphatic fluid. Also, lymph vessels called lacteals are the channels for the absorption of fats from the small intestine into the bloodstream, as well as a passageway for toxic or disease substances which leave tissue spaces and get trapped in **lymph nodes** (6).

A lymph node contains lymphocytes and lymphatic channels which are held together by a fibrous connective tissue capsule. The lymph nodes have many functions. They trap and filter toxic and malignant substances from inflammatory and cancerous lesions. There are also special cells in lymph nodes which can phagocytize foreign substances and digest them. These phagocytic cells are called **histiocytes** (a type of **reticuloendothelial** cell). Lymph nodes also produce lymphocytes, which fight disease by producing antibodies.

The major sites of lymph node concentration are the **cervical** (7), **axillary** (8), **inguinal** (9), and **mediastinal** (10) regions of the body.

B. Related Lymphatic Organs

The **spleen** and **thymus gland** are organs composed of lymphatic tissue.

Spleen

The spleen (pictured in Figure 14–10) is located in the upper left quadrant of the abdomen, adjacent to the stomach. While the spleen is not essential to life, it has several important functions:

1. Destruction of old erythrocytes by reticuloendothelial cells. Because of hemolytic activity in the spleen, bilirubin is formed there and added to the bloodstream.

2. Filtration of microorganisms and other foreign material from the blood.

3. Production of antibodies and immunity, chiefly by leukocytes.

4. Storage of blood, especially red blood cells. Blood is released by the spleen as the body needs it.

5. Production of blood cells such as lymphocytes and monocytes. Also, the spleen seems to have a stimulatory effect on the production of blood from the bone marrow.

Thymus

The thymus gland (pictured in Figure 14–11) is located in the mediastinum, posterior to the breast bone and between the lungs. It plays an important role in the body's immunologic system, especially in fetal life and the early years of growth. It is known that thymectomy performed in animals during the first few weeks of life

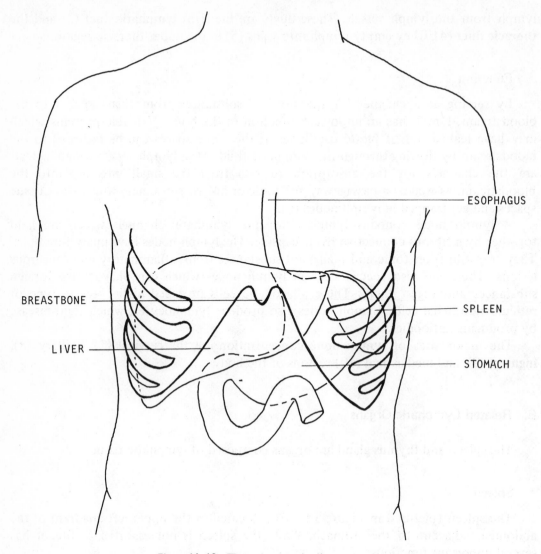

Figure 14–10 The spleen and adjacent organs.

impairs the ability of the animal to make antibodies to fight against foreign antigens and impairs the animal's ability to reject skin grafts.

The thymus manufactures special lymphocytes called **T-cells**. These T-cells migrate to the site of antigens and phagocytize the antigen to destroy it. Other types of lymphocytes are called **B-cells**. These are produced in the bone marrow, and they destroy antigens by producing antibodies which neutralize or inactivate the antigen.

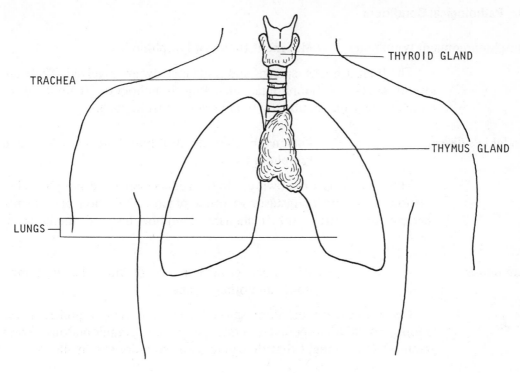

Figure 14–11 The thymus gland.

C. Combining Forms

Combining Form	Structure or Substance	Terminology	Meaning
lymph/o	lymph	lymphocytosis _____	
		lymphopoiesis _____	
		lymphoid _____	
lymphaden/o	lymph gland	lymphadenopathy _____	
lymphangi/o	lymph vessels	lymphangiogram _____	
splen/o	spleen	splenomegaly _____	
		hypersplenism _____	
		splenosis _____	
thym/o	thymus gland	thymectomy _____	
		thymoma _____	

D. Pathological Conditions

lymphosarcoma or **lymphoma**   Malignant tumor of lymph nodes.

> The lymph nodes, spleen, and bone marrow are involved. There are several types of lymphoma, including lymphocytic (composed of lymphocytes) and histiocytic (composed of histiocytes).

Hodgkin's disease   Malignant enlargement of lymph nodes, spleen, and lymphoid tissue.

> This disease of unknown etiology produces enlarged lymph nodes, splenomegaly, and metastases to other organs. Radiation and chemotherapy to destroy the malignant lymphocytes are methods of treatment.

sarcoidosis   Abnormal growth of small tubercles in lymph nodes and other organs.

> Lesions develop on skin, spleen, liver, and lymph nodes. These lesions resemble tubercular nodes and are granulomatous (form granules). It is thought that the etiology of sarcoidosis is an allergy.

myasthenia gravis   Disease of severe muscle weakness.

> This condition is often associated with benign tumors of the thymus (thymoma). Symptoms often disappear with resection of the tumor.

lymphadenitis   Inflammation of lymph nodes, usually due to infection.

lymphocytosis   Increased numbers of lymphocytes in the blood or bone marrow, owing to lymphocytic leukemia or lymphoma, or in response to certain types of infection.

V. EXERCISES

A. Build medical terms:

1. Lack of neutrophils (deficiency) _____

2. Enlargement of the spleen _____

3. Dilation of lymph vessels _____

4. Destruction of blood _____

5. Embryonic monocyte _____

6. Formation of bone marrow _____

7. Slight increase in white blood cells _____

8. Disease condition of platelets _____

9. Stop, or control, blood _____

10. Abnormal condition of cells of unequal sizes _____

B. *Give the meaning of the following:*

1. splenic atrophy _____

2. plateletpheresis _____

_____

3. anticoagulant _____

4. embolus _____

5. bleeding time _____

6. electrophoresis _____

_____

7. T-cells _____

8. clotting time _____

9. B-cells _____

10. reticuloendothelial cells _____

_____

11. polymorphonuclear leukocytes _____

12. eosinophilia _____

C. *Arrange the following terms in order of their developmental stages of growth in the bone marrow:*

1. normoblast, erythrocyte, erythroblast, stem cell, reticulocyte

    a. _____

    b. _____

    c. _____

    d. _____

    e. _____

2. promyelocyte, myeloblast, neutrophilic band, neutrophilic metamyelocyte, stem cell, myelocyte, segmented neutrophil

    a. _____

    b. _____

    c. _____

    d. _____

    e. _____

    f. _____

    g. _____

3. lymphocyte, stem cell, prolymphocyte, lymphoblast

    a. _____

    b. _____

    c. _____

    d. _____

4. promonocyte, stem cell, monocyte, monoblast

    a. _____

    b. _____

    c. _____

    d. _____

5. megakaryocyte, stem cell, thrombocyte, megakaryoblast, promegakaryocyte

    a. _____

    b. _____

    c. _____

    d. _____

    e. _____

D. *Use the following terms to fill in the blanks for the sequence of events that takes place in clotting:*

    prothrombin, thrombin, thromboplastin, fibrinogen, fibrin

Platelets disintegrate + plasma factors $\xrightarrow[\text{release of}]{\text{cause}}$ (1) _____

(2) _____ $\xrightarrow[\text{calcium}]{\text{thromboplastin}}$ (3) _____

(4) _____ $\xrightarrow{\text{thrombin (enzyme)}}$ (5) _____

Which of the above substances are plasma proteins?

_____ and _____

E. *Provide the answers requested:*

1. What is an isoantigen? _____

_____

_____

What is an agglutinin? _____

_____

_____

2. Give the isoantigens and agglutinins in the 4 blood types:

Blood Type	Isoantigen	Agglutinin
A		
B		
AB		
O		

3. Will agglutination result from the following donor-to-recipient blood transfusions?

	Donor	Recipient	
(a)	A	AB	_____
(b)	B	A	_____
(c)	O	B	_____
(d)	AB	O	_____

F. *Give the meaning of the following medical terms:*

1. differentiated _____

2. plasma _____

3. lacteal _____

4. poikilocytosis _____

5. bilirubin _____

6. blood dyscrasia _____

7. chyle _____

8. axillary _____

9. serum _____

10. spleen _____

_____

11. acute myelogenous leukemia _____

_____

12. spherocytosis _____

13. heparin _____

14. reticulocytosis _____

G. *Match the blood and lymph disorders given below with their associated symptoms:*

1. purpura

2. pernicious anemia

3. polycythemia

4. hemophilia

5. aplastic anemia

6. mononucleosis

7. thalassemia

8. sickle cell anemia

9. granulocytosis

10. sarcoidosis

_____ A. pancytopenia

_____ B. eosinophilia

_____ C. lack of plasma clotting factor

_____ D. monocytosis

_____ E. inherited defect in hemoglobin synthesis

_____ F. vitamin B_{12} cannot be absorbed into the body

_____ G. erythremia

_____ H. granulomatous tubercles in lymph nodes, spleen, liver, and skin

_____ I. crescent-shaped erythrocytes; reticulocytosis

_____ J. multiple pinpoint hemorrhages and accumulation of blood under the skin

ANSWERS

A.
1. neutropenia
2. splenomegaly
3. lymphangiectasis
4. hemolysis
5. monoblast
6. myelopoiesis
7. leukocytosis
8. thrombocytopathy
9. hemostasis
10. anisocytosis

B.
1. Wasting away, deterioration of the spleen.
2. Separation or removal of platelets from other blood constituents; use of a centrifuge to spin down blood and separate out platelets from plasma and other cells.
3. Chemical which prevents coagulation, or clotting, of blood.
4. Floating clot or other material.
5. Time it takes platelets to plug up a small puncture.
6. Transmission of electricity through a plasma solution to separate out the various plasma components.
7. Lymphocytes made in the thymus gland.
8. Time it takes for blood clot (fibrin threads) to form.
9. Lymphocytes formed in the bone marrow.
10. Type of phagocytic cell found in lymph nodes, spleen, liver, bone marrow, and other locations.
11. Granulocytic leukocytes having nuclei with many shapes; neutrophils.
12. Increase in eosinophils.

C.
1. a. stem cell
   b. erythroblast
   c. normoblast
   d. reticulocyte
   e. erythrocyte

2. a. stem cell
   b. myeloblast
   c. promyelocyte
   d. myelocyte
   e. metamyelocyte
   f. neutrophilic band
   g. segmented neutrophil

3. a. stem cell
   b. lymphoblast
   c. prolymphocyte
   d. lymphocyte

4. a. stem cell
   b. monoblast
   c. promonocyte
   d. monocyte

5. a. stem cell
   b. megakaryoblast
   c. promegakaryocyte
   d. megakaryocyte
   e. thrombocyte

D.
1. thromboplastin
2. prothrombin
3. thrombin
4. fibrinogen
5. fibrin

Prothrombin and **fibrinogen** are plasma proteins.

E.
1. An **isoantigen** (agglutinogen) is a substance which causes the production of an agglutinin (type of antibody). Some isoantigens are naturally found in red blood cells. These are called A and B type isoantigens.

   An **agglutinin** is an antibody in plasma which is capable of causing agglutination, or clumping together, of cells. Two types in human plasma are anti-A and anti-B agglutinins.

2.

Type	Isoantigen	Agglutinin
A	A	anti-B
B	B	anti-A
AB	AB	no agglutinins
O	no isoantigens	anti-A and anti-B

3. (a) no
   (b) yes (anti-B agglutinin of the recipient will clump with B-type isoantigen of the donor)
   (c) no
   (d) yes (anti-A and anti-B agglutinins in type O blood will clump with A- and B-type isoantigens of the AB donor)

F. 1. Change in structure and function which is different from the original type (specialization).
  2. Liquid portion of blood; contains proteins and water and various salts, wastes, nutrients, hormones, and vitamins.
  3. Lymph vessel in villi of small intestine; absorbs fats from the intestinal tract.
  4. Abnormal condition of varied, irregularly shaped red blood cells.
  5. Pigment in bile which is produced when hemoglobin is destroyed.
  6. Any blood abnormality or pathological condition.
  7. Milky lymph substance in the lacteals of small intestine; consists largely of digested fats.
  8. Pertaining to the armpit.
  9. Plasma after the plasma clotting proteins and factors have been removed.
  10. An oval body lying near the stomach. It is composed of reticuloendothelial tissue which destroys worn-out red cells and bacteria; stores blood cells; forms blood cells in the embryo.
  11. Abnormal proliferation of immature granulocytic leukocytes called myeloblasts.
  12. Abnormal condition of having oval or round red blood cells as opposed to those with the normal biconcave shape. This makes the erythrocyte fragile and likely to hemolyze.
  13. An anticoagulant substance.
  14. Abnormal condition of increase of reticulocytes, which are immature red blood cells.

G. 1. J 5. A 9. B
  2. F 6. D 10. H
  3. G 7. E
  4. C 8. I

REVIEW SHEET 14

Combining Forms

agglutin/o	micr/o
bas/o	mon/o
chrom/o	morph/o
eosin/o	myel/o
erythr/o	neutr/o
fibrin/o	norm/o
granul/o	nucle/o
hem/o	phag/o
hemat/o	poikil/o
immun/o	reticul/o
is/o	sider/o
kary/o	spher/o
leuk/o	splen/o
lymphaden/o	thromb/o
lymphangi/o	thym/o
macr/o	

Suffixes

-blast	-genic
-cytosis	-globin
-emia	-globulin

-penia _____   -phoresis _____

-pheresis _____   -poiesis _____

-philia _____   -stasis _____

Additional Terms

agglutinins _____

_____

agglutinogens _____

_____

albumin _____

anemia _____

antibodies _____

_____

antigens _____

aplastic anemia _____

basophil _____

B-cell lymphocyte _____

bilirubin _____

bleeding time _____

blood dyscrasia _____

chyle _____

coagulation time _____

corpuscle _____

differentiation _____

electrophoresis _____

eosinophil _____

fibrin _____

fibrinogen _____

formed elements _____

globulin _____

granulocytes _____

hemoglobin _____

hemolytic anemia _____

hemophilia _____

heparin _____

histiocyte _____

Hodgkin's disease _____

immune reaction _____

infectious mononucleosis _____

interstitial fluid _____

isoantigen _____

lacteals _____

leukemia _____

lymphosarcoma _____

megakaryocyte _____

monocyte _____

myasthenia gravis _____

neutrophil _____

normoblast _____

pernicious anemia _____

plasma _____

plasmapheresis _____

platelets _____

polycythemia vera _____

prothrombin _____

purpura _____

reticulocytes _____

reticuloendothelial cells _____

Rh factor _____

sarcoidosis _____

serum _____

sickle cell anemia _____

spleen _____

stem cell _____

T-cell lymphocytes _____

thalassemia _____

thrombin _____

thromboplastin _____

thymus gland _____

type A blood group _____

type B blood group _____

type AB blood group _____

type O blood group _____

CHAPTER 15

MUSCULOSKELETAL SYSTEM

In this chapter you will:

Learn the terms relating to the structure and function of bones, joints, and muscles;

Understand the process of bone formation and growth;

Locate and name the major bones of the body;

Make words with and analyze the combining forms, prefixes, and suffixes used to describe bones, joints, and muscles; and

Learn the terminology relating to the major types of musculoskeletal disease conditions.

This chapter is divided into the following sections:

I. INTRODUCTION

The musculoskeletal system includes the bones, muscles, and joints. Each has several important functions in the body. **Bones**, by providing the framework around which the body is constructed, protect and support our internal organs. Also, by serving as a point of attachment for muscles, bones assist in body movement. The inner core of bones is composed of hematopoietic tissue (red bone marrow manufactures blood cells), while other parts are storage areas for minerals necessary for growth, such as calcium and phosphorus.

Joints are the places where bones come together. Several different types of joints are found within the body. The type of joint found in any specific location is determined by the need for greater or lesser flexibility of movement.

Muscles, whether attached to bones or to internal organs and blood vessels, are responsible for movement. Internal movement involves the contraction and relaxation of muscles which are a part of viscera, and external movement is accomplished by the contraction and relaxation of muscles which are attached to bones.

II. VOCABULARY

This list omits names of specific bones. The bones are defined according to location in section III of this chapter.

acetabulum	Rounded depression, or socket, in the pelvic bone. Named because of its resemblance to a rounded cup the Romans used for vinegar (acetum). The acetabulum is where the thigh bone joins with the pelvis.
acromion	Outward extension (process) of the shoulder bone forming the point of the shoulder.
amphiarthrosis	Joint which permits slight movement, but in all directions. The joints between the vertebrae are examples.
aponeurosis	Flat, fibrous connective tissue (tendon) which attaches muscles to bones or other tissue.
articulation	Joint.

bone process	Extension or outgrowth of bone tissue.
bursae (singular: bursa)	Sacs of fluid located at and around joints which act as cushions and reduce friction.
calcium	One of the mineral matter constituents of bone.
cancellous bone	Porous bone tissue found in the epiphyses of long bones and other bones as well.
cartilage tissue	Flexible, rubbery connective tissue found at the ends of bones, forming the joint surface; also found in the embryonic skeleton, and in the ribs, nasal septum, external ear, and respiratory tubes of the adult.
compact bone	Hard, dense tissue, also called cortical bone, found under the periosteum layer of all bones.
condyle	Knuckle-like process at the end of the bone near the joint.
decalcified bone	Bone from which calcium has been removed.
diaphysis	Shaft, or midportion, of long bone.
diarthrosis	Freely movable joint; a hinge joint.
epiphyseal plate	Area at the ends of long bones in which growth takes place.
epiphysis	Each end of a long bone.
false ribs	Last five pairs of ribs (8 to 12). The rib cartilages of the 8th, 9th, and 10th pairs are attached to the cartilages of the rib above, and not directly to the breastbone.
fascia	Fibrous bands of connective tissue binding muscles together.
fissure	Narrow slitlike opening.
flat bones	Found in shoulder, pelvis, and ribs; protect soft body parts.
floating ribs	Last two pairs (11 and 12) of the false ribs. These ribs are not attached to the breastbone at all.

fontanelle	Soft spot (incomplete bone formation) between the bones of the skull of an infant.
foramen	Opening for passage of blood vessels and nerves into and from bone.
fossa	Depression or cavity in bone.
haversian canals	Minute canals filled with blood vessels; found in compact bone.
intervertebral cartilaginous disks	Cartilage tissue between the vertebrae to absorb shocks and provide flexibility of movement.
joint	Area of connection between two or more bones; an articulation.
ligaments	Connective tissue binding bones to bones.
long bones	Found in extremities; examples are thigh bone and lower leg bone.
mastoid process	Rounded projection on the skull bone behind the ear.
medullary cavity	Central, hollowed out cavity in shaft of bones; contains bone marrow within a network of cancellous bone.
olecranon	Process on the medial lower arm bone (ulna) which extends behind the elbow joint.
osseous tissue	Bone tissue.
ossification	Process of bone formation.
palliative	Relieving symptoms; not a cure.
phosphorus	Mineral substance found in bones in combination with calcium (calcium phosphate).
red bone marrow	Found in porous, cancellous tissue of bones; site of hemopoiesis.
sarcolemma	Delicate membrane surrounding each skeletal muscle fiber.
sequestrum	Dead bone tissue.

sinus	Air cavity within bone.
skeletal muscles	Muscles which are attached to bones; also called voluntary or striated muscle.
smooth muscles	Involuntary muscles in viscera and blood vessels.
spur	Outgrowth from bone (pathological).
striated muscles	Voluntary, skeletal muscles.
sulcus	Groovelike depression.
suture	Juncture line where two bones form a synarthrosis.
synarthrosis	Joint which does not permit any movement.
synovial membrane	Surrounds a freely movable joint and secretes a fluid (synovial fluid) which lubricates the joint cavity.
tendon	Connective tissue binding muscles to bones.
trochanter	Large process below the neck of the femur for muscle attachments.
true ribs	First seven pairs of ribs, which articulate with the sternum.
tubercle	Small, rounded process on a bone; serves for attachment of muscles or tendons.
tuberosity	Large, rounded process on bone; serves for attachment of muscles or tendons.
vertebral arch	Posterior part of the vertebra consisting of several processes which aid in muscle and bone attachment.
vertebral column (backbone)	Twenty-six bone segments enclosing and protecting the spinal cord.
xiphoid process	Lower, narrow portion of the breastbone.
yellow bone marrow	Found in the diaphyses of long bones; composed of fatty tissue.

III. BONES

A. Formation and Structure

Formation

Bones are complete organs, chiefly composed of connective tissue called **osseous** (bony) **tissue** plus a rich supply of blood vessels and nerves. Osseous tissue is a dense connective tissue which consists of **osteocytes** (bone cells) surrounded by a hard, intercellular substance filled with calcium salts.

During fetal development, the bones of the fetus are composed of **cartilage tissue**, which resembles osseous tissue but is more flexible and less dense because of a lack of calcium salts in its intercellular spaces. As the embryo develops, the process of depositing calcium salts in the soft, cartilaginous bones occurs, and continues throughout the life of the individual after birth. The gradual replacement of cartilage and its intercellular substance by immature bone cells and calcium deposits is called **ossification** (bone formation).

Osteoblasts are the immature bone cells which produce the bony tissue that replaces cartilage during ossification. **Osteoclasts** (-clast means to break) are large cells which function in bone to reabsorb, or digest, bony tissue. Osteoclasts are called bone phagocytes.

A bone grows in width through the action of osteoclasts within which dissolve out the inner walls and make the interior hollow wider. At the same time, osteoblasts add layers of bony tissue to the outer surface. When a bone breaks, osteoblasts lay down the mineral bone matter (calcium salts) and osteoclasts remove excess bone debris (smooth out the bone).

The formation of bone is dependent to a great extent on a proper supply of **calcium** and **phosphorus** to the bone tissue. These minerals must be taken into the body along with a sufficient amount of vitamin D. Vitamin D helps the passage of calcium through the lining of the small intestine and into the bloodstream. Once calcium and phosphorus are in the bones, osteoblastic activity produces an enzyme which splits phosphorus substances and causes the formation of a calcium-phosphate compound giving bone its characteristic hard quality.

Not only are calcium and phosphorus part of the hard, bony structure of bone tissue, but calcium is also stored in bones and small quantities are present in the blood. If the proper amount of calcium is lacking in the blood, nerve fibers are unable to transmit impulses effectively to muscles; heart muscle becomes weak and muscles attached to bones undergo spasms.

The necessary level of calcium in the blood is maintained by the parathyroid gland, which secretes a hormone to release calcium from bone storage. Excess of the hormone (caused by tumor or other pathological process) will raise blood calcium at the expense of the bones, which become weakened by the loss of calcium.

Structure

Bones all over the body are of several different types. **Long bones** are found in the thigh, lower leg, and upper and lower arm. These bones are very strong, are broad at the ends where they join with other bones, and have large surface areas for muscle attachment.

Short bones are found in the wrist and ankle and have small, irregular shapes. **Flat bones** are found covering soft body parts. These are the shoulder bone, ribs, and pelvic bones. **Sesamoid bones** are small, rounded bones resembling a grain of sesame in shape. They are found near joints; the knee cap is the largest example of this type of bone.

Figure 15–1 shows the anatomical divisions of a long bone such as the thigh bone or upper arm bone. Label the figure as you read the following.

The shaft, or long middle region, of a long bone is called the **diaphysis** (1). Each end of a long bone is called an **epiphysis** (2). The **epiphyseal line** or **plate** (3) represents an area of cartilage tissue in the bone which is constantly being replaced by new bony tissue as the bone grows. Cartilage cells (chondrocytes) slowly migrate away from the region of the plate. Lack of blood supply to the area triggers formation of calcium deposits in the bone. The epiphyseal plate closes up and disappears as new bone tissue completely replaces cartilage tissue. When a long bone has achieved its full growth, an x-ray of the epiphysis shows no evidence of the epiphyseal plate.

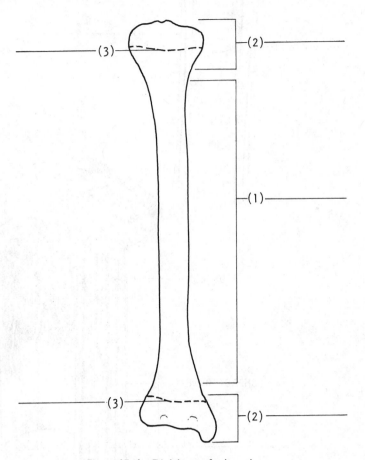

Figure 15–1 Divisions of a long bone.

Figure 15–2 shows some of the structures which are part of the composition of the epiphysis and diaphysis. The **periosteum** (1) is a strong, fibrous, vascular membrane that covers the surface of a long bone, except at the ends of the epiphyses. Bones other than long bones are completely covered by the periosteum as well. Beneath the periosteum is the layer of immature cells (osteoblasts) which deposit calcium-phosphorus compounds in the bony tissue.

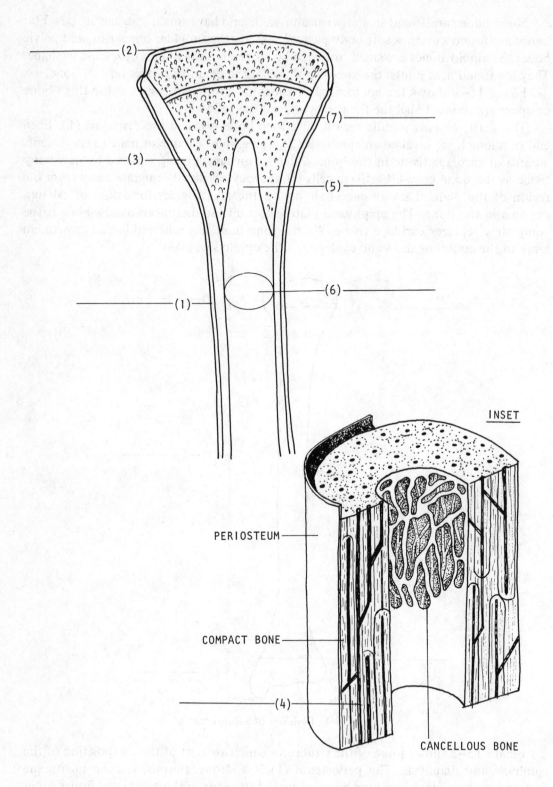

Figure 15-2 Interior bone structure.

INSET

PERIOSTEUM

COMPACT BONE

CANCELLOUS BONE

The ends of long bones are covered by a thin layer of cartilage called **articular cartilage** (2). This cartilage layer cushions the bones at the place where they meet with other bones (joints).

Compact (cortical) bone (3) is a layer of hard, dense tissue which lies under the periosteum in all bones and chiefly around the diaphysis of long bones. Within the compact bone is a system of small canals containing blood vessels which bring oxygen and nutrients to the bone and remove waste products such as carbon dioxide. The inset in Figure 15–2 shows these channels, called **haversian canals** (4), in the compact bone. Compact bone is tunneled out in the shaft of long bones by a central **medullary cavity** (5) which contains **yellow bone marrow** (6). Yellow bone marrow is chiefly composed of fatty connective tissue.

Cancellous bone (7), sometimes called spongy bone, is much more porous and less dense than compact bone. The mineral matter in it is laid down in a series of separated bony fibers called a spongy latticework. It is found largely in the epiphyses of long bones and in the middle portion of most other bones of the body as well. Spaces in cancellous bone contain **red bone marrow**. This marrow, as opposed to yellow marrow which is fatty tissue, is richly supplied with blood and consists of immature and mature blood cells in various stages of development.

In an adult, the ribs, pelvic bone, sternum (breastbone), and vertebrae, as well as the epiphyses of long bones, contain red bone marrow within cancellous tissue. The red marrow in the long bones is plentiful in young children, but decreases through the years and is replaced by yellow marrow.

B. Processes and Depressions in Bones

Bone processes are enlarged tissue which normally extend out from bones. Label Figure 15–3 which shows the shapes of some of the common bony processes:

(1) **bone head** – rounded end of a bone separated from the body of the bone by a neck.

(2) **tubercle** – small, rounded process which serves as a site of tendon or muscle attachment.

(3) **trochanter** – large projection on the femur which serves as a site of attachment for muscle.

(4) **tuberosity** – large, rounded process which serves as a site of muscle or tendon attachment.

(5) **condyle** – rounded, knuckle-like process at the joint.

Bone depressions are the openings or hollow regions in a bone which, like the processes, help to join one bone to another. In addition, depressions serve as a passageway for blood vessels and nerves. The names of some common depressions in bone are:

fossa – furrow or hollow area in a bone.

foramen – opening for blood vessels and nerves.

fissure – a narrow, deep, slitlike opening.

sulcus – a groove.

sinus – air cavity within a bone.

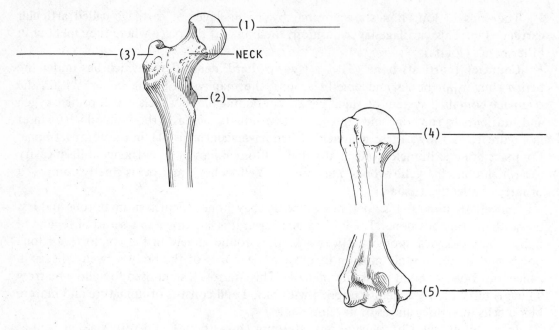

Figure 15-3 Bone processes.

C. Cranial Bones

The bones of the skull, or cranium, protect the brain and structures related to it, such as the sense organs. Muscles for controlling head movements and chewing motions are connected to the cranial bones. Sinuses, or air cavities, are located in specific places within the cranial bones to lighten the cranium and warm and moisten air as it passes through.

The cranial bones of a newborn child are not completely joined. There are gaps of unossified tissue in the skull at birth. These are called soft spots, or fontanelles (little fountains). The pulse of blood vessels can be felt under the skin in those areas.

Figure 15-4 illustrates the bones of the cranium. Label them as you read the following descriptions:

(1) **frontal bone** – forms the forehead and bony sockets which contain the eyes.

(2) **parietal bone** – there are two parietal bones which form the roof and upper part of the sides of the cranium.

(3) **temporal bone** – two temporal bones form the lower sides and base of the cranium. Each bone encloses an ear and contains a fossa for joining with the mandible (lower jaw bone). The **mastoid process** is a round process of the temporal bone behind the ear.

(4) **occipital bone** – forms the back and base of the skull and joins the parietal and temporal bones, forming a suture (juncture line of cranial bones). The inferior portion of the occipital bone has an opening called the **foramen magnum** through which the spinal cord passes.

(5) **sphenoid bone** – this bat-shaped bone extends behind the eyes and forms part of the base of the skull. Because it joins with the frontal, occipital, and ethmoid bones, it serves as an anchor to hold those skull bones together. (Sphen/o means wedge.)

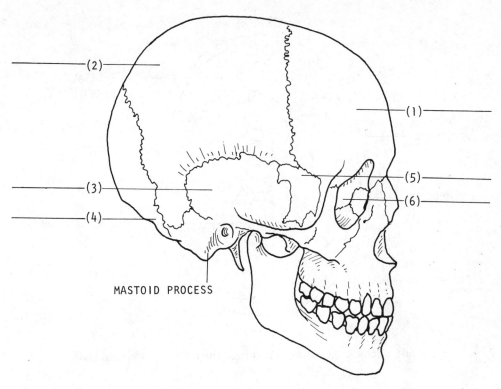

Figure 15-4   Cranial bones, lateral view.

(6) **ethmoid bone** – this delicate bone is composed primarily of spongy, cancellous bone. It supports the nasal cavity and forms part of the orbits of the eyes. (Ethm/o means sieve.)

Study Figure 15–5 which shows the above-mentioned cranial bones as viewed through the floor of the cranial cavity. Note the foramen magnum.

D.   Facial Bones

All of the facial bones, except one, are joined together by sutures so that they are immovable. The mandible (lower jaw bone) is the only facial bone capable of movement. This ability is necessary for activities such as mastication (chewing) and speaking.

Figure 15–6 shows the facial bones; label it as you read the following descriptions of the facial bones:

(1)   **nasal bones** – two slender nasal (nas/o = nose) bones support the bridge of the nose. They join with the frontal bone superiorly and form part of the nasal septum.

(2)   **lacrimal bones** – two paired lacrimal (lacrim/o = tear) bones are located one at the corner of each eye. These thin, small bones contain fossae for the lacrimal gland (tear gland) and canals for the passage of the lacrimal duct.

(3)   **maxillary bones** – two large bones compose the massive upper jaw bones (maxillae). They are joined by a suture in the median plane. If the two bones do not come together normally before birth, the condition known as cleft palate results.

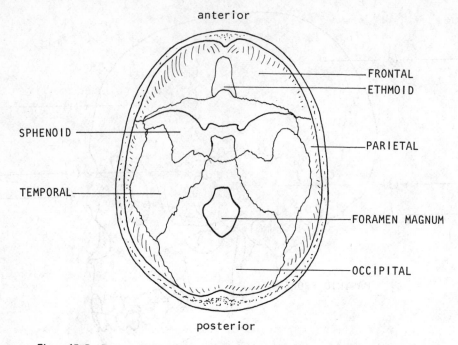

Figure 15-5   Bones of the skull viewed from the floor of the cranial cavity.

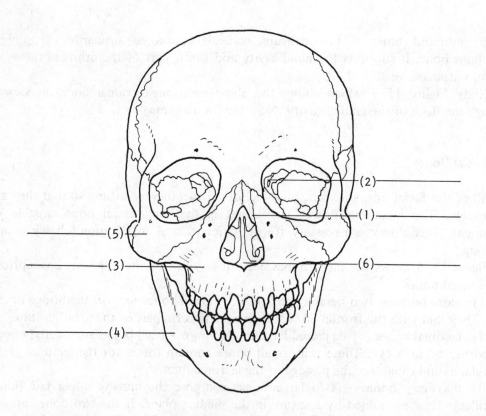

Figure 15-6   Facial bones.

(4) **mandibular bone** — this is the lower jaw bone. Both the maxilla and mandible contain the sockets called alveoli in which the teeth are embedded.

(5) **zygomatic bones** — two bones, one on each side of the face, form the high portion of the cheek.

(6) **vomer** — this thin, single, flat bone forms the lower portion of the nasal septum.

E. Vertebral Column

The **vertebral**, or spinal, **column** is composed of 26 bone segments, called vertebrae, which are arranged in five divisions from the base of the skull to the tailbone.

Figure 15–7 illustrates these divisions of the vertebral column; label it as you read the following:

> The first seven bones of the vertebral column, forming the neck bone, are the **cervical (Cl-C7) vertebrae** (1). These vertebrae do not articulate (join) with the ribs.

> The second set of 12 vertebrae are known as the **thoracic (T1-T12 or Dl-D12) vertebrae** (2). These vertebrae articulate with the 12 pairs of ribs.

> The third set of five vertebral bones are the **lumbar (L1-L5) vertebrae** (3). They are the strongest and largest of the backbones.

> The **sacrum** (4) is a slightly curved, triangularly shaped bone. At birth it is composed of five separate segments; these gradually become fused in the young child.

> The **coccyx** (5) is the tailbone, and it, too, is a fused bone, having been formed from four small bones.

Figure 15–8 illustrates the general structure of a vertebra. Although the individual vertebrae in the separate regions of the spinal column are all slightly different in structure, they do have several parts in common.

A vertebra is composed of an inner, thick, disk-shaped portion called the **vertebral body** (1). Between the body of one vertebra and the bodies of vertebrae lying beneath and above are **cartilaginous disks** which help to provide flexibility and cushion most shocks to the vertebral column.

The **vertebral arch** (2) is the posterior part of the vertebra, and consists of a **spinous process** (3), **transverse processes** (4), and **laminae** (5). The **neural canal** (6) is the space between the vertebral body and the vertebral arch through which the spinal cord passes.

F. Bones of the Thorax, Pelvis, and Extremities

Label Figure 15–9 as you read the following descriptions of the bones of the thorax (chest cavity), pelvis (hip bone), and extremities (arms and legs):

Bones of the Thorax

(1) **clavicle** — collar bone; a slender bone, one on each side of the body, connecting the breastbone to each shoulder bone.

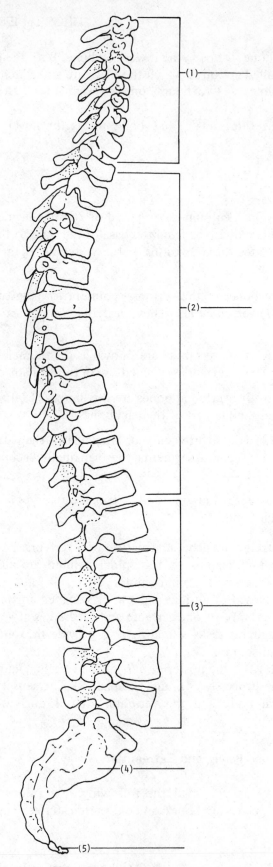

Figure 15-7 Vertebral column.

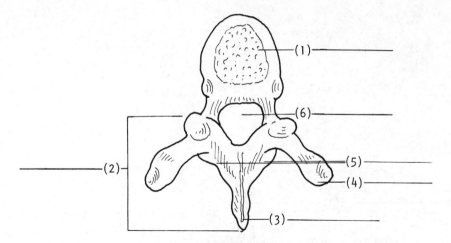

Figure 15-8   General structure of a vertebra.

(2) **scapula** – shoulder bone; two flat, triangular bones, one on each dorsal side of the thorax. The extension of the scapula which joins with the clavicle to form the joint of the shoulder is called the **acromion**.

(3) **sternum** – breastbone; a flat bone extending down the midline of the chest. The uppermost part of the sternum articulates on the sides with the clavicle and ribs, while the lower, narrower portion is attached to the diaphragm and abdominal muscles. The lower portion of the sternum is called the **xiphoid process**.

(4) **ribs** – there are 12 pairs of ribs. The first seven pairs articulate with the sternum anteriorly through cartilaginous attachments called costal cartilages. These ribs join in the back with the vertebral column and are called the **true ribs**. The last five pairs are called **false ribs** because instead of joining the sternum directly they converge and join the seventh rib at a point before the sternum is reached. The **floating ribs** are the last two pairs of false ribs, which are completely free at their anterior extremities. The floating ribs do not complete their curve, but come to an end in the midchest. All the ribs are attached to the vertebral column dorsally, creating a cagelike structure which encloses the heart, lungs, and other vital thoracic structures.

Bones of the Arm and Hand

(5) **humerus** – upper arm bone; the large head of the humerus is rounded and joins with the scapula and clavicle.

(6) **ulna** – medial lower arm bone; the proximal bony process of the ulna at the elbow is called the **olecranon** (elbow bone).

(7) **radius** – lateral lower arm bone.

(8) **carpals** – wrist bones; there are two rows of four bones each in the wrist.

(9) **metacarpals** – these are five radiating bones to the fingers.

(10) **phalanges** (singular: phalanx) – finger bones; each finger (except the thumb) has three phalanges: a proximal, middle, and distal phalanx. The thumb has only two phalanges.

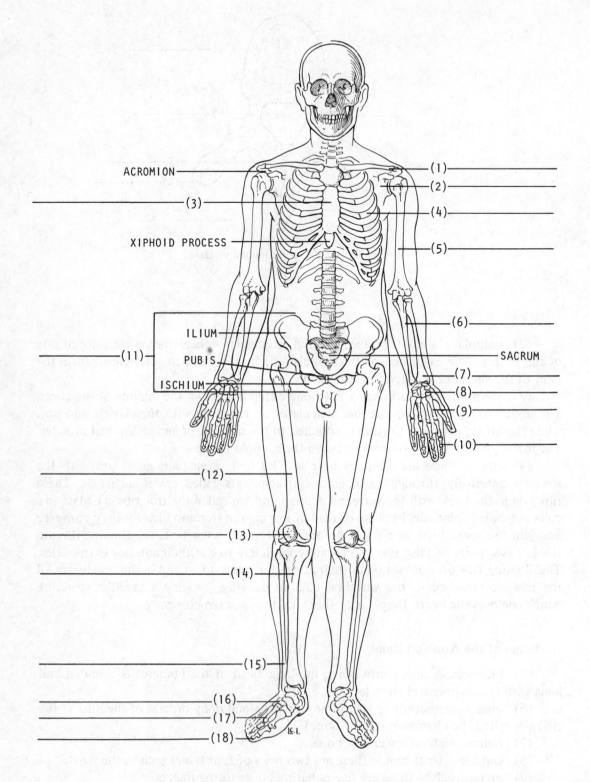

ACROMION —————————— (1) ——————

—————————— (2) ——————

—————— (3) —————— (4) ——————

XIPHOID PROCESS —————— (5) ——————

—————— (6) ——————

ILIUM —————— (11) —————— SACRUM

PUBIS —————— (7) ——————

ISCHIUM —————— (8) ——————

—————— (9) ——————

—————— (10) ——————

—————— (12) ——————

—————— (13) ——————

—————— (14) ——————

—————— (15) ——————

—————— (16) ——————
—————— (17) ——————
—————— (18) ——————

Figure 15–9 Bones of the thorax, pelvis, and extremities.

Bones of the Pelvis

(11) **pelvic girdle** – hip bone; this large bone supports the trunk of the body and articulates with the leg bones and sacrum. The adult pelvic bone is composed of three pairs of fused bones: the ilium, ischium, and pubis.

The **ilium** is the uppermost and largest portion. Dorsally, the two parts of the ilium do not meet. Rather, they join the sacrum on either side. The connection between the iliac bones and the sacrum is so firm that they are commonly spoken of as one bone: the sacroiliac. The superior part of the ilium is known as the iliac crest. It is filled with red bone marrow, and serves as an attachment for abdominal wall muscles.

The **ischium** is the posterior part of the pelvis. The ischium and the muscles attached to it are what you sit on.

The **pubis** is the anterior part and contains suture marks where the two pubes join by way of a cartilaginous disk. This area of fusion is called the **pubic symphysis**.

The region within the ring of bone formed by the pelvic girdle is called the pelvic cavity. The rectum, sigmoid colon, bladder, and female reproductive organs lie within the pelvic cavity.

Bones of the Leg and Foot

(12) **femur** – thigh bone; this is the longest bone in the body. At its proximal end it has a rounded head which fits into a depression, or socket, in the hip bone. This socket is called the **acetabulum**.

(13) **patella** – kneecap; this is a small, flat bone which lies in front of the articulation between the femur and one of the lower leg bones called the tibia. It is surrounded by protective tendons and held in place by muscle attachments.

(14) **tibia** – largest of two lower bones of the leg; the tibia (meaning "flute") runs under the skin in the front part of the leg. It joins with the femur at the patella, and at its distal end (ankle) forms a swelling which is the bony prominence at the inside of the ankle. The tibia is commonly called the **shin bone**.

(15) **fibula** – smaller of two lower leg bones; this thin bone, well hidden under the leg muscles, joins at its proximal end with the tibia laterally, and joins at its distal end with the tibia and ankle bones to form the bony prominence on the outside of the ankle.

(16) **tarsals** – ankle bones; these are seven short bones which resemble the carpal bones of the wrist but are larger. The **calcaneus** is the largest of these bones and is also called the heel bone.

(17) **metatarsals** – there are five metatarsal bones—each leads to the phalanges of the toes.

(18) **phalanges of the toes** – there are two phalanges in the big toe and three in each of the other four toes.

Figure 15–10 illustrates the bones of the foot.

G. Combining Forms and Suffixes

These are divided into two groups: general terms and terms related to specific bones.

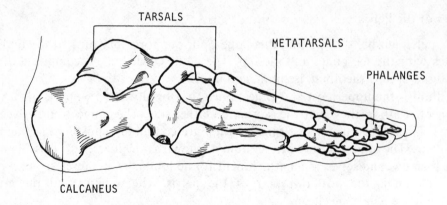

Figure 15–10 Bones of the foot, lateral view.

General Terms

Combining Form	Definition	Terminology	Meaning
oste/o	bone	osteitis _____	
		osteotome _____	
		osteomalacia _____	
		osteoma _____	
		osteogenic _____	
calci/o	calcium	calcification _____	
-physis	to grow, growth	epiphysis _____	
		diaphysis _____	
		symphysis _____	
vertebr/o *(used to describe the structure)*	vertebra	vertebral _____	
spondyl/o *(used to make words about conditions of the structure)*	vertebra	spondylosis _____	
		spondylitis _____	
		spondylolysis _____	

rachi/o	spinal column, vertebrae	rachialgia _____
		rachiotomy _____
lamin/o	lamina *(part of the vertebral arch)*	laminectomy _____ *An operation often performed to relieve the symptoms of a ruptured intervertebral disk.*
kyph/o	humpback *(posterior curvature in the thoracic region)*	kyphosis _____
lord/o	curve, swayback *(anterior curvature in the lumbar region)*	lordosis _____ *This term is used to describe both the normal anterior curvature of the spinal column in the lumbar region and an excessive, abnormal anterior curvature, or swayback, condition.*
scoli/o	crooked, bent *(lateral curvature)*	scoliosis _____
myel/o	bone marrow, spinal cord	myeloma _____
		myelopoiesis _____
cervic/o	neck	cervical _____
thorac/o	chest	thoracic _____
lumb/o	loins, lower back	lumbar _____
		lumbodynia _____
-blast	embryonic or immature cell	osteoblast _____
-clast	to break	osteoclast _____
-desis	to bind	spondylosyndesis _____ _____ *Spinal fusion.*
-malacia	softening	osteomalacia _____ *A condition in which vitamin D deficiency leads to decalcification of bones.*

-porosis	passage	osteoporosis _____

This failure of osteoblasts to lay down bone matrix may result from poor supply of calcium to bones, hormone and nutritional disorders, or the natural process of aging.

Specific Bones

crani/o	skull bones	craniotomy _____
maxill/o	upper jaw bone	maxillary _____
submaxill/o	lower jaw bone	submaxillary _____
mandibul/o	lower jaw bone	mandibular _____
clavicul/o	clavicle *(collar bone)*	clavicular _____
scapul/o	scapula, shoulder bone	scapular _____
cost/o	ribs	costal _____
		chondrocostal _____
		_____
		costoclavicular _____
		costovertebral _____
		_____
stern/o	sternum, breastbone	sternal _____
humer/o	humerus	humeral _____
uln/o	ulna *(medial lower arm bone)*	ulnar _____
olecran/o	elbow	olecranal _____

radi/o	radius; ray *(lateral lower arm bone)*	radial _____
carp/o	carpus, wrist bones	carpal _____
metacarp/o	metacarpals *(hand bones)*	metacarpectomy _____
phalang/o	phalanges *(finger and toe bones)*	phalangeal _____
pelv/i	pelvic bone	pelvimetry _____
ili/o	ilium *(superior portion of the hip bone)*	iliac _____
ischi/o	ischium *(inferior, dorsal part of the hip bone)*	ischial _____
pub/o	pubis *(anterior, inferior part of the hip bone)*	pubic _____
acetabul/o	acetabulum *(socket of hip bone into which the head of the thigh bone fits)*	acetabular _____
femor/o	femur *(thigh bone)*	femoral _____
patell/o	patella *(kneecap)*	patellar _____
tibi/o	tibia *(shin bone)*	tibial _____
fibul/o	fibula *(smaller of the two leg bones)*	fibular _____

perone/o	fibula	peroneal	_____
calcane/o	calcaneus	calcaneal	_____
	(heel bone)		

H. Pathological Conditions

osteodystrophy   Bad development of bone.

> This pathological condition can arise from a variety of disease processes. Vitamin D deficiency and overproduction of hormones are common etiological factors. Some types of osteodystrophies are:

osteitis fibrosa cystica   Inflammation of bone with fibrous changes in the bone tissue.

> When the parathyroid gland produces an excess of parathyroid hormone (hyperparathyroidism), calcium is removed from the bones and appears in the blood. The bones become porous (osteoporosis) and decalcified, leading to curvature and cyst formation as well as fractures. Blood calcium accumulation may lead to renal and cystic calculi (stones).

rickets (rachitis)   Inflammation of the spinal column.

> Rickets is an osteodystrophy characterized by **osteomalacia**. It is primarily a disease of infancy and childhood when bones are forming but fail to receive important minerals for growth. The bones become soft and bend easily, leading to kyphosis as well as other bone curvatures.
> The etiology of rickets is usually related to dietary deficiency of vitamin D. Vitamin D is necessary for the proper absorption of calcium and phosphorus from the small intestine into the blood. Bone formation is dependent upon a sufficient amount of calcium and phosphorus, especially during the early years of bone growth. Infants and young children whose diets are lacking in foods which supply vitamin D to the body (milk, egg yolks, butter, cod liver oil) may thus develop rickets.

osteomyelitis   Inflammation of the bone and bone marrow.

> This inflammation involves the soft parts of the bone, especially the bone marrow in the medullary cavity of the bone. The hard, calcified part of the bone becomes softened as well, as a result of the inflammation.
> The etiology of osteomyelitis is bacterial. Staphylococci invade the bloodstream after gaining access to the body through the skin. Sometimes trauma to the skin and bone leads to rupture of blood

vessels so that the staphylococci begin to grow in blood clots and injured tissue.

The clinical course involves bone abscess (inflammation and pus collection) and eventually death of bone tissue with thrombosis of blood vessels in the bone marrow. **Sequestrum** is the term used to describe a piece of dead bone tissue. The entire body may become involved in the disease if the thrombi carrying staphylococci spread to the organs and pyemia develops.

Antibiotic therapy can correct the condition once a correct diagnosis is made so that the abscess and thrombosis formation can be averted.

osteogenic sarcoma	Flesh (connective tissue) tumor arising from bone.

This is the most common of the malignant bone tumors. Osteoblasts multiply without control and form large tumors, especially at the ends of long bones.

Ewing's tumor	Malignant bone tumor.

This tumor, arising in bone, is highly malignant, but may be cured with surgery, radiation therapy, and chemotherapy.

multiple myeloma	Malignant tumor of bone marrow.

This is a highly malignant tumor of bone marrow cells. Anemia is usually present and pain and pathological fractures are common. Because the proliferating tumor cells are plasma cells which produce plasma proteins called globulins, hyperglobulinemia is a valuable diagnostic aid.

Treatment of malignant bone tumors such as osteogenic sarcoma, Ewing's tumor, and multiple myeloma usually consists of amputation in the hope of preventing spread of the tumor (metastasis). Radiation and chemotherapy are **palliative** (relieving) agents for widespread tumor, but may be curative if treatment is begun when the tumor is localized.

IV. JOINTS

A. Classification of Joints

A joint (articulation) is a coming together of two or more bones. There are three types of joints in the body. They are classified according to the degree of movement which the bone permits:

Synarthrosis

A **synarthrosis** is a joint which does not permit movement at all. Bones come together and are bound, or united, by a layer of fibrous tissue which does not permit movement. Examples of synarthroses are suture joints of the skull.

Amphiarthrosis

An **amphiarthrosis** is an articulation which permits slight movement. The bone surfaces of the joint are connected by elastic fibrocartilage and are partially movable. This type of joint is found between the vertebrae and between the small bones of the ankle and wrist.

Diarthrosis

A **diarthrosis** is a freely movable joint. Label the structures in Figure 15–11 as you read the following description of a diarthrotic joint:

The bones in a diarthrotic joint are separated by a **joint capsule** (1) composed of fibrous cartilage tissue. **Ligaments** (fibrous bands, or sheets, of connective tissue) often anchor the bones together around the joint capsule to strengthen it. The surface of the bones at the joint is covered with a smooth cartilage surface called the **articular cartilage** (2). The **synovial membrane** (3) lies under the joint capsule and lines the **synovial cavity** (4) between the bones. The synovial cavity is filled with a special lubricating fluid produced by the synovial membrane. This **synovial fluid** contains water and nutrients which nourish as well as lubricate the joints so that friction on the articular cartilage is minimal.

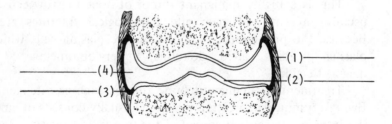

Figure 15–11 Diarthrosis (freely movable joint).

B. Bursae

Bursae are closed sacs of synovial fluid lined with a synovial membrane. They are formed in the spaces between **tendons** (connective tissue binding muscles to bones), **ligaments** (connective tissue binding bones to bones), and bones. Bursae lubricate these areas where friction would normally develop close to the joint capsule.

Some common bursae locations are at the elbow joint (olecranon bursa), knee joint (patellar bursa), and shoulder joint (subacromial bursa).

C. Combining Forms

Combining Form	Definition	Terminology	Meaning
arthr/o	joint	arthropyosis _____	
		hydroarthrosis _____	
		arthrorrhagia _____	
		arthrodesis _____	
articul/o	joint	articulation _____	
		articular surface _____	
synovi/o	synovia *(fluid which lubricates joints)*	synovial membrane _____	
		synovitis _____	
burs/o	bursa *(sac of synovial fluid near joints)*	bursitis _____	
chondr/o	cartilage	chondrocostal _____	
		chondromalacia _____	
		achondroplasia _____	
		chondrogenesis _____	
fibros/o	fibrous connective tissue	fibrositis _____ *Also called rheumatism.*	
ten/o tend/o tendin/o	tendons *(fibrous bands connecting muscles to bones)*	tenodesis _____	
		tendoplasty _____	
		tenosynovitis _____	
		tendinitis _____	
ligament/o	ligaments *(fibrous bands connecting bones to other bones)*	ligamentous _____	

syndesm/o	ligament	syndesmoplasty _____
		syndesmorrhaphy _____
ankyl/o	crooked, bent, stiff	ankylosis _____
amphi-	on both sides	amphiarthrosis _____
syn-	together	synarthrosis _____
di-, dia-	complete	diarthrosis _____

D. Pathological Conditions

arthritis   Inflammation of joints.

> There are many different types of arthritis. Some of the more common forms are:

rheumatoid arthritis   Chronic joint inflammation, stiffness, and swelling; of unknown cause.

> This is a chronic inflammatory condition affecting primarily the small joints of the hands and feet at first and then larger joints later. Women in young adulthood are primarily afflicted. The course of the disease involves thickening and inflammation of the synovial membranes of the joint and damage to the articular cartilage. The inflammatory tissue is then covered with thick tissue which adheres and prevents easy joint movement. This is called **ankylosis** (stiffness). The fibrous tissue thus formed may even calcify and form a bony ankylosis, a bony union of the joint which prevents any movement. The joint during the course of the disease is swollen and painful. In acute stages of the illness, pyrexia (fever) is present. Treatment consists of local applications of heat, and drugs to reduce inflammation and pain.

gouty arthritis   Inflammation of joints caused by excessive uric acid in the blood.

> The etiology of this condition is an inborn error of metabolism. Individuals afflicted with gout form too much uric acid (nitrogenous waste) in the body. Large amounts of uric acid are unable to be metabolized and removed from the body. Uric acid accumulates in the blood, joints, and soft tissues near the joints. The uric acid crystals destroy the articular cartilage and damage the synovial membrane of the joint. Osteoarthritis develops as the cartilage disappears, and the underlying bone atrophies as well as forming ossified outgrowths (**spurs**) which limit the movement of the joint.

The joints chiefly affected are the big toe, fingers, and knee. Treatment consists of drugs to prevent joint inflammation and a special diet which avoids foods that increase the tendency to accumulate uric acid in the body (red wine, beer, meat).

protrusion of an intervertebral disk   Abnormal position of a cartilaginous segment separating the vertebrae.

This condition is known as "slipped disk." The intervertebral disk protrudes or slips out of its normal position between the vertebrae and may press on nerves in the spinal cord or nerves leading to other parts of the body. The most common areas for slippage to occur are the regions of L5-S1 (between the 5th lumbar and 1st sacral vertebrae) and C5-C6 (between the 5th and 6th cervical vertebrae). Low back pain or cervical pain are clinical symptoms, along with **sciatica** (pain radiating down the leg along the path of the sciatic nerve). Muscle spasms may contribute to discomfort as well. If bed rest and avoidance of trauma to the afflicted area are not helpful, then surgery may be indicated. **Laminectomy** or **spondylosyndesis** may be advised to remove the disk and bind the vertebrae together.

V. MUSCLES

A. Types of Muscles

There are three types of muscles in the body. Label Figure 15–12 as you read the following descriptions of the various types of muscles:

Striated muscles (1), also called **voluntary** or **skeletal** muscles, are the muscle fibers which move all bones, as well as the face and eyes. We have conscious control over the activity of this type of muscle. Striated muscle fibers (cells) contain many nuclei and have a pattern of dark and light bands, or fibrils, in their cytoplasm. A delicate membrane called a **sarcolemma** surrounds each skeletal muscle fiber.

Smooth muscles (2), also called **involuntary** or **visceral** muscles, are those muscle fibers which move our internal organs such as the digestive tract, blood vessels, and

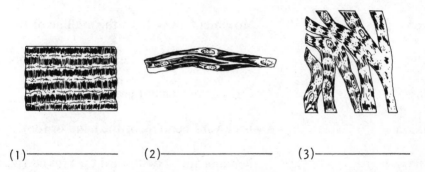

(1)—————— (2)—————— (3)——————

Figure 15-12 Types of muscles.

secretory ducts leading from glands. We have no conscious control over these muscles. They are called "smooth" because they have no dark and light fibrils in their cytoplasm. There is also only one nucleus to a cell in smooth muscle fibers. While skeletal muscle fibers are arranged in bundles, smooth muscle forms sheets of fibers as it wraps around tubes and vessels.

Cardiac muscle (3) is striated in appearance but like smooth muscle in its action. Its movement cannot be consciously controlled. The fibers of cardiac muscle are branching fibers and are found in the heart.

B. Actions of Skeletal Muscles

Skeletal (striated) muscles are the muscles which move the bones of our body. When a muscle contracts, one of the bones to which it is joined remains virtually stationary as a result of other muscles which hold it in place. The point of attachment of the muscle to the stationary bone is called the **origin** (beginning) of that muscle. However, when the muscle contracts, another bone to which it is attached does move. The point of junction of the muscle to the bone that moves is called the **insertion** of the muscle.

There can be more than one origin for a muscle, as is the case with the upper arm muscle (biceps brachii) where one origin is at the upper end of the humerus near the shoulder joint and a second origin is above the scapula. The insertion of the biceps brachii is at the upper end of the radius near the elbow.

Near the point of insertion, a muscle narrows and is connected to the bone by way of a tendon (stringy, cordlike sheath of connective tissue). One type of tendon which helps attach muscles to bones, as well as to their tissues, is called an **aponeurosis** (apo = upon).

Muscles can perform a variety of actions. Some of the terms used to describe those actions are listed below with a short description of the specific type of movement performed:

Action	*Meaning*
Flexion	Bending, decreasing the angle at the joint between bones.
Extension	Straightening of a flexed limb.
Abduction	Movement away from the midline of the body.
Adduction	Movement toward the midline of the body.
Rotation	Circular movement around an axis.
Dorsiflexion	Backward bending of the hand or foot.
Plantar flexion	Bending the foot toward the ground (plant/o = the sole of the foot).

Supination	Facing upward; as applied to the hand, the act of turning the palm forward (anteriorly) or upward.
Pronation	Facing downward; as applied to the hand, the act of turning the palm backward posteriorly.

Your medical dictionary will have a complete list of the muscles of the body, with a description of their origin, insertion, and various actions.

C. Combining Forms

Combining Form	Definition	Terminology	Meaning
my/o	muscle	myalgia _____	
myos/o	muscle	myositis _____	
leiomy/o	smooth, visceral muscle	leiomyoma _____	
rhabdomy/o	skeletal, striated muscle	rhabdomyoma _____	
sarc/o	flesh *(connective tissue)*	leiomyosarcoma _____	
myocardi/o	heart muscle	myocardial _____	
		myocarditis _____	
fibr/o	fibers or fibrous tissue	myofibrosis _____	
fasci/o	fascia *(fibrous membrane separating and enveloping muscle tissue)*	fasciotomy _____	
aponeur/o	aponeurosis *(type of tendon)*	aponeurorrhaphy _____	
-sthenia	strength	myasthenia _____	
-trophy	development, nourishment	hypertrophy _____	
		atrophy _____	

C. Pathological Conditions

myasthenia gravis   Lack of muscle strength marked by paralysis.

This condition affects the voluntary muscles of the body, especially those of the face. The etiology of myasthenia is unknown, but it is thought that there is some defect at the myoneural junction where the nerve enters the muscle fiber to stimulate muscle contraction. There is either a lack of **acetylcholine** to help transmit the impulse across the myoneural junction or an increase in **cholinesterase**, which is an enzyme released at the junction to destroy whatever acetylcholine remains after the impulse has passed. Treatment consists of giving a drug to interfere with cholinesterase production. In some cases, thymectomy (removal of thymus gland) is beneficial, but the reason for this is unknown.

muscular dystrophy   Poor muscle development.

This disease usually begins in childhood and seems to affect only young males. Muscle structure and metabolism are changed so that while the muscle becomes enlarged and bulges it is not a true growth of parenchymal tissue related to improving muscle functioning. Muscle tissue is replaced by interstitial fat tissue (**pseudohypertrophy**) and the muscle cells themselves lose their functional ability and display atrophy.

VI. EXERCISES

A. Give the meaning of the following:

1. calcium _____

_____

2. osteoclasts _____

3. ossification _____

4. medullary cavity _____

5. cancellous bone _____

6. aponeurosis _____

7. articular cartilage _____

8. diaphysis _____

9. epiphyseal plate _____

10. haversian canals _____

B. *Match the following bone processes and depressions with their proper meaning:*

1. fissure	_____	air cavity within bone.
2. sulcus	_____	opening for nerves and blood vessels in bone.
3. tubercle		
	_____	large process on femur for muscle attachment.
4. sinus		
5. trochanter	_____	large rounded process.
6. fossa	_____	narrow slitlike opening.
7. condyle	_____	groovelike depression in bone surface.
8. foramen	_____	knuckle-like process at end of bone.
9. tuberosity	_____	small rounded process.
	_____	furrow or cavity in bone.

C. *Build medical terms:*

1. Immature bone cell _____

2. Membrane close around bone tissue _____

3. Softening of cartilage _____

4. Pertaining to the sacrum and the ilium _____

5. Abnormal condition of vertebrae _____

6. Instrument to cut bone _____

7. Humpback _____

8. Pertaining to the tailbone _____

9. Inflammation of bone and joints _____

10. Removal of the laminae of a vertebral arch _____

D. *Match the cranial bone with its location:*

1. parietal _____ lower sides and base of the cranium.

2. occipital _____ forehead and part of eye sockets.

3. frontal _____ bat-shaped bone behind the eyes and part of base of skull.

4. temporal

_____ delicate bone supporting the nasal cavity

5. ethmoid and orbits of eyes.

6. sphenoid _____ upper part of sides of the skull and roof.

_____ back and base of the skull.

E. *Identify the following facial bones:*

1. mandible _____

2. nasal _____

3. maxilla _____

4. lacrimal _____

5. vomer _____

6. zygomatic _____

F. *Match the following medical terms for bones with their locations in the body:*

Bones		*Locations*
1. humerus	_____	breastbone.
2. clavicle	_____	ankle bones.
3. scapula	_____	posterior part of pelvic bone.
4. sternum	_____	upper arm bone.
5. ulna	_____	kneecap.

6. carpals   _____   finger or toe bones.

7. radius   _____   uppermost part of the pelvic bone.

8. phalanges   _____   medial lower arm bone.

9. fibula   _____   wrist bones.

10. femur   _____   shoulder bone.

11. patella   _____   largest of two bones of the lower leg.

12. tibia   _____   thigh bone.

13. tarsals   _____   smaller of two bones of the lower leg.

14. ilium   _____   collar bone.

15. ischium   _____   lateral lower arm bone.

G. *Give the meaning of the following:*

1. pubic symphysis _____

2. acetabulum _____

3. floating ribs _____

4. olecranon _____

5. acromion _____

6. xiphoid process _____

7. mastoid process _____

8. suture _____

9. neural canal _____

10. false ribs _____

11. calcaneus _____

12. scoliosis _____

13. rachiotomy _____

14. lordosis _____

15. costochondral _____

H. *Give the combining form for the following bones:*

1. lower jaw bone _____

2. thigh bone _____

3. heel bone _____

4. upper jaw bone _____

5. breastbone _____

6. collar bone _____

7. shoulder bone _____

8. bones of finger and toes _____

9. kneecap _____

10. fibula _____

I. *Build medical terms:*

1. Binding together of vertebrae _____

2. Abnormal condition of porous bones _____

3. Bad bone development _____

4. Inflammation of bone and bone marrow _____

5. Dead bone tissue _____

6. Tumor of bone marrow _____

7. Surgical repair of a ligament _____

8. Inflammation of a tendon and synovial membrane _____

9. Abnormal condition of pus in a joint _____

10. Lack of cartilage formation _____

J. *Give the meaning of the following medical terms:*

1. ankylosis _____

2. palliative _____

3. diarthrosis _____

4. sarcolemma _____

5. ligament _____

6. bursa _____

7. synovial fluid _____

8. striated muscle _____

9. tendon _____

10. smooth muscle _____

11. decalcification _____

12. fascia _____

13. insertion of a muscle _____

14. origin of a muscle _____

K. *Describe some of the characteristics of the following musculoskeletal disorders:*

1. rickets _____
_____

2. gout _____
_____

3. muscular dystrophy _____
_____

4. rheumatoid arthritis _____

_____

5. osteomyelitis _____

_____

6. multiple myeloma _____

_____

7. osteitis fibrosa cystica _____

_____

8. myasthenia gravis _____

_____

L. *Match the term for muscle action with its meaning:*

1. extension

_____ movement away from the midline.

2. rotation

_____ facing downward; in the hand, turning the palm downward, or posteriorly.

3. flexion

_____ facing upward; in the hand, turning the palm forward, or anteriorly.

4. adduction

5. supination

_____ straightening a flexed limb.

6. abduction

_____ bending the sole of the foot downward toward the ground.

7. pronation

_____ circular movement around an axis.

8. dorsiflexion

_____ bending (decreasing the angle between a joint).

9. plantar flexion

_____ movement toward the midline.

_____ backward bending of the hand or foot.

ANSWERS

A.
1. Mineral substance necessary for the formation of bony tissue. Combined in bones with phosphorus in the form of calcium-phosphate compound.
2. Bone cells which reabsorb bony tissue.
3. Process of forming bone tissue; cells and hard calcium-phosphate matrix (intercellular material).
4. Hollowed-out cavity in the diaphysis of long bone; contains yellow bone marrow.
5. Spongy bone found in the epiphyses of long bone and other bones as well; contains red bone marrow.
6. Fibrous sheath of connective tissue (tendon) which attaches muscles to bones.
7. Smooth connective tissue found on bones at the joint surface.
8. Shaft of a long bone.
9. Cartilaginous area, in epiphysis of long bones, which is the region of active bone growth.
10. Canal in compact bone tissue containing blood vessels and nerves.

B. 4
8
5
9
1
2
7
3
6

C.
1. osteoblast
2. periosteum
3. chondromalacia
4. sacroiliac
5. spondylosis
6. osteotome
7. kyphosis
8. coccygeal
9. osteoarthritis
10. laminectomy

D. 4
3
6
5
1
2

E.
1. lower jaw bone.
2. bone of the nose.
3. upper jaw bone.
4. bone located at the corner of the eye; contains fossae for tear glands.
5. lower portion of the nasal septum.
6. cheek bone.

F. 4
13
15
1
11
8
14
5
6
3
12
10
9
2
7

G.
1. Anterior portion of pelvic bone; where pubic bones have grown together (amphiarthrotic joint).
2. Socket in the pelvic girdle for head of femur to articulate with pelvic bone.
3. Last two false ribs; not attached to sternum.
4. Elbow joint.
5. Extension of the scapula which forms the point of the shoulder.
6. Lower, narrow portion of breastbone (sternum).
7. Bulge in the temporal bone of the skull just behind the ear.
8. Place of union of two bones in a synarthrotic joint.
9. Cavity between the vertebral arch and vertebral body through which spinal cord passes.
10. Last five pairs of ribs; the first three of these attach to the sternum indirectly through cartilaginous extensions.
11. Heel bone.
12. Abnormal condition of lateral curvature of the spinal column in the thoracic region.
13. Incision into the spinal column.
14. Swayback; anterior curvature of the spine in the lumbar region. Also may refer to the normal anterior curvature of the lumbar spine.
15. Pertaining to the rib cartilage.

H. 1. mandibul/o
    2. femor/o
    3. calcane/o
    4. maxill/o
    5. stern/o
    6. clavicul/o
    7. scapul/o
    8. phalang/o
    9. patell/o
   10. fibul/o

I. 1. spondylosyndesis
    2. osteoporosis
    3. osteodystrophy
    4. osteomyelitis
    5. sequestrum
    6. myeloma
    7. syndesmoplasty
    8. tenosynovitis
    9. arthropyosis
   10. achondroplasia

J. 1. Abnormal condition of stiffness.
    2. To relieve symptoms, not cure.
    3. Fully movable joint.
    4. Delicate membrane surrounding a striated muscle fiber.
    5. Connective tissue binding bones to bones.
    6. Sacs filled with synovial fluid, located at or near joints.
    7. Fluid in joints and bursae for lubrication.
    8. Voluntary, skeletal muscle.
    9. Connective tissue binding muscles and bones.
   10. Involuntary, visceral muscle.
   11. Lack of calcium in tissue such as bones or teeth.
   12. Fibrous connective tissue binding bundles of muscles together.
   13. Point of attachment of muscle to the bone which it moves.
   14. Point of attachment of muscle to a bone which remains fixed and stationary.

K. 1. Bone-softening disease (osteomalacia) caused by vitamin D deficiency.
    2. Metabolic disorder; causes accumulation of uric acid in joints, blood, and soft tissues of the body, and osteoarthritis develops.
    3. Poor muscle development owing to faulty metabolism and structure within the muscle.
    4. Chronic inflammatory condition of joints involving damage to the synovial membrane and articular cartilage.
    5. Inflammation of bone marrow due to bacterial invasion of bone.
    6. Malignant tumor of bone marrow tissue; anemia and hyperglobulinemia are symptoms.
    7. Form of osteodystrophy caused by excess of parathyroid hormone leading to loss of calcium from bones (osteoporosis).
    8. Lack of strength in voluntary muscles of the body, especially the face. Etiology is unknown, but the condition represents a defect at the myoneural junction.

L. 6
   7
   5
   1
   9
   2
   3
   4
   8

REVIEW SHEET 15

Combining Forms

acetabul/o	_____	humer/o	_____
acromi/o	_____	ili/o	_____
ankyl/o	_____	ischi/o	_____
aponeur/o	_____	kyph/o	_____
articul/o	_____	lamin/o	_____
arthr/o	_____	leiomy/o	_____
burs/o	_____	ligament/o	_____
calcane/o	_____	lord/o	_____
calci/o	_____	lumb/o	_____
carp/o	_____	mandibul/o	_____
cervic/o	_____	maxill/o	_____
chondr/o	_____	metacarp/o	_____
clavicul/o	_____	my/o	_____
coccyg/o	_____	myel/o	_____
cost/o	_____	myocardi/o	_____
crani/o	_____	myos/o	_____
fasci/o	_____	olecran/o	_____
femor/o	_____	oste/o	_____
fibr/o	_____	patell/o	_____
fibros/o	_____	pelv/o	_____
fibul/o	_____	perone/o	_____

phalang/o _____

pub/o _____

pubi/o _____

pyr/o _____

rachi/o _____

radi/o _____

rhabdomy/o _____

sacr/o _____

sarc/o _____

scapul/o _____

scoli/o _____

spondyl/o _____

stern/o _____

submaxill/o _____

syndesm/o _____

synovi/o _____

ten/o _____

tend/o _____

tenon/o _____

thorac/o _____

tibi/o _____

uln/o _____

vertebr/o _____

Suffixes

-blast _____

-clast _____

-desis _____

-lemma _____

-malacia _____

-physis _____

-porosis _____

-sthenia _____

-trophy _____

Prefixes

amphi- _____

de- _____

di- _____

peri- _____

sym- _____

syn- _____

Additional Terms Related to Bones

acetabulum _____

acromion _____

bone head _____

bone process _____

calcium _____

cancellous bone _____

compact bone _____

condyle _____

diaphysis _____

epiphyseal plate _____

epiphysis _____

Ewing's sarcoma _____

false ribs _____

fissure _____

flat bones _____

floating ribs _____

fontanelle _____

foramen _____

fossa _____

haversian canals _____

mastoid process _____

medullary cavity _____

multiple myeloma _____

olecranon _____

osseous tissue _____

ossification _____

osteitis fibrosa cystica _____

osteoclast _____

osteodystrophy _____

osteogenic sarcoma _____

osteomyelitis _____

palliative _____

phosphorus _____

red bone marrow _____

rickets _____

sequestrum _____

sinus _____

spur _____

sulcus _____

trochanter _____

true ribs _____

tubercle _____

tuberosity _____

vertebral arch _____

vertebral column _____

xiphoid process _____

yellow bone marrow _____

Name the six cranial bones:

_____   _____

_____   _____

_____   _____

Name the six facial bones:

_____   _____

_____   _____

_____   _____

Name the five divisions of the vertebral column:

_____   _____

_____   _____

_____

Give the medical term for the following bones:

collar bone   _____

shoulder bone   _____

breastbone   _____

upper arm bone   _____

medial lower arm bone   _____

lateral lower arm bone   _____

wrist bone   _____

bones between wrist and fingers   _____

hip bone   _____

thigh bone   _____

knee bone   _____

shin bone   _____

smaller lower leg bone   _____

ankle bones   _____

heel bone   _____

bones between ankle and toes   _____

Additional Terms Related to Joints

amphiarthrosis

articular cartilage

articulation

bursae

cartilage tissue

condyle

diarthrosis

gouty arthritis

intervertebral disk

ligaments

rheumatoid arthritis

suture

synarthrosis

synovial membrane

tendons

Additional Terms Related to Muscles

abduction _____

adduction _____

aponeurosis _____

dorsiflexion _____

extension _____

fascia _____

flexion _____

insertion of a muscle _____

muscular dystrophy _____

myasthenia gravis _____

origin of a muscle _____

plantar flexion _____

pronation _____

rotation _____

sarcolemma _____

skeletal muscle _____

supination _____

visceral muscle _____

CHAPTER 16

SKIN

In this chapter you will:

Identify the layers of the skin and the accessory structures which are associated with the skin;

Build medical words using the combining forms which are related to the specialty of dermatology; and

Become familiar with terms used to describe lesions, symptoms, and pathological conditions which relate to the skin.

The chapter is divided into the following sections:

I. INTRODUCTION

The skin and its accessory organs (hair, nails, and glands) are known as the **integumentary system** of the body. Integument means covering, and the skin is the outer covering for the body. It is, however, more than a simple body covering. The skin, as a complex system of specialized tissues, contains glands which secrete several types of fluids, nerves which carry impulses, and blood vessels which aid in the regulation of the body temperature. The following paragraphs review the many important functions of the skin.

First, as a protective membrane over the entire body, the skin guards the deeper tissues of the body against excessive loss of water, salts, and heat and against invasion by pathogens and their toxins. Secretions from the skin are slightly acid in nature and this contributes to the skin's ability to prevent bacterial invasion.

Second, the skin contains two types of glands which produce important secretions. These glands under the skin are the **sebaceous** and **sweat glands**. The sebaceous glands produce an oily secretion called **sebum**, while the sweat glands produce a watery secretion called **sweat**. Sebum and sweat are carried to the outer edges of the skin by ducts, and excreted from the skin through openings, or pores. Sebum helps to lubricate the surface of the skin, and sweat helps to cool the body as it evaporates from the skin surface.

Third, nerve fibers located under the skin act as receptors for sensations such as pain, temperature, pressure, and touch. The adjustment of an individual to his or her environment is thus dependent on the sensory messages relayed to the brain and spinal cord by the sensitive nerve endings in the skin.

Fourth, several different tissues in the skin aid in maintaining the body temperature (thermoregulation). Nerve fibers coordinate thermoregulation by carrying messages to the skin from heat centers in the brain which are sensitive to increases and decreases in body temperature. Impulses from these fibers cause blood vessels to dilate to bring blood to the surface and cause sweat glands to produce the watery secretion which carries heat away.

II. VOCABULARY

basal layer	The deepest region of the epidermis (outer layer of the skin). The basal layer contains actively dividing skin cells and gives rise to all the cells of the epidermis.
collagen	A protein found in the connective tissue of the middle layer of the skin. Collagen is also found in cartilage, bone, and ligaments.
comedo	Blackhead; plug of protein and sebum within an opening in the skin.
corium	Middle layer of the skin, beneath the epidermis (outer layer). It is composed of glands, blood vessels, lymphatics, and nerve endings surrounded by loose connective tissue. The corium is also called the dermis.
dermis	Middle layer of the skin; also called the corium.
epidermis	Outermost layer of the skin.
epithelium	The covering of the internal and external surfaces of the body. It consists of tightly joined cells.
fibroblast	A cell which secretes collagen; found in the corium layer of the skin.

hair	An outgrowth from the skin which is composed of a protein called keratin.
hair follicle	Sac or tube within which each hair grows.
histiocyte	Connective tissue cell found in the corium. This cell is phagocytic (protects the body by engulfing and destroying foreign material).
horny cell	Cell in the epidermis which is filled with a hard protein substance called keratin.
integumentary system	The skin and its accessory structures, including hair and nails.
keratin	A hard protein material found in the epidermis of the skin as well as the hair and nails. Keratin means "horn," apparently because it occurs in animal horns.
lipocyte	A fat cell; found in the subcutaneous (innermost) layer of the skin.
lunula	Half-moon shaped white arch near the root of a nail.
mastocyte	Connective tissue cell found in the corium. It contains substances which when released account for allergic responses in skin, and aid in blood coagulation. A mastocyte is also known as a mast cell.
melanin	Black pigment formed by special cells (melanocytes) in the epidermis and other parts of the body.
melanocyte	A cell which contains and synthesizes melanin.
nail	Outgrowth of the skin which is attached to the distal end of each phalanx (finger and toe bone). A nail is composed of keratin.
sebaceous gland	Oil-secreting gland in the corium layer of the skin. Sebaceous glands are associated with hair follicles.
sebum	Oily substance secreted by the sebaceous glands of the skin.
squamous epithelium	Flat, scalelike cells composing the epidermis.

strata	Layers.
stratified	Arranged in layers (as are the layers of epithelial cells in the epidermis).
stratum corneum	Outermost layer of the epidermis; consists of flattened, keratinized (horny) cells.
subcutaneous tissue	Innermost layer of the skin, below the corium. It contains primarily fat tissue.
sweat glands	Glands found in the corium of the skin. They secrete a watery fluid called sweat.

III. STRUCTURE OF THE SKIN

Figure 16–1 shows the three layers of the skin. Label these layers from the outer surface inward:

(1) **Epidermis** – a thin, cellular membrane layer.

(2) **Corium** or **dermis** – dense, fibrous, connective tissue layer.

(3) **Subcutaneous tissue** – thick, fat-containing tissue.

Epidermis

The epidermis is the outermost, totally cellular layer of the skin. It is composed of **squamous epithelium**. Epithelium is the covering of both the internal and external surfaces of the body. Squamous epithelial cells are flat and scalelike. In the outer layer of the skin, these cells are arranged in several layers (**strata**) and are, therefore, called **stratified squamous epithelium**.

The epidermis lacks blood vessels, lymphatic vessels, and connective-type tissue (elastic fibers, cartilage, fat) and is, therefore, dependent on the deeper corium layer and its rich network of capillaries for nourishment. In fact, oxygen and nutrients seep out of the capillaries in the corium, pass through tissue fluid, and supply nourishment to the deeper layers of the epidermis.

Figure 16–2 illustrates the multilayered cells of the epidermis. The deepest layer is called the **basal layer** (1). The cells in the basal layer are constantly growing and multiplying and give rise to all the other cells in the epidermis. As the basal layer cells divide, they are pushed upward and away from the blood supply of the corium layer by a steady stream of younger cells. In their movement toward the most superficial layer of the epidermis, called the **stratum corneum** (2), the cells flatten, shrink, lose their nuclei, and die, becoming filled with a protein called **keratin**. The cells are then called **horny cells**, reflecting their composition of keratin, which is a hard, protein material. Finally, within 3 to 4 weeks after beginning as a basal cell in the deepest part of the epidermis, the horny, keratinized cell is sloughed off from the surface of the

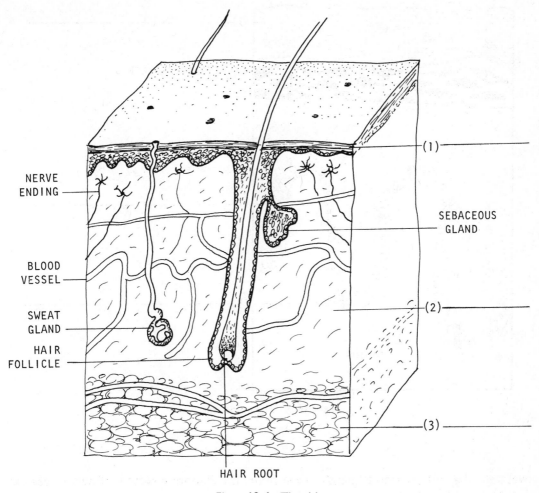

NERVE ENDING

SEBACEOUS GLAND

BLOOD VESSEL

SWEAT GLAND

HAIR FOLLICLE

(1)

(2)

(3)

HAIR ROOT

Figure 16–1   The skin.

skin. The epidermis is thus constantly renewing itself, cells dying at the same rate at which they are born.

The basal layer of the epidermis contains special cells called **melanocytes** (3). Melanocytes form and contain a black pigment called **melanin**. The amount of black pigment accounts for the color differences among the races of man. Also, the presence of melanin in the epidermis is vital for protection against the harmful effects of ultraviolet radiation which can manifest themselves as skin cancer. Individuals who, through a flaw in their chemical makeup, are incapable of forming melanin at all are called **albino** (meaning "white"). Skin and hair are white, and the eyes are red because in the absence of pigment the tiny blood vessels are visible in the iris (normally pigmented portion) of the eye.

Corium

The corium layer, directly below the epidermis, is also called the **dermis**. In contrast to the epidermis, it is living tissue composed of blood and lymph vessels and nerve fibers, as well as the accessory organs of the skin, which are the hair follicles,

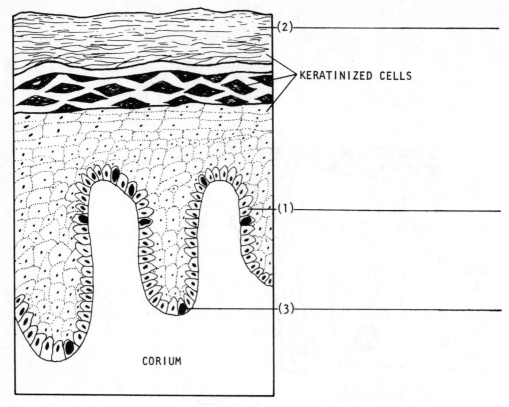

KERATINIZED CELLS

CORIUM

Figure 16-2 The epidermis.

sweat glands, and sebaceous glands. To support the elaborate system of nerves, vessels, and glands, the corium contains cells and fibers.

There are several types of connective tissue cells in the corium: **fibroblasts**, **histiocytes**, and **mastocytes**. Fibroblasts are supportive cells which produce a fibrous protein material called **collagen**. **Histiocytes** are phagocytic cells which protect the body by engulfing foreign materials. **Mastocytes** (mast cells) are specialized cells which contain quantities of histamine (a substance released in allergies which produces itching) and heparin (a blood clotting substance).

The fibers in the dermis, or corium, are mainly composed of collagen. Collagen is a protein which is tough and resistant but also flexible. In the infant, collagen is loose and delicate, and it becomes harder as the body ages. The collagen fibers support and protect the blood and nerve networks which pass through the corium.

Subcutaneous Layer

The subcutaneous layer of the skin is another connective tissue layer which specializes in the formation of fat. **Lipocytes** (fat cells) are predominant in the subcutaneous layer and they manufacture and store large quantities of fat. Obviously, areas of the body and individuals vary as far as fat deposition is concerned. Functionally, this layer of the skin is important in protection of the deeper tissues of the body and as a heat insulator.

IV. ACCESSORY ORGANS OF THE SKIN

A. Hair

A hair fiber is composed of a tightly fused meshwork of horny cells filled with the hard protein called keratin. Hair growth is similar to the growth of the epidermal layer of the skin. Deep-lying cells in the hair root (see Figure 16–1) produce horny cells which move upward through the **hair follicles** (shafts or sacs which hold the hair fibers). Melanocytes are located at the root of the hair follicle and they supply the melanin pigment for the horny cells of the hair fiber. Hair turns gray when the melanocytes stop producing melanin.

B. Nails

Nails are hard, keratin plates covering the dorsal surface of the last bone of each toe and finger. They are composed of horny cells which are cemented together tightly and can extend indefinitely unless cut or broken. A nail grows in thickness and length as a result of division of cells in the region of the nail root which is at the base (proximal portion) of the nail plate.

Most nails grow about 1 mm. a week, which means that fingernails may regrow in 3 to 5 months. Toenails grow more slowly than fingernails.

The **lunula** is a semilunar (half-moon) white region at the base of the nail plate, and is generally found in the thumbnail of most people and in varying degrees in lateral fingers. It is white because the keratinizing cells in that area reflect white light.

C. Glands

Sebaceous Glands

Sebaceous glands are located in the corium layer of the skin, and secrete an oily substance called **sebum**. Sebaceous glands are closely associated with hair follicles, and their ducts open into the hair follicle through which the sebum is released. Figure 16–1 shows the relationship of the sebaceous gland to the hair follicle. The sebaceous glands are influenced by sex hormones which cause them to hypertrophy at puberty and atrophy in old age.

Sweat Glands

Sweat glands are tiny, coiled glands found on almost all body surfaces. Figure 16–1 illustrates how the coiled sweat gland originates deep in the corium and straightens out to extend up through the epidermis. The tiny opening on the surface is called a pore.

Sweat, or perspiration, is almost pure water, with dissolved materials such as salt making up less than 1 per cent of the total composition. It is colorless and odorless. The odor produced when sweat accumulates on the skin is due to the action of bacteria on the sweat.

Sweat cools the body as it evaporates into the air. Perspiration is controlled by the sympathetic nervous system whose nerve fibers are activated by the heat regulatory center in the hypothalamic region of the brain which stimulates sweating.

A special variety of sweat gland, active only from puberty onward and larger than the ordinary kind, is concentrated in a few areas of the body near the reproductive organs and in the armpits. These glands secrete an odorless sweat, but it contains certain substances which are easily broken down by bacteria on the skin. The breakdown products are responsible for the characteristic human body odor. The milk-producing mammary gland is another type of modified sweat gland; it secretes milk only after the birth of a child.

V. COMBINING FORMS

Combining Form	Definition	Terminology	Meaning
derm/o dermat/o	skin	hypodermic _____	
		dermatorrhagia _____	
		dermatitis _____	
		dermatoplasty _____	
		erythroderma _____	
		epidermolysis _____	
cutane/o	skin	subcutaneous _____	
xer/o	dry	xeroderma _____	
pachy/o	thick, heavy	pachyderma _____	
xanth/o	yellow	xanthoderma _____	
		xanthoma _____	
melan/o	black	melanocyte _____	
leuk/o	white	leukoderma _____	
alb/o	white	albinism _____	
erythem/o	flushed, redness	erythema _____	
kerat/o	horny, hard (also used to describe the cornea of the eye)	keratosis _____	

acanth/o	thorny, spiny	acanthosis _____
		Thickening of the epidermis.
onych/o	nail	epionychium _____
	(used to describe nail conditions)	onychophagia _____
		onychodystrophy _____
ungu/o	nail	subungual _____
myc/o	fungus, a type of plant	onychomycosis _____
		dermatomycosis _____
seb/o	sebum	seborrhea _____
diaphor/o	sweat	diaphoresis _____
hidr/o	sweat	anhidrosis _____
	(used more commonly to make words)	hidradenitis _____
squam/o	scale	squamous _____
histi/o	tissue	histiocyte _____
adip/o	fat	adipose _____
lip/o	fat	lipoid _____
trich/o	hair	trichomycosis _____
caus/o	burn	causalgia _____
		caustic _____

VI. LESIONS, SYMPTOMS, AND PATHOLOGICAL CONDITIONS OF THE SKIN

Cutaneous Lesions

A lesion is a pathological or traumatic discontinuity in tissue. The following are terms describing common skin lesions:

macules   Flat lesions which change the color of the skin.

Freckles, tattoo marks, and flat moles are examples.

papules   Solid elevations of the skin.

Warts (verrucae), which are caused by a virus infection, are an example. Papules differ in size and location within the corium and subcutaneous tissue.

wheals   Smooth, slightly elevated areas which are redder or paler than the surrounding skin.

A wheal is a type of papule which may be circumscribed, as in a mosquito bite, or involve a wide area, as in allergic reactions. Wheals are commonly known as **hives**, and are often accompanied by itching.

vesicles   Circumscribed collections of clear fluid (blisters).

Vesicles are found in burns, allergy, and dermatitis. **Bullae** (singular: bulla) are large vesicles.

pustules   Circumscribed collections of pus (abscess of the skin).

Since vesicles commonly coexist with pustules, the term vesico-pustular is common.

nevus   Proliferation of blood vessels or pigmented cells on
(plural: nevi)   the skin surface.

Birthmarks (hemangiomas) and moles (pigmented cells) are nevi.

Symptoms

alopecia   Baldness.

This condition can result normally from the aging process, or be induced by drugs, illness, or forms of dermatitis. It occurs when replacement of hair fibers fails to keep up with normal hair loss. Hair of the eyebrows normally lasts 3 to 5 months; that of the scalp, 2 to 5 years.

urticaria   Hives.

This condition is basically a localized edema (swelling) in association with itching. Etiology may be allergy to foods or drugs or psychological stimuli.

pruritus   Itching.

Pruritus is associated with most forms of dermatitis, and other conditions as well. It arises as a result of stimulation of the nerve network in the skin by enzymes released in allergic reactions and by irritations caused by substances from the blood or foreign bodies.

ecchymosis   Purplish, macular patch.

Ecchymoses are caused by hemorrhages into the skin. They are commonly known as black and blue marks or bruises.

petechiae   Small, pinpoint hemorrhages.

Petechiae are smaller versions of ecchymoses.

purpura   Merging ecchymoses and petechiae over any part of the body.

Pathological Conditions

acne   Inflammatory papular and pustular eruption of the skin.

Acne begins with the building up of sebum and keratin in the form of a blackhead (**comedo**). Bacteria (staphylococci) break down the fat molecules in sebum, producing irritant substances which cause inflammation of the surrounding tissue. Treatment consists of long-term antibiotic use and topical medications to dry the skin and remove the fatty substances produced in the hair follicles.

burns   Lesion caused by heat contact.

Burn lesions are usually classified into three types: **first degree burns** (no blisters; superficial lesions mainly in the epidermis; hyperesthesia; and erythema); **second degree burns** (damage to the epidermis and corium; blisters; erythema; and hyperesthesia); and **third degree burns** (both the epidermis and corium are destroyed and subcutaneous layer is damaged, leaving charred, white tissue).
Burns may be due to caustic chemicals, radiation, heat, or the rubbing of objects against the skin.

tinea   Infection of the skin caused by a fungus (a type of plant).

There are many different forms of this fungus skin disease. Examples are ringworm and athlete's foot. Scaling, pruritus, and red patches on the skin are symptoms. Fungistatic preparations for application on the skin can be helpful.

gangrene

Death of tissue associated with loss of blood supply.

In this condition, ischemia resulting from injury, inflammation, frostbite, diseases such as diabetes, or arteriosclerosis can lead to necrosis of tissue, followed by bacterial invasion and putrefaction.

eczema

Inflammatory skin disease.

This condition of unrecognized cause may be chronic or acute dermatitis with a variety of skin lesions—erythematous, vesicular, papular, or pustular. It is often accompanied by pruritus.

psoriasis

Chronic, recurrent dermatosis marked by silvery gray scales covering red patches on the skin.

Psoriasis commonly occurs at the knee, elbow, or scalp. It is neither contagious nor infectious, but is due to an increased rate of growth of the basal layer of the epidermis. Its etiology is unknown.

impetigo

Bacterial inflammatory skin disease characterized by pustules.

This is a contagious pyoderma and is usually caused by staphylococci or streptococci. The common course of this skin condition is to progress from vesicles to a pustular phase and then to crust over.

pemphigus

Blistering (bullous) eruptions affecting the skin and mucous membranes.

The bullous lesions appear asymptomatically and absorb into the skin, leaving pigmented spots. In severe cases, the disorder may require treatment by anti-inflammatory drugs such as a corticosteroid (hormone from the adrenal gland).

systemic lupus erythematosus (systemic L.E.)

Inflammatory disease of the joints and collagen of the skin, as well as any organ of the body.

Lupus (meaning "wolflike") produces a characteristic "butterfly" pattern of redness over the cheeks and nose. In more severe cases, the extent of erythema increases and all exposed areas of the skin may be involved. Alopecia is common. Systemic L.E. is treated with anti-inflammatory drugs such as corticosteroids to control symptoms.

Systemic L.E. should be differentiated from chronic discoid lupus erythematosus, which is a milder scaling plaquelike eruption of the skin confined to the face, scalp, ears, chest, and arms.

Skin Neoplasia

Benign Neoplasms

keratoses   Thickened areas of the epidermis.

Keratoses may be caused by old age or excessive exposure to sunlight.

leukoplakia   White, thickened patches on mucous membrane tissue.

This may be a precancerous lesion. It is common in smokers, and may be caused by chronic inflammation. Gums and tongue are often affected.

Cancerous Lesions

basal cell carcinoma   Malignant tumor of the basal cell layer of the epidermis.

This is the most frequent type of skin cancer. It is a slow-growing tumor of the basal layer of the epidermis. It usually occurs on the upper half of the face, near the nose, and is nonmetastasizing.

squamous cell carcinoma   Malignant tumor of the squamous epithelial cells of the epidermis.

This type of cancerous lesion is a hyperplasia of a layer of the epidermis which is closer to the surface of the skin than the basal layer. The tumor may also grow in places other than the skin, wherever squamous epithelium is found (mouth, larynx, bladder, esophagus, and so forth). It is most common in old age, and its growth is more rapid than that of basal cell carcinoma. Metastasis to the regional lymph nodes may occur. Leukoplakia may precede the formation of the carcinoma.

malignant melanoma   Cancerous tumor composed of melanin-pigmented cells.

Melanomas are literally "black tumors." They arise from pigment-producing cells in the epidermis called **melanoblasts**. A malignant melanoma is one of the most malignant of all cancerous tumors. It usually occurs on the face, neck, and extremities at first and metastasizes via the blood vessels and lymphatics, proceeding toward the lungs, liver, and brain.

Benign melanomas are called pigmented nevi and are found in almost every person. Nevi grow to a specific size and then stop growing. If a nevus is in a particular area of the body which is subjected to trauma and friction, it is usually resected to prevent it from becoming a malignant melanoma.

mycosis fungoides   Rare, chronic skin disease caused by the infiltration of malignant lymphocytes.

Mycosis fungoides is characterized by generalized erythroderma and large reddish raised areas (tumors) that spread and ulcerate (produce disintegration of tissue). In some cases, the malignant cells may involve lymph nodes and other organs.

VII. EXERCISES

A. *Build medical words:*

1. Surgical repair of the skin _____

2. Inflammation of the nails _____

3. Dry skin _____

4. Yellow tumor _____

5. Tissue cell _____

6.` Redness, flushing _____

7. Under the nail _____

8. Abnormal condition of lack of sweat _____

9. Fat cell _____

10. Abnormal condition of a fungus in the hair _____

B. *Give the meaning of the following medical terms:*

1. integument _____

2. collagen _____

3. mastocytes (mast cells) _____

_____

4. basal layer _____

5. keratin _____

6. melanin _____

_____

7. squamous cell epithelium _____

_____

8. corium _____

9. lunula _____

10. sebaceous glands _____

_____

11. histiocyte _____

12. stratum corneum _____

C. *Match the cutaneous lesion with its description:*

1. pustule   _____   hive.

2. macule   _____   raised or flat pigmented area on the skin.

3. vesicle   _____   localized abscess; area of suppuration (pus formation).

4. wheal

    _____   discolored spot or patch on the skin; no elevation or depression in skin.

5. papule

6. nevus   _____   raised lesion with collection of clear fluid; a blister.

    _____   solid, red, elevated area on the skin.

D. *Name the dermatological symptoms:*

1. baldness _____

2. itching _____

3. localized swelling with itching _____

4. black and blue marks _____

5. small pinpoint hemorrhages _____

6. white plaques on mucous membrane tissue _____

7. hardened, thickened areas of the epidermis _____

8. widespread hemorrhages and ecchymoses over the body _____

E. *Match the pathological skin condition with its description:*

1. gangrene   _____   bullous eruptions affecting the skin and
                                           mucous membranes.

2. tinea
                                _____   scaly eruption, commonly on elbows, scalp,
3. eczema   or knee.

4. impetigo   _____   black pigment cells which become cancer-
                                           ous and metastasize all over the body.

5. psoriasis
                                _____   contagious, infectious pyoderma.

6. melanoma
                                _____   necrosis of skin tissue.

7. basal cell
    carcinoma   _____   malignant neoplasm originating in scalelike
                                           cells of the epidermis.

8. squamous cell
    carcinoma   _____   widespread inflammatory disease of the
                                           joints and skin, with "butterfly" pattern of
9. systemic lupus   redness over the cheeks and nose.
    erythematosus
                                _____   malignant growth of cells from the basal
10. pemphigus   layer of the epidermis.

                                _____   chronic form of dermatitis which may
                                           involve erythematous, pustular, or papular
                                           lesions.

                                _____   fungal skin disease.

F. *Give the combining forms for the following:*

1. yellow _____

2. horny _____

3. thorny, spiny _____

4. fat (2) _____

_____

5. hair _____

6. sweat (2) _____

_____

7. fungus _____

8. nail (2) _____

_____

9. burn _____

10. white (2) _____

_____

ANSWERS

A.
1. dermatoplasty
2. onychitis
3. xeroderma
4. xanthoma (composed of fatty tissue)
5. histiocyte
6. erythema
7. subungual
8. anhidrosis
9. lipocyte
10. trichomycosis

B.
1. Covering; the skin.
2. A fibrous protein found in the connective tissue of the corium.
3. Connective tissue cells found in the corium. They contain substances which can cause allergic responses and help in blood coagulation.
4. Deepest layer of the epidermis. It is the actively dividing layer of the epidermis.
5. Tough protein substance in hair, nails, and epidermis of the skin.
6. Black pigment which gives color to hair and skin. It is made by special cells called melanocytes which are located in the basal layer of epidermis.
7. Flat, scalelike cells which compose the epidermis of the skin, as well as line the body cavities and form portions of glands and ducts.
8. Layer of the skin beneath the epidermis; largely connective tissue surrounding blood vessels, lymphatics, and nerve endings; dermis.
9. Half-moon shaped white area near the root of the nail.
10. Oil- (sebum-) secreting glands of the skin. They are found in the corium, and most have a hair follicle associated with them.
11. Connective tissue cell in the corium; phagocytic in function.
12. Outermost layer of the epidermis.

C. 4
6
1
2
3
5

D.
1. alopecia
2. pruritus
3. urticaria
4. ecchymoses
5. petechiae
6. leukoplakia
7. keratoses
8. purpura

E. 10   8
5   9
6   7
4   3
1   2

F. 1. xanth/o
     2. kerat/o
     3. acanth/o
     4. lip/o, adip/o
     5. trich/o
     6. hidr/o, diaphor/o
     7. myc/o
     8. onych/o, ungu/o
     9. caus/o
    10. leuk/o, alb/o

REVIEW SHEET 16

Combining Forms

acanth/o	_____	lip/o	_____
adip/o	_____	melan/o	_____
alb/o	_____	myc/o	_____
caus/o	_____	onych/o	_____
cutane/o	_____	pachy/o	_____
derm/o	_____	py/o	_____
dermat/o	_____	seb/o	_____
diaphor/o	_____	squam/o	_____
erythem/o	_____	trich/o	_____
hidr/o	_____	ungu/o	_____
histi/o	_____	xanth/o	_____
kerat/o	_____	xer/o	_____
leuk/o	_____		

Additional Terms

acne _____

alopecia _____

basal cell carcinoma _____

bullae _____

burn _____

collagen _____

comedo _____

corium _____

dermis _____

ecchymosis _____

eczema _____

epidermis _____

fibroblast _____

gangrene _____

histiocyte _____

impetigo _____

integumentary system _____

keratin _____

keratoses _____

leukoplakia _____

lunula _____

macules _____

malignant melanoma _____

mastocyte _____

melanin _____

mycosis fungoides _____

nevi _____

papules _____

petechiae _____

pemphigus _____

pruritus _____

psoriasis _____

pustules _____

sebaceous glands _____

sebum _____

squamous cell carcinoma _____

stratified _____

subcutaneous tissue _____

systemic lupus erythematosus _____

tinea _____

urticaria _____

verrucae _____

wheals _____

CHAPTER 17

SENSE ORGANS: THE EYE AND THE EAR

In this chapter you will:

Learn the location and function of the major parts of the eye and the ear;

Recognize and work with the combining forms, prefixes, and suffixes most commonly used to describe these organs and their parts; and

Understand the terminology related to the pathological conditions which may affect the eye and ear.

This chapter is divided into the following sections:

I. INTRODUCTION

In the previous chapter, we noted that the sensitive nerve endings in the corium (dermis) layer of the skin receive impulses from various stimuli applied to the external surfaces of the body. These nerve endings transmit electrical messages, initiated by the stimuli, to regions of the brain (cerebrum and thalamus) so that we can recognize sensations such as temperature, touch, pain, and pressure. In Chapter 11 (Nervous

System), we learned that nerve cells which carry impulses from a sense organ or sensory receptor area, such as the skin, taste buds, and olfactory regions (centers of smell in the nose) to the brain are called **afferent sensory neurons**.

The **eye** and the **ear** are sense organs, like the skin, taste buds, and olfactory regions. As such, they are receptors whose sensitive cells may be activated by a particular form of energy or stimulus in the external or internal environment. The sensitive cells in the eye and ear respond to the stimulus by initiating a series of nerve impulses along afferent sensory neurons which lead to the brain.

No matter what kind of stimulus is applied to a particular receptor, the sensation felt is determined by the regions in the brain which are connected to that receptor. Thus, mechanical injury which might stimulate receptor cells in the eye and the ear would produce sensations of vision (flashes of light) and sound (ringing in the ears). Similarly, if one could make a nerve connection between the sensitive receptor cells of the ear and the area in the brain associated with sight, it would be possible to perceive, or "see," sounds.

Figure 17–1 is a flow diagram recapitulating the general pattern of events when such stimuli as light and sound are applied to sense organs such as the eye and ear.

STIMULUS $\xrightarrow[\text{to}]{\text{applied}}$ RECEPTOR CELLS IN EAR AND EYE $\xrightarrow[\text{excite}]{\text{which}}$ AFFERENT NERVE FIBERS $\xrightarrow[\text{impulse to}]{\text{which carry}}$ BRAIN $\}$ where nerve impulses are translated into sound sensations and visual images

Figure 17–1 Pattern of events in stimulation of a sense organ.

The first part of this chapter investigates the eye and the terminology related to its anatomy, function, and pathological conditions. The second part of the chapter investigates in a similar fashion the terminology of the ear.

II. THE EYE

A. Vocabulary

accommodation	Adjustment which makes the lens of the eye fatter or thinner in order to bring an object into focus on the retina (sensitive innermost layer of the eye).
aqueous humor	Watery, transparent liquid circulating through the anterior and posterior chambers of the eye.
biconcave lens	Lens having two depressed, hollow, bowl-like sides.
biconvex lens	Lens having two sides which are rounded, elevated, and curved evenly, like part of a sphere.

choroid layer	Layer of the eye which contains blood vessels.
ciliary body	Structure on each side of the lens of the eye; contains muscles which control the shape of the lens.
cones	Photosensitive receptor cells of the retina which change light energy into a nerve impulse.
conjunctiva	Mucous membrane over anterior surface of eyeball and eyelid.
cornea	Fibrous layer of clear tissue over anterior portion of eyeball.
fovea centralis of the retina	Tiny pit or depression in the retina which is the region of clearest vision.
iris	Colored part of the eye.
lens of the eye	Transparent, biconvex structure which has the ability of bending light rays to bring them in focus on the sensitive, innermost layer of the eye (retina).
macula lutea	A yellowish region on the retina which contains the fovea centralis.
miotics	Drugs which constrict the pupil of the eye.
optic chiasma	Point at which the fibers of the optic nerve, which carries impulses from the retina, cross in the brain. (Chiasma means "a crossing.")
optic disk	Region in the eye where the optic nerve meets the retina.
pupil	Opening of the eye, surrounded by the iris, through which light rays pass.
receptor	Group of cells which receive the impulses from a stimulus. A sense organ is a receptor.
refraction	To break back; bending of light rays by the cornea, lens, and fluids of the eye, bringing the rays into focus on the sensitive receptor cells of the retina.
retina	Sensitive nerve cell layer of the eye; contains receptor cells called rods and cones.

rods   Light-sensitive receptor cells of the retina.

sclera   White of the eye.

vitreous humor   Soft, jelly-like material filling the large inner
                                  chamber of the eye. (Vitreous means "glassy.")

B. Anatomy and Physiology

Label Figure 17–2 as you read the following:

Light rays enter the dark center of the eye, the **pupil** (1), after passing through a mucous membrane called the **conjunctiva** (2) and a transparent fibrous membrane called the **cornea** (3). The cornea covers the anterior portion of the eyeball, and its function is to bend, or refract, the rays of light so that they are focused properly on the sensitive receptor cells in the posterior region of the eye. The **sclera** (4), or white of the eye, is a tough and fibrous supportive tissue and is continuous with the cornea on the anterior surface of the eyeball.

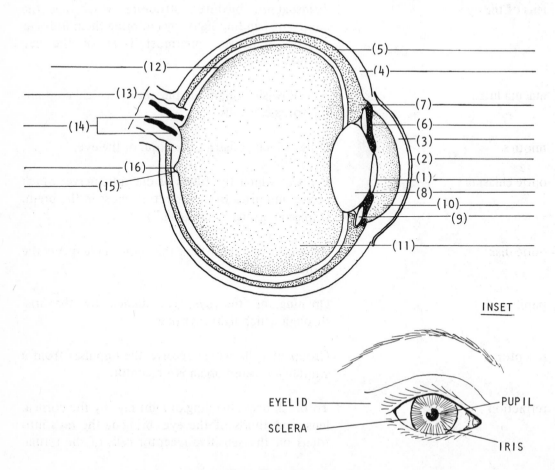

Figure 17–2 The eye.

The **choroid** (5) is a membranous lining inside the sclera and contains many blood vessels which supply nutrients to the eye. This vascular layer is continuous with the **iris** (6) and the **ciliary body** (7) on the anterior surface of the eye.

The iris is the colored portion of the eye which surrounds the pupil. Two sets of iris muscles (circular and radial) respond to bright and dim light by contracting. The circular muscles constrict the pupil in bright light, and the radial muscles dilate the pupil in dim light, thereby regulating the amount of light admitted to the interior of the eyeball. The inset in Figure 17–2 shows the iris and its relationship to the pupil.

The ciliary body, on each side of the **lens** (8), contains ciliary muscles which can adjust the shape and thickness of the lens. These changes in the shape of the lens (which lies posterior to the iris) aid in the refraction (bending) of light rays. When objects are less than 20 feet away, the rays of light coming from them would tend to be focused improperly if only the cornea were to bend the light rays. The cornea's refractive powers are not adequate to properly focus the image directly on the sensitive receptor cells at the back of the eye. Therefore, the lens is constricted and thickened by the ciliary body and further refracts the rays of light so that the image is properly focused. This refractive power of the lens is called **accommodation**.

Besides regulating the shape of the lens, the ciliary body also secretes a fluid called **aqueous humor**, which flows through the **posterior chamber** (9) and **anterior chamber** (10) of the eye. The fluid is constantly produced and leaves the eye through veins which carry it into the bloodstream. Another cavity of the eye is called the **vitreous chamber** (11), which is a large region behind the lens filled with a soft jelly-like material, the **vitreous humor**. Vitreous humor is not constantly reformed and its escape from the eye can cause blindness. Both the aqueous and vitreous humors function to further refract light rays.

The **retina** (12) is the sensitive nerve layer of the eye. As light energy, in the form of waves, travels through the eye, it is refracted (by the cornea, lens, and fluids) so that it focuses on sensitive receptor cells of the retina called the **rods** and **cones**. There are approximately 6 million cones and 120 million rods in the retina. The cones are more sensitive in light than the rods, and sharpness of vision depends on the cone cells. Rods function better in dim light and are helpful in night vision.

Light energy, when focused on the retina, causes a chemical change in the rods and cones, initiating nerve impulses which then travel from the eye to the brain via the **optic nerve** (13). The region in the eye where the optic nerve meets the retina is called the **optic disk** (14). The **macula lutea** (15) is a yellow spot in the center of the retina which contains a pit, or depression, called the **fovea centralis** (16). This section of the retina, largely composed of cones, functions as the area of sharpest vision. Figure 17–3 shows the retina of a normal eye as seen through an ophthalmoscope.

Figure 17–4 illustrates the pathway of the light-stimulated nervous impulse from the sensitive cells of the retina to the visual region of the cerebral cortex in the brain. Label this figure as you read the following paragraph:

The rods and cones in the **retina** (A) synapse (meet) with neurons which lead to the **optic nerve fibers** (B). As the optic nerve fibers travel into the brain, the fibers located more medially cross in an area called the **optic chiasma** (C). Nerve fibers from the right half of each retina now form an **optic tract** (D), synapsing in the **thalamus** (E) of the brain and ending in the right visual region of the **cerebral cortex** (F). Similarly, fibers from the left half of each retina merge to form the optic tract and pass from the thalamus to the left region of the **cerebral cortex** (G).

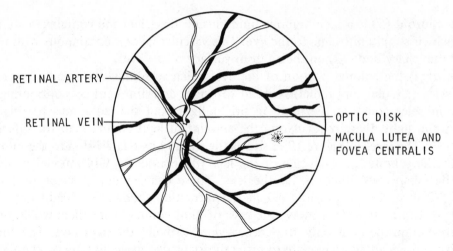

Figure 17-3   Retina of a normal eye seen through an ophthalmoscope.

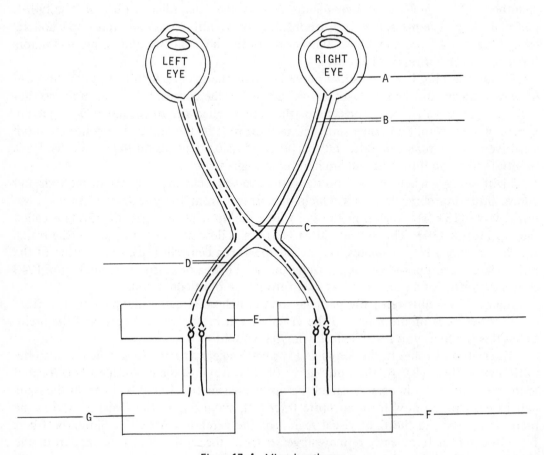

Figure 17-4   Visual pathway.

Study Figure 17–5, which summarizes the pathway of light rays from the conjunctival membrane to the inner visual region in the cerebral cortex of the brain.

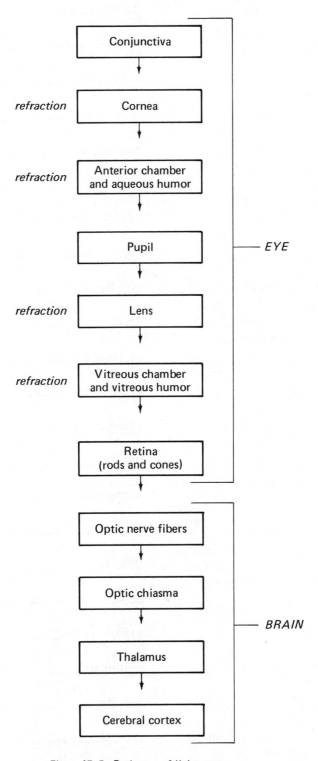

Figure 17–5 Pathway of light rays.

C. Combining Forms and Suffixes

Combining Form	Definition	Terminology	Meaning
ophthalm/o	eye	ophthalmoscope _____	
		ophthalmia _____	
ocul/o	eye	intraocular _____	
core/o cor/o	pupil	corectopia _____	
		anisocoria _____	
		coreometer _____	
		corectasis _____	
pupill/o	pupil	pupillary _____	
kerat/o	cornea, horny substance	keratitis _____	
		keratoplasty _____	
		keratomalacia _____	
corne/o	cornea	corneal dystrophy _____	
scler/o	sclera *(white of the eye)*	scleritis _____	
		scleromalacia _____	
ir/o irid/o	iris *(colored portion of the eye on either side of the pupil)*	iritis _____	
		iridectomy _____	
		iridoplegia _____	
		iridokeratitis _____	
retin/o	retina	retinopathy _____	
		retinitis _____	
cycl/o	ciliary body of the eye	cycloplegia _____	
		cyclitis _____	

uve/o	vascular layer of the eye *(the lens, ciliary body, and choroid)*	uveitis _____
lacrim/o	tear, tear duct, lacrimal duct	lacrimation _____ lacrimal _____ lacrimotomy _____
dacry/o	tear	dacryolith _____
dacryoaden/o	tear gland	dacryoadenectomy _____
dacryocyst/o	lacrimal sac, tear sac *(See Fig. 17–6 for illustration of the lacrimal sac, nasolacrimal duct, and lacrimal ducts)*	dacryocystitis _____ _____ dacryocystotome _____ _____ dacryocystorhinostomy _____ _____

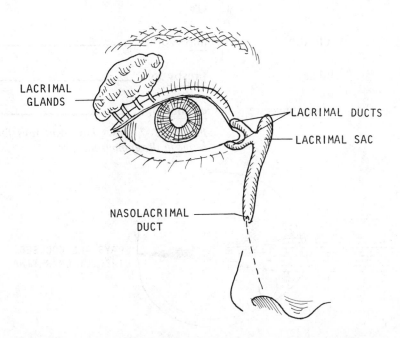

Figure 17–6   Lacrimal sac, nasolacrimal duct, and lacrimal ducts.

conjunctiv/o	conjunctiva	conjunctivitis _____
		subconjunctival _____
blephar/o	eyelid	blepharoptosis _____
		blepharospasm _____
		symblepharosis _____
aque/o	water	aqueous humor _____
vitre/o	glassy	vitreous humor _____
xer/o	dry	xerophthalmia _____
phot/o	light	photophobia _____
is/o	equal	anisocoria _____
mi/o	smaller, less	miotic _____
myc/o	fungus (immature plant)	keratomycosis _____
glauc/o	gray	glaucoma _____

From the dull gray-green gleam of the affected eye.

ambly/o	dull, dim	amblyopia _____
presby/o	old age	presbyopia _____
emmetr/o	in due measure	emmetropia _____

Figure 17–7 shows how light rays focus on the retina in the emmetropic eye.

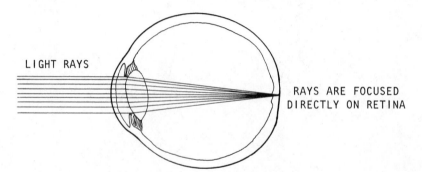

LIGHT RAYS

RAYS ARE FOCUSED
DIRECTLY ON RETINA

Figure 17–7 Emmetropia.

-opia	vision	diplopia _____
-tropia	to turn	esotropia _____

D. Errors of Refraction

myopia   Nearsightedness.

Figure 17–8 illustrates this condition which occurs when the eyeball is too long and light rays do not properly focus on the retina. The image perceived is blurred because the light rays are focused in front of the retina. Concave glasses (thicker at the periphery than in the middle) correct this condition because the lenses spread the rays out before they reach the cornea and thus they can be properly focused directly on the retina.

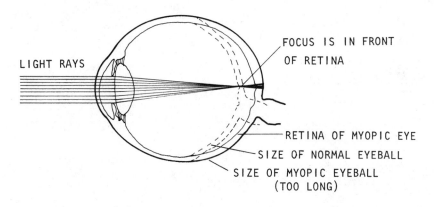

MYOPIC EYE

LIGHT RAYS

FOCUS IS IN FRONT
OF RETINA

RETINA OF MYOPIC EYE
SIZE OF NORMAL EYEBALL
SIZE OF MYOPIC EYEBALL
(TOO LONG)

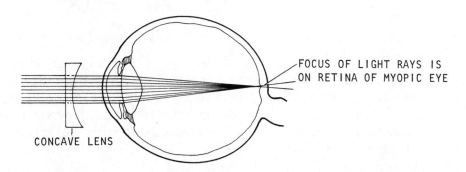

CORRECTION FOR MYOPIA

FOCUS OF LIGHT RAYS IS
ON RETINA OF MYOPIC EYE

CONCAVE LENS

Figure 17–8 Myopia and its correction.

hyperopia   Farsightedness.
   (hypermetropia)

      As Figure 17–9 illustrates, the eyeball in this condition is too short. Parallel rays of light tend to focus behind the retina, and this results in a blurred image. A convex lens (thicker in the middle than at the sides) bends the rays inward before they reach the cornea, and thus the rays can be focused properly.

HYPEROPIC EYE

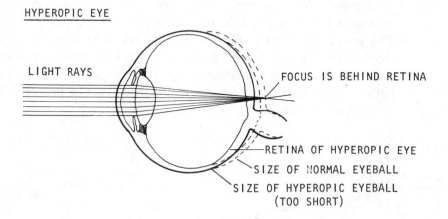

CORRECTION FOR HYPEROPIA

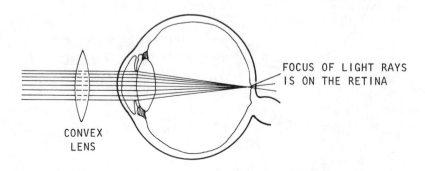

Figure 17–9 Hyperopia and its correction.

presbyopia   Impairment of vision due to old age.

      With increasing age, loss of elasticity of the ciliary body impairs its ability to adjust the lens for accommodation to near vision. The lens of the eye cannot become fat to bend the rays coming from near objects (less than 20 feet). The light rays focus behind the retina, as in hyperopia. Therefore, a convex lens is needed to refract the rays coming from objects closer than 20 feet.

astigmatism   Defective curvature of the cornea of the eye.

This problem results from one or more abnormal curvatures of the cornea. This causes light rays to be unevenly and not sharply focused on the retina so that the image is distorted. Lenses placed in the proper position in front of the eye correct this corneal problem.

E. Pathological Conditions

glaucoma

Increased intraocular pressure results in the lens becoming opaque (impenetrable by light).

In this disease condition, intraocular pressure in the anterior and posterior chambers is elevated because of inability of aqueous humor to leave the eye and enter the bloodstream. If it is not treated, blindness can result. Sometimes glaucoma is associated with such conditions as iridocyclitis, iritis, and certain neoplasms. Treatment with **miotics** (drugs which constrict the pupil so that aqueous humor can escape) or surgery to achieve drainage of the fluid may be effective.

cataract

Clouding of the lens, causing decreased vision.

The etiology of a cataract is unknown, but it is thought to be linked to the process of aging and heredity. There are many types of cataracts, all of which in one form or another involve loss of transparency of the lens. Vision appears blurred as the lens clouds over and becomes opaque. Surgical removal of the lens, and eyeglasses to help in refraction, constitute effective treatment for cataracts.

nystagmus

Rapidly jerking movement of the eye from side to side.

There are various forms of this condition, and many causes, including neurologic diseases, inner ear disorders, occupational hazards (working in darkness for long periods or constantly watching moving objects), and congenital disorders.

strabismus

Abnormal deviations of the eye.

This condition is also called **squint** or cross-eye. It is a failure of the eyes to "look" in the same direction because of weakness of a muscle controlling the position of one eye. It is usually correctable with surgery. Different forms of strabismus include **esotropia** (convergent squint), when the eyes turn inward toward each other, and **exotropia** (divergent squint), when the eyes turn outward (laterally) from each other.

macular degeneration

Deterioration of the macula lutea of the retina.

This condition may be inherited or drug-induced, and it leads to a severe loss of central vision. Peripheral vision (using the part of the retina outside the macular region) may be retained.

retinitis pigmentosa	Progressive retinal sclerosis, pigmentation, and atrophy.

The major characteristic of this condition is the deposition of pigmented scar on the retina. This is an inherited disease associated with decreased vision, especially night blindness (nyctalopia).

scotoma	Area of depressed vision surrounded by an area of normal vision.

A restricted area of loss of vision caused by damage to the retina or optic nerve; a "blind spot." Scot/o means darkness.

hemianopsia	Loss of one-half of the visual field (the space of vision of each eye).

This symptom is usually due to a stroke or damage to a portion of the optic nerve or its connecting fibers.

III. THE EAR

A. Vocabulary

auricle	The protruding part of the external ear, not contained within the head; the flap of the ear.
cerumen	Waxy substance secreted by the external ear; also called ear wax.
cochlea	A spirally wound (snail-shaped) tube in the inner ear; contains sensitive hearing receptor cells.
cilia	Hairlike processes on cells.
endolymph	Fluid contained in the inner ear.
eustachian tube	Canal leading from the middle ear to the pharynx (throat). It is also called the auditory (hearing) tube.
fenestration	Surgical creation of a window-like opening. Used to restore hearing by creating a new opening into the inner ear.
graft	A substitute or replacement for a damaged or missing part.

incus

The second conducting bone (ossicle) of the middle ear; also called the anvil.

labyrinth

The mazelike series of canals which compose the inner ear. The bony labyrinth contains the cochlea and organs of balance (equilibrium).

malleus

The first conducting ossicle of the middle ear; also called the hammer because of its characteristic shape.

meatus

Opening or canal. The auditory meatus is a canal leading from the external ear (auricle) to the middle ear.

organ of Corti

Found in the cochlea of the inner ear; contains sensitive auditory receptor cells.

ossicle

Small bone; used to describe the small bones of the middle ear (malleus, incus, and stapes).

oval window

Membrane between the middle and inner ears.

perilymph

Auditory fluid contained in the labyrinth of the inner ear.

pinna

The auricle, or flap of the ear.

prosthesis

To put or place before; an artificial part.

purulent

Pus-forming; suppurative.

saccule

An organ in the inner ear associated with maintaining balance and equilibrium; means "little bag."

semicircular canals

Passages in the inner ear associated with balance and equilibrium.

stapes

Third ossicle of the middle ear; stapes means "stirrup."

tympanic membrane

A membrane between the outer and middle ear; also called the eardrum.

utricle

A tiny, saclike structure in the inner ear which, along with the saccule and semicircular canals, is associated with the maintenance of balance and equilibrium.

B. Anatomy and Physiology

Sound waves are received by the outer ear, conducted to special receptor cells within the ear, and transmitted by those cells to nerve fibers which lead to the auditory region of the brain in the cerebral cortex. It is within the nerve fibers of the cerebral cortex that the sensations of sound are perceived.

Label Figure 17–10 as you read the following paragraphs describing the anatomy and physiology of the ear.

The ear can be divided into three separate regions—outer ear, middle ear, and inner ear. The outer and middle ears function in the conduction of sound waves through the ear, while the inner ear contains structures which receive the auditory waves and relay them to the brain.

Outer Ear

Sound waves enter the ear through the **pinna**, also called the **auricle** (1), which is the projecting part, or flap, of the ear. The **external auditory meatus (auditory canal)** (2) leads from the pinna and is lined with numerous glands which secrete a yellowish brown, waxy substance called **cerumen**. Cerumen lubricates and protects the ear.

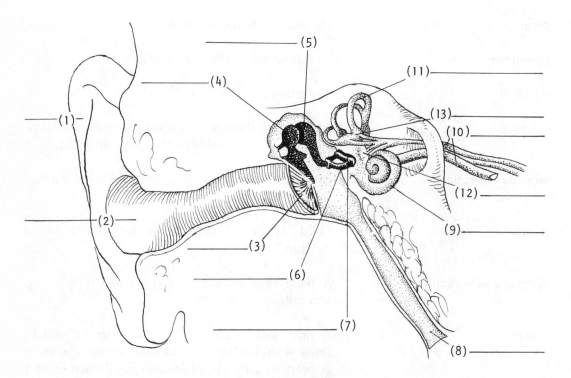

Figure 17–10 The ear.

Middle Ear

Sound waves travel through the auditory canal and strike a membrane between the outer and middle ear. This is the **tympanic membrane**, or **eardrum** (3). As the eardrum vibrates, it moves three small bones, or **ossicles**, which conduct the sound waves through the middle ear. These bones, in the order of their vibration, are the **malleus** (4), the **incus** (5), and the **stapes** (6). As the stapes moves, it touches a membrane called the **oval window** (7) which separates the middle from the inner ear.

Before proceeding with the pathway of sound conduction and reception into the inner ear, an additional structure which affects the middle ear should be mentioned. The **eustachian tube** (8) is a canal leading from the middle ear to the pharynx. It is normally closed but opens upon swallowing. In an efficient way, this tube can prevent damage to the eardrum and shock to the middle and inner ears. Normally the pressure of air in the middle ear is equal to the pressure of air in the external environment. However, if you ascend in the atmosphere, as in flying an airplane, climbing a high mountain, or riding a fast elevator, the atmospheric pressure, and that in the outer ear, will drop, while that in the middle ear remains the same—greater than that in the outer ear. This inequality of air pressure on the inside and outside of the eardrum forces the eardrum to bulge outward and eventually to burst. Swallowing will open the eustachian tube so that air can leave the middle ear and enter the throat until the atmospheric and middle ear pressures are balanced. The eardrum then relaxes and the danger of its bursting is averted.

Inner Ear

Sound vibrations, having been transmitted by the movement of the eardrum to the bones of the middle ear, reach the inner ear via the fluctuations of the oval window which separates the middle and inner ears. The inner ear is also called the **labyrinth** because of its circular, mazelike structure. The part of the labyrinth which leads from the oval window is a bony, snail-shaped structure called the **cochlea** (9). The cochlea contains special auditory liquids called **perilymph** and **endolymph** through which the vibrations travel. Also present in the cochlea is a sensitive auditory receptor called the **organ of Corti**. In the organ of Corti, tiny hair cells called **cilia** receive vibrations from the auditory liquids and relay the sound waves to **auditory nerve fibers** (10) which end in the auditory center of the cerebral cortex, where these impulses are interpreted and "heard."

Study Figure 17–11, which is a schematic representation of the pathway of sound vibrations from the outer ear to the brain.

The ear is an important organ of equilibrium (balance), as well as an organ for hearing. Within the inner ear are three organs responsible for equilibrium. Refer back to Figure 17–10 and label these three organs: **semicircular canals** (11), **utricle** (12), and **saccule** (13). These organs contain the fluid called endolymph, as well as sensitive hair cells. In an intricate manner, the fluid and hair cells fluctuate in response to the movements of the head. This sets up impulses in nerve fibers which lead to the brain. Messages are then sent to muscles in all parts of the body to assure that equilibrium is maintained.

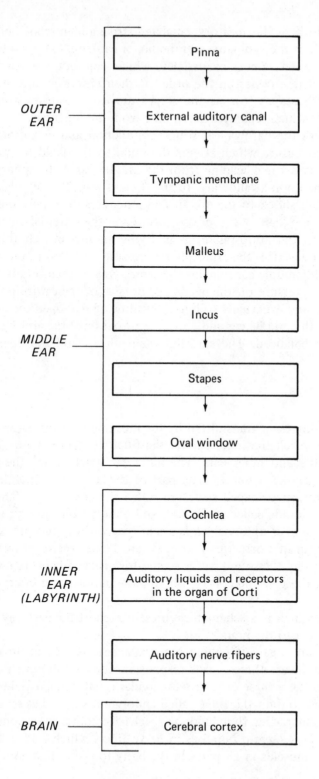

Figure 17–11 Pathway of sound vibrations.

C. Combining Forms and Suffixes

Combining Form	Definition	Terminology	Meaning
audi/o	hearing	audiometer _____	
		audiogram _____	
acou/o	hearing	acoustic _____	
ot/o	ear	otitis media _____	
		otoscope _____	
		otorrhea _____	
aur/o aur/i	ear	aural discharge _____	
		auricle _____	
cerumin/o	cerumen *(wax in the outer ear)*	ceruminal _____	
staped/o	stapes *(3rd ossicle of the middle ear)*	stapedial _____	
		stapedectomy _____	
		Prosthesis is used to connect incus and oval window.	
myring/o	eardrum	myringoplasty _____	
		myringotomy _____	
tympan/o	eardrum, middle ear	tympanic _____	
		tympanoplasty _____	
salping/o *(in gynecological context, this term refers to the fallopian tubes)*	eustachian tube	salpingoscope _____	
		salpingopharyngeal _____	
		_____	

mastoid/o	mastoid process *(posterior portion of the temporal bone of the skull which extends downward behind the external auditory meatus)*	mastoidectomy _____
-emphraxis	obstruction, blockage	salpingoemphraxis _____ _____
-cusis	hearing	presbycusis _____
-phonia	sound	dysphonia _____

D. Pathological Conditions

macrotia Abnormal enlargement of the pinnae.

microtia Abnormally small pinnae.

Surgery can be performed to correct both of these congenital anomalies.

suppurative otitis media Bacterial infection of the middle ear.

Staphylococcus, streptococcus, or pneumococcus can be the infecting organism. Antibiotics are an excellent treatment. Surgical evacuation of the purulent (pus) material through the tympanic membrane will prevent hearing loss and mastoiditis. This procedure is called a myringotomy.

otosclerosis Hardening of the bony tissue of the labyrinth.

This condition is a bone disease of the labyrinth. Spongy bone forms around the oval window and may lead to the fixation or ankylosis (stiffening) of the stapes bone. This causes hearing loss and progressive deafness. Treatment is surgical. Stapedectomy with replacement by a tissue graft (fatty tissue from the ear lobe) and a prosthesis (stainless steel wire) is effective in overcoming deafness. In order to do this operation, the oval window must be **fenestrated** (opened) so that the otosclerotic areas of the stapes can be removed.

presbycusis Hearing loss occurring with old age.

This is the most common form of nerve deafness. It is usually the result of the physiological process of aging.

Deafness is also commonly caused as a result of an infectious illness such as mumps. Total irreversible unilateral loss of hearing may occur.

vertigo
Sensation of irregular or whirling motion either of oneself or of external objects.

Vertigo is dizziness often associated with nausea, and is due to a severe disturbance of the equilibrium organs in the labyrinth. The etiology is varied. It is most commonly caused by a viral illness. Cerebral concussion (brain injury), toxicity due to use of certain drugs, and syphilis (a contagious venereal disease) are other conditions leading to vertigo, and in some cases deafness.

tinnitus
Ringing sound in the ears.

The cause and mechanism of this auditory symptom are unknown. It may be associated with chronic otitis, myringitis, or labyrinthitis, as well as other disorders.

Meniere's syndrome
Vertigo, nausea, vomiting, and tinnitus, leading to progressive deafness.

This syndrome is caused by rapid, violent firing of the fibers of the auditory nerves and brings on attacks of vertigo. Nausea, vomiting, tinnitus, and unilateral deafness are symptoms. If degeneration of the organ of Corti occurs, progressive deafness is the result. Treatment is bed rest and administration of drugs to dilate blood vessels and reduce spasm of vessels in the ear.

acoustic neuroma
Malignant tumor arising from the acoustic nerve in the brain.

This tumor causes tinnitus, vertigo, and decreased hearing as its initial symptoms.

IV. EXERCISES

A. *Match the structure in the eye with its description:*

1. pupil

2. conjunctiva

3. cornea

4. sclera

5. choroid

6. iris

7. ciliary body

8. lens

9. retina

10. vitreous humor

_____ Contains sensitive cells called rods and cones which transmit light energy to nerve fibers.

_____ Muscles which control the shape of the lens.

_____ Transparent body which lies behind the iris and in front of the vitreous humor; it refracts light rays onto the retina.

_____ Jelly-like material behind the lens which helps to maintain the shape of the eyeball.

_____ Dark center of the eye through which light rays enter the eye.

_____ Vascular layer of the eyeball which is continuous with the iris.

_____ Mucous membrane over the outside of the eye and under the eyelid.

_____ Transparent fibrous membrane which refracts light.

_____ Colored portion of the eye; surrounds the pupil.

_____ White of the eye; fibrous supportive tissue.

B. *Build medical terms:*

1. Incision of a muscle of the eye _____

2. Paralysis of the eye (muscles) _____

3. Unequal (size of) pupils _____

4. Abnormal fungus condition of the eye _____

5. Softening of the cornea _____

6. Inflammation of the ciliary body _____

7. Incision into a tear duct _____

8. Instrument to visually examine the eye _____

9. Condition of disease of the retina _____

10. Prolapse of the eyelid _____

C. *Give the meaning of the following medical terms:*

1. macula lutea _____

2. refraction _____

3. accommodation _____

4. rods and cones _____

5. optic chiasma _____

6. intraocular _____

7. scleral icterus _____

8. uveitis _____

9. xerophthalmia _____

10. iridokeratitis _____

11. diplopia _____

12. miotic _____

13. coreometer _____

14. lacrimal _____

15. corneal dystrophy _____

16. conjunctivitis _____

17. photophobia _____

18. emmetropia _____

19. biconvex _____

20. biconcave _____

D. *Match the medical term for the eye disorder with its proper definition:*

1. nystagmus   _____   Any abnormal deviation of the eye; squint.

2. amblyopia   _____   Nearsightedness; eyeball is too long.

3. cataract   _____   Turning inward of eye.

4. hyperopia   _____   Defective vision or blindness in half of the
                                    visual field.
5. esotropic
                       _____   Abnormal curvature of the cornea, leading
6. myopic   to blurred vision.

7. presbyopia   _____   Lens clouds over with opaque film and
                                    vision is impaired.
8. exotropia
                       _____   Blockage of circulation of aqueous humor
9. astigmatism   leads to increased intraocular pressure.

10. glaucoma   _____   Quick, jerky movement of the eye from
                                    side to side.
11. macular degeneration
                       _____   Farsightedness; eyeball is too short.
12. retinitis pigmentosa
                       _____   Dull, dim vision.
13. strabismus
                       _____   Tendency of the eye to turn outward.
14. scotoma
                       _____   Defect of vision of old age due to loss of
15. hemianopsia   elasticity of the lens.

                       _____   Blind spot; area of depressed vision sur-
                                    rounded by an area of less depressed or
                                    normal vision.

                       _____   Progressive sclerosis; pigmentation and
                                    atrophy of the inner lining of the eye.

                       _____   Deterioration of the macula lutea of the
                                    retina.

E. Explain the difference between concave and convex lenses and how they can correct refraction for conditions such as hyperopia and myopia:

_____

_____

_____

_____

_____

_____

F. Arrange the following terms in the correct order to indicate their sequence in the transmission of sound waves to the brain from the outer ear:

incus, tympanic membrane, pinna, cochlea, malleus, oval window,

external auditory canal, auditory liquids and receptors, stapes,

auditory nerve fibers, cerebral cortex

1. _____   7. _____

2. _____   8. _____

3. _____   9. _____

4. _____   10. _____

5. _____   11. _____

6. _____

G. Give the meaning of the following medical terms:

1. labyrinth _____

2. semicircular canals _____

3. eustachian tube _____

4. stapes _____

5. organ of Corti _____

6. perilymph and endolymph _____

7. cerumen _____

8. utricle _____

_____

9. oval window _____

10. tympanic membrane _____

H. *Build medical terms:*

1. Instrument to examine the ear _____

2. Removal of the third bone of middle ear _____

3. Pertaining to the eustachian tube and throat _____

4. Flow of pus from the ear _____

5. Instrument to measure hearing _____

6. Incision of the eardrum _____

7. Surgical repair of the eardrum _____

8. Deafness due to old age _____

9. Small ear _____

10. Inflammation of the middle ear _____

I. *Give the meaning of the following medical terms:*

1. vertigo _____

2. Meniere's syndrome _____

3. otosclerosis _____

4. tinnitus _____

5. labyrinthitis _____

6. salpingoemphraxis _____

7. ankylosis _____

8. acoustic neuroma _____

ANSWERS

A. 9
7
8
10
1
5
2
3
6
4

B.
1. ophthalmomyotomy
2. ophthalmoplegia
3. anisocoria
4. ophthalmomycosis
5. keratomalacia

6. cyclitis
7. lacrimotomy
8. ophthalmoscope
9. retinopathy
10. blepharoptosis

C.
1. Yellow spot in the retina which contains the fovea centralis (area of clearest vision).
2. The bending of light rays by the cornea, lens, and fluids of the eye.
3. The adjustment which the lens of the eye normally makes to bring an object into focus on the retina.
4. Photosensitive cells of the retina.
5. The crossing point of the fibers of the optic nerve in the brain.
6. Within the eye.
7. Abnormal yellow coloration of the white of the eye.
8. Inflammation of the vascular layer of the eyeball (the choroid and iris).
9. Condition of dryness of the eye.
10. Inflammation of the iris and the cornea.
11. Double vision.
12. An agent that causes the pupil to contract.
13. Instrument to measure the pupil.
14. Pertaining to tears.
15. Poor development of the cornea.
16. Inflammation of the conjunctiva.
17. Fear of light.
18. Condition of normal vision ("in proper measure").
19. Having two convex (rounded, elevated) surfaces.
20. Having two concave (rounded, depressed) surfaces.

D. 13
6
5
15
9
3
10
1
4
2
8
7
14
12
11

E. A concave lens has a depressed or hollowed-out central region, while a convex lens is curved evenly and resembles a sphere by bulging outward. Hyperopia is farsightedness due to shortness of the eyeball, which causes the images to be refracted behind the retina. Convex lenses when placed in front of the eye will bend or refract the rays inward so they focus more nearly in the retina. Myopia is nearsightedness and results when the eyeball is too long, causing the image to be focused in front of the retina. Concave lenses in front of the eye will help to spread the rays so that they can be properly focused on the retina.

F. 1. pinna
2. external auditory canal
3. tympanic membrane
4. malleus
5. incus
6. stapes

7. oval window
8. cochlea
9. auditory liquids and receptors
10. auditory nerve fibers
11. cerebral cortex

G. 1. Cochlea and organs of equilibrium (semicircular canals, saccule, and utricle).
2. Organ of equilibrium in the inner ear.
3. Passageway between the middle ear and the throat.
4. Third ossicle (little bone) of the middle ear.
5. Region in the cochlea which contains auditory receptors.
6. Auditory fluids circulating within the inner ear.
7. Wax in the external auditory meatus.
8. Tiny sac in the inner ear associated with the semicircular canals and important in maintaining equilibrium and balance.
9. Delicate membrane between the middle and inner ears.
10. Eardrum.

H. 1. otoscope
2. stapedectomy
3. salpingopharyngeal
4. otopyorrhea

5. audiometer
6. myringotomy (tympanotomy)
7. tympanoplasty (myringoplasty)

8. presbycusis
9. microtia
10. otitis media

I. 1. Sensation of irregular or whirling motion either of oneself or of external objects.
2. Syndrome consisting of vertigo, nausea, vomiting, and ringing in the ears, leading to progressive deafness.
3. Abnormal condition of hardening of the bony structure of the inner ear.
4. Ringing sensation in the ears.
5. Inflammation of the labyrinth of the inner ear.
6. Obstruction of the eustachian tube.
7. Stiffness or immobility between bones.
8. Malignant tumor arising from the acoustic nerve in the brain.

REVIEW SHEET 17

Combining Forms

acou/o	_____	kerat/o	_____
ambly/o	_____	lacrim/o	_____
aque/o	_____	mastoid/o	_____
audi/o	_____	mi/o	_____
aur/o	_____	myc/o	_____
auri/o	_____	myring/o	_____
blephar/o	_____	ocul/o	_____
cerumin/o	_____	ophthalm/o	_____
conjunctiv/o	_____	ot/o	_____
cor/o	_____	phot/o	_____
core/o	_____	presby/o	_____
corne/o	_____	pupill/o	_____
cycl/o	_____	retin/o	_____
dacry/o	_____	salping/o	_____
dacryoaden/o	_____	scler/o	_____
dacryocyst/o	_____	staped/o	_____
emmetr/o	_____	tympan/o	_____
glauc/o	_____	uve/o	_____
ir/o	_____	vitre/o	_____
irid/o	_____	xer/o	_____
is/o	_____		

Suffixes

-cusis _____   -phonia _____

-emphraxis _____   -tropia _____

-opia _____

Additional Terms Relating to the Eye

accommodation _____

aqueous humor _____

astigmatism _____

biconcave lens _____

biconvex lens _____

cataract _____

choroid layer _____

ciliary body _____

cones _____

conjunctiva _____

cornea _____

esotropia _____

exotropia _____

fovea centralis _____

glaucoma _____

hemianopsia _____

hyperopia _____

iris _____

lens of the eye _____

macula lutea _____

macular degeneration _____

miotics _____

myopia _____

nystagmus _____

optic chiasma _____

optic disk _____

presbyopia _____

pupil _____

receptor _____

refraction _____

retina _____

retinitis pigmentosa _____

rods _____

sclera _____

scotoma _____

strabismus _____

vitreous humor _____

Additional Terms Relating to the Ear

acoustic neuroma _____

auditory meatus (canal) _____

auricle _____

cerumen _____

cochlea _____

cilia _____

endolymph _____

eustachian tube _____

fenestration _____

graft _____

incus _____

labyrinth _____

macrotia _____

malleus _____

microtia _____

organ of Corti _____

ossicle _____

otosclerosis _____

oval window _____

perilymph _____

pinna _____

presbycusis _____

prosthesis _____

purulent _____

saccule _____

semicircular canals _____

stapes _____

suppurative otitis media _____

tinnitus _____

tympanic membrane _____

utricle _____

vertigo _____

CHAPTER 18

THE ENDOCRINE SYSTEM

In this chapter you will:

Learn the names of the endocrine glands and their hormones;

Understand the functions of the various hormones and how they affect the body;

Analyze medical terms related to the endocrine glands and their hormones; and

Learn the terms which describe the pathological conditions resulting from excessive and deficient secretions of the endocrine glands.

This chapter is divided into the following sections:

I. INTRODUCTION

The endocrine system is composed of **glands** located in many different regions of the body, all of which release specific chemical substances directly into the bloodstream. These chemical substances, called **hormones,** can regulate the many and varied functions of an organism. For example, one hormone stimulates the growth of bones, another causes the maturation of sex organs and reproductive cells, and another controls the metabolic rate (metabolism) within all the individual cells of the body. In addition, one powerful endocrine gland in the brain secretes a wide variety of different hormones which travel through the bloodstream and regulate the activities of other endocrine glands.

All the **endocrine** glands, no matter which hormones they produce, secrete their hormones directly into the bloodstream rather than into ducts leading to the exterior of the body. Those glands which send their chemical substances into ducts and out of the body are called **exocrine** glands. Examples of exocrine glands are sweat, mammary, mucous, salivary, and lacrimal (tear) glands.

The ductless, internally secreting **endocrine glands** are listed below. Locate these glands on Figure 18–1.

(1) thyroid gland

(2) parathyroid glands (four glands)

(3) adrenal glands (one pair)

(4) pancreas

(5) pituitary gland

(6) ovaries in female (one pair)

(7) testes in male (one pair)

(8) pineal gland

(9) thymus gland

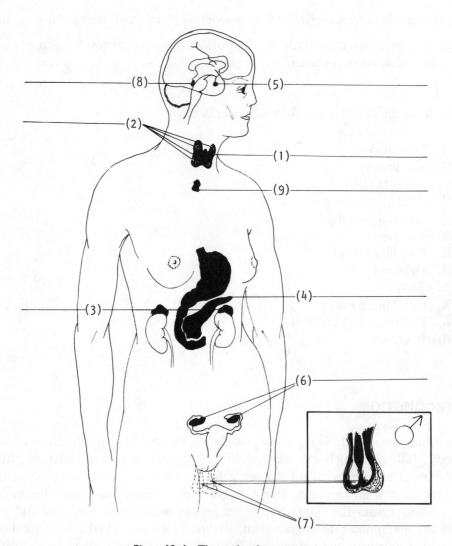

Figure 18–1   The endocrine system.

The last two glands on this list, the pineal and thymus glands, are included as endocrine glands because they are ductless, although little is known about their endocrine function in the human body. The pineal gland, located in the central portion of the brain, is believed to secrete a substance called **melatonin**. Melatonin contributes to the process of skin pigmentation. The pineal is also known to regulate the estrus (reproductive) cycle in lower animals. The thymus gland, located behind the sternum and extending into the neck, is large in childhood but shrinks in size in adults. Its structure, although ductless, resembles a lymph gland (contains lymphatic tissue and antibody-producing lymphocytes), and it is thought that the thymus might play a role in the immune process (antibody-antigen reactions) in the body. Although the exact functions of the thymus are not known, it may also be involved in various disease processes; for example, removal of the thymus gland is found to be helpful in treating a muscular-neurological disorder called myasthenia gravis.

II. VOCABULARY

adrenocorticotropic hormone (ACTH)	Hormone secreted by the anterior lobe of the pituitary gland in the brain. ACTH stimulates the outer section of the adrenal glands to secrete hormones.
adenohypophysis	Anterior lobe of the pituitary gland (endocrine gland at the base of the brain). It is derived from the pharynx, or throat, during development of the embryo.
adrenal cortex	The outer section of the adrenal gland. This region of the gland secretes three different types of hormones, called glucocorticoids, mineralocorticoids, and androgens.
adrenal medulla	The inner section of the adrenal gland. This region produces two hormones called epinephrine (adrenaline) and norepinephrine (noradrenaline).
adrenaline	Epinephine.
aldosterone	Hormone secreted by the adrenal cortex; stimulates the kidney tubules to retain salts in the body.
androgens	Male hormones secreted primarily by the testes, and to a lesser extent by the adrenal cortex. Androgens stimulate the development of male secondary sex characteristics.

antidiuretic hormone (ADH)	Hormone secreted by the posterior lobe of the pituitary gland. ADH stimulates the kidney tubules to retain water in the body, and constricts arterioles to increase blood pressure; it is also called vasopressin.
catecholamines	Complex substances derived from an amino acid. Catecholamines have actions resembling sympathetic nervous impulses. They cause stimulation of blood pressure, metabolic rate, and heart rate. Examples of catecholamine substances are the hormones epinephrine and norepinephrine.
cortisol	One of the hormones secreted by the adrenal cortex. Cortisol (also called hydrocortisone) regulates the proper metabolism of sugars, fats, and proteins in cells.
cortisone	A substance derived from cortisol which has identical action. Cortisone is useful in treating inflammatory conditions in the body.
endocrine glands	Ductless glands which secrete substances (hormones) directly into the bloodstream.
epinephrine	Hormone produced by the adrenal medulla. Its action mimics the responses of the sympathetic nervous system, producing tachycardia, bronchodilation, hypertension, and so forth. Epinephrine is also called adrenaline.
estrogen	A female hormone secreted by the ovaries. Estrogen causes the development of female sex characteristics and proliferation of the lining of the uterus.
exocrine glands	Glands which secrete substances through ducts to body surfaces or into tubes and cavities. Examples are mammary, lacrimal, salivary, mucous, and sweat glands.
fasting blood sugar (FBS)	Determination of amount of sugar in the bloodstream after patient has fasted for several hours.
follicle-stimulating hormone (FSH)	This hormone is secreted by the anterior pituitary gland (adenohypophysis). It stimulates the development of the egg in the ovary and the production of the hormone estrogen.

glucagon	Hormone produced by cells in the pancreas called the islets of Langerhans. Glucagon stimulates an increase of glucose in the bloodstream by releasing sugar from glycogen (a starch storage substance) in the liver.
glucocorticoids	Group of hormones secreted by the adrenal cortex; cortisol is an example. These hormones stimulate the production of glucose in the liver.
glucose tolerance test (GTT)	Test which measures the ability of a patient to utilize glucose in the body. A GTT is used to detect pathological conditions such as diabetes mellitus, hypoglycemia, and liver and adrenal cortex dysfunctions.
gonadotropic hormones	These hormones are secreted by the adenohypophysis, and they stimulate the development and functioning of the gonads, which are the testes in the male and the ovaries in the female.
homeostasis	A tendency in an organism to return to stability or a uniform state.
hormones	Chemical substances originating in a ductless gland and conveyed through the bloodstream to another part of the body.
hydrocortisone	Cortisol; a glucocorticoid hormone secreted by the adrenal cortex.
hypophysis	An endocrine gland at the base of the brain. It is composed of two lobes, an anterior lobe (adenohypophysis) and a posterior lobe (neurohypophysis). The hypophysis is also called the pituitary gland.
hypothalamus	Region of the brain which lies in close proximity to the hypophysis. It is believed to stimulate the hypophysis to secrete its hormones.
insulin	Hormone secreted by cells in the pancreas called the islets of Langerhans. Insulin is essential for the proper uptake and metabolism of sugar in cells.
iodine	A chemical element which composes a large part of the hormone produced by the thyroid gland.

islets of Langerhans

Endocrine cells of the pancreas. These cells produce hormones called insulin and glucagon.

isthmus

A narrow strip of tissue connecting two parts. The isthmus of the thyroid gland is a narrow band joining the lobes of the gland.

luteinizing hormone (LH)

This gonadotropic hormone is produced by the anterior lobe of the pituitary gland. It stimulates the development and maintenance of the corpus luteum within the ovary. The corpus luteum secretes progesterone, a hormone which is important in sustaining pregnancy.

melatonin

A hormone secreted by the pineal gland; its body function is unknown, but it is believed to have some effect on skin pigmentation and ovarian function.

mineralocorticoids

Salt-retaining hormones secreted by the adrenal cortex. Aldosterone is an example.

neurohypophysis

Posterior lobe of the pituitary gland. It is derived from nerve tissue.

norepinephrine

Hormone secreted by the adrenal medulla. Its action is similar to that of epinephrine but mainly centers on vasoconstriction (narrowing of blood vessels). It is also called noradrenaline.

oxytocin

This hormone is secreted by the neurohypophysis (posterior lobe of the pituitary gland). Oxytocin stimulates the uterus to contract during labor.

parathyroid hormone (PTH)

Hormone which is secreted by the parathyroid glands (four small glands near the thyroid glands). Parathyroid hormone regulates the amount of calcium in the blood and bones.

pineal gland

Endocrine gland located in the middle of the brain. It secretes a hormone called melatonin, which is believed to affect skin pigmentation and regulate the estrus cycle in lower animals.

pituitary growth hormone (GH)

Hormone secreted by the adenohypophysis. It stimulates the growth of long bones in the body. Pituitary growth hormone is also called somatotropin.

progesterone	A female hormone secreted by the ovaries. Progesterone is important in sustaining the uterine lining during pregnancy.
prolactin (LTH)	Hormone secreted by the adenohypophysis. Prolactin stimulates the secretion of milk from the mammary glands.
somatotropin	Pituitary growth hormone.
steroids	Complex molecules containing carbon atoms in ring structure. Cholesterol is the main building block of steroids.
suprarenal glands	Adrenal glands; endocrine organs, one situated on top of each kidney.
sympathomimetic	Producing effects similar to that produced by the sympathetic nervous system.
testosterone	The major type of androgen (male hormone) secreted by the testes. Testosterone stimulates the development of male secondary sex characteristics.
tetany	Continuous contraction of muscles; associated with low levels of parathyroid hormone.
thymus gland	Ductless gland located in the mediastinum. The thymus has the internal structure of a lymph gland and may play a role in the body's immune response.
thyroid-stimulating hormone (TSH)	Hormone secreted by the adenohypophysis. TSH stimulates the thyroid gland to secrete thyroxine.
thyroxine	Hormone secreted by the thyroid gland. Thyroxine increases the general rate of metabolism within the cells of the body.
vasopressin	Antidiuretic hormone.

III. THYROID GLAND

A. Location and Structure

Label Figure 18–2:

The thyroid gland is composed of a **right** and **left lobe** (1) on either side of the **trachea** (2), just below a large piece of cartilage called the **thyroid cartilage** (3). The **isthmus** (4) of the thyroid gland is a narrow strip of glandular tissue which connects the two lobes on the ventral surface of the trachea.

B. Function

The hormone secreted by the thyroid gland is called **thyroxine**. Thyroxine is synthesized in the thyroid gland from **iodine**, which is picked up from the bloodstream circulating through the gland, and from an amino acid called tyrosine.

Thyroxine is necessary in the body to maintain a normal level of metabolism in all body cells. Cells need oxygen to carry on metabolic processes, one aspect of which is the burning of food to release the energy stored within the food. Thyroxine aids cells in their uptake of oxygen and thus supports the metabolic rate in the body. Injections of thyroxine will raise the metabolic rate, while removal of the thyroid gland, diminishing thyroxine content in the body, will result in a lower metabolic rate, heat loss, and poor physical and mental development.

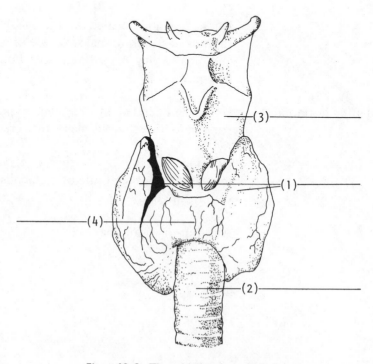

Figure 18–2 Thyroid gland, ventral view.

A radioactive iodine substance is used to trace the ability of the thyroid gland to make thyroxine. This form of iodine which gives off radioactive rays is traced as it passes to the thyroid gland through the bloodstream.

IV. PARATHYROID GLANDS

A. Location and Structure

Label Figure 18–3:
The **parathyroid glands** are four small oval bodies (1) located on the dorsal aspect of the **thyroid gland** (2).

B. Function

Parathyroid hormone (PTH) is secreted by the parathyroid glands. This hormone regulates the amount of calcium in the blood in a homeostatic manner (**homeostasis** refers to a state of equilibrium or constancy in the internal environment of the body). Low levels of calcium in the blood stimulate the parathyroid glands to secrete parathyroid hormone. The hormone causes calcium to leave bone tissue and enter the bloodstream, thereby restoring blood calcium levels to normal. In a similar manner, homeostasis is reached when high concentrations of calcium in the blood cause the parathyroid to turn off its secretion of hormone. Calcium then remains in bones and does not enter the bloodstream, where the level is already too high.

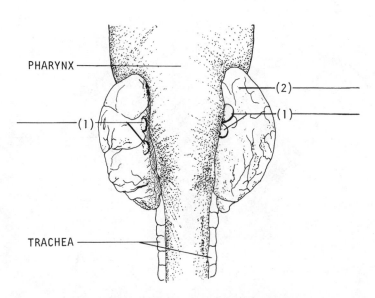

Figure 18-3 Parathyroid glands, dorsal view.

Calcium is important in bone formation, blood coagulation, and the maintenance of normal neuromuscular functioning. Excesses of parathyroid hormone, which pulls calcium out of bones, can then lead to softening or weakening of bones, fractures, and deformity, as well as formation of calcium stones in the urinary tract. Deficiency of parathyroid hormone, which leads to low levels of calcium in the blood, is associated with muscular excitability, spasms, and twitching. This condition of continuous muscle contraction is known as **tetany**.

V. ADRENAL GLANDS

A. Location and Structure

Label Figure 18–4:

The adrenal glands, also called the **suprarenal glands**, are two small glands situated one on top of each **kidney** (1). Each gland consists of two parts, an outer portion called the **adrenal cortex** (2) and an inner portion called the **adrenal medulla** (3). The cortex and medulla are two glands in one, each secreting its own different endocrine hormones. The cortex secretes hormones called **steroids** (complex chemicals derived from cholesterol), and the medulla secretes hormones called **catecholamines** (chemicals derived from an amino acid).

B. Function

The adrenal cortex secretes three types of steroid hormones:

1. **Mineralocorticoids** – These hormones are essential to life because they regulate the amount of mineral salts (also called **electrolytes**) which are retained in the

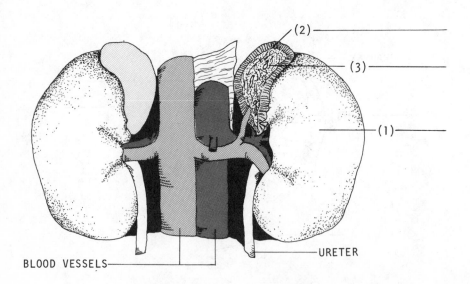

Figure 18–4 The adrenal glands.

body. A proper balance of water and salts in the blood and tissues is essential to the normal functioning of the body.

The most important mineralocorticoid hormone is called **aldosterone**. The secretion of aldosterone by the adrenal cortex increases the reabsorption of sodium (a mineral electrolyte commonly found in salts) by the kidney tubules. At the same time, aldosterone stimulates the excretion of another electrolyte called potassium.

The secretion of aldosterone increases manyfold in the face of a severe sodium-restricted diet, thereby enabling the body to hold needed salt in the bloodstream.

2. **Glucocorticoids** – These hormones have an important influence on the metabolism of sugars, fats, and proteins within all body cells.

Cortisol (also called **hydrocortisone**) is the most important glucocorticoid hormone. Cortisol increases the ability of cells to make new sugars out of fats and proteins (gluconeogenesis) and regulates the quantity of sugars, fats, and proteins in the blood and cells.

Cortisone is a hormone very similar to cortisol which can be prepared synthetically. Cortisone is useful in treating inflammatory ailments such as rheumatoid arthritis.

3. **Androgens, Estrogens, and Progestins** – These are male and female hormones which maintain the secondary sex characteristics, such as beard and breast development, and are necessary for reproduction. Most of these hormones are also produced in the ovaries and testes. Excess adrenal androgen secretion in females leads to virilism, and excess adrenal estrogen and progestin secretion in males produces abnormal feminine characteristics.

The adrenal medulla secretes two types of catecholamine hormones:

1. **Epinephrine (adrenaline)** – This hormone increases cardiac activity, dilates bronchial tubes, and stimulates the production of glucose from a storage substance called glycogen when glucose is needed by the body.

2. **Norepinephrine (noradrenaline)** – This hormone constricts vessels and raises blood pressure.

Both epinephrine and norepinephrine are called **sympathomimetic** agents because they mimic, or copy, the actions of the sympathetic nervous system. During times of stress, these hormones are secreted by the adrenal medulla in response to nervous stimulation. They help the body respond to crisis situations by raising blood pressure, increasing heartbeat and respiration, and bringing sugar out of storage in the cells.

VI. PANCREAS

A. Location and Structure

Label Figure 18–5:

The **pancreas** (1) is an endocrine gland located behind the **stomach** (2) in the region of the 1st and 2nd lumbar **vertebrae** (3). The specialized cells in the pancreas which produce hormones are called the **islets of Langerhans**.

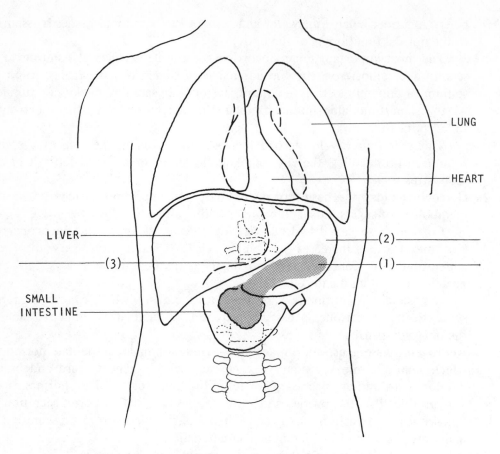

Figure 18-5   The pancreas.

B.   Function

The islets of Langerhans produce two hormones called **insulin** and **glucagon**. Both of these hormones play a role in the proper metabolism of sugars and starches in the body. Insulin is necessary in the bloodstream so that sugars can pass from the blood into the cells of the body where they are burned to release energy. Glucagon stimulates the breakdown in the liver of a glucose storage substance called glycogen. When glycogen is broken down (glycogenolysis), glucose is released by the liver cells, thereby causing an increase in blood sugar.

A **glucose tolerance test (GTT)** measures the way sugars are handled by the body. The test involves intravenous or oral administration of a measured amount of glucose and then a test of blood and urine sugar levels to see how quickly the body disposes of sugar. **Fasting blood sugar (FBS)** level refers to the amount of sugar in the blood after the patient has fasted for several hours.

VII. PITUITARY GLAND

A. Location and Structure

Label Figure 18–6:

The pituitary gland, also called the **hypophysis**, is a small, pea-sized gland located at the base of the brain and composed of two distinct lobes. The anterior lobe is known as the **adenohypophysis** (1) and is composed of glandular tissue which is an outgrowth of the throat during the development of the embryo. The posterior lobe is called the **neurohypophysis** (2) and is derived from nerve tissue of the brain during the development of the embryo. The **hypothalamus** (3) is a region of the brain which is in close proximity to the pituitary gland. It is believed that special hormones from the hypothalamus control the many secretory activities of the pituitary gland.

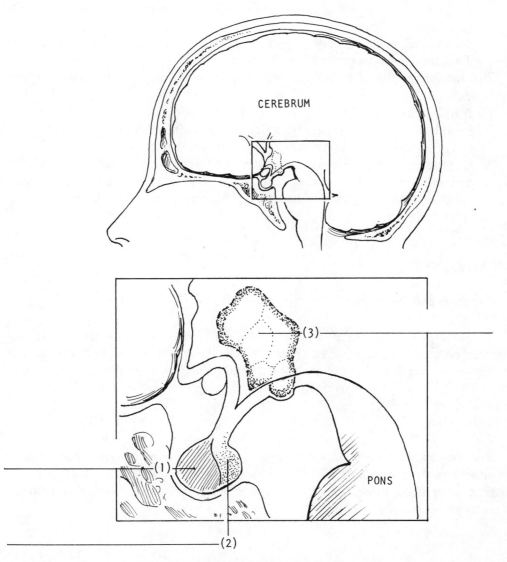

Figure 18–6 Pituitary gland.

B. Function

The hormones of the **adenohypophysis** are:
1. **Pituitary growth hormone (GH**; also called **somatotropin, STH)** — This hormone acts on bone tissue to accelerate its growth in the body.
2. **Thyroid-stimulating hormone (TSH)** — This hormone stimulates the growth of the thyroid gland and its secretion of thyroxine.
3. **Adrenocorticotropic hormone (ACTH)** — This hormone stimulates the growth of the adrenal cortex and increases its secretion of steroid hormones (primarily cortisol).
4. **Gonadotropic hormones** — There are several gonadotropic hormones which influence the growth and hormone secretion of the ovaries in females and testes in males. In the female, **follicle-stimulating hormone (FSH)** stimulates the growth of eggs in the ovaries; **luteinizing hormone (LH)** induces the secretion of progesterone (pregnancy-sustaining hormone) from the ovaries; and **prolactin (LTH)** promotes the growth of breast tissue and maintains lactation (production of milk).

   In the male, gonadotropins from the adenohypophysis influence the development of spermatozoa and testes.

The **neurohypophysis** is not as well understood, but secretes two important hormones:
1. **Antidiuretic hormone (ADH)** — This hormone, also known as **vasopressin,** stimulates the reabsorption of water by the kidney tubules. In addition, ADH can also increase blood pressure by constricting arterioles.
2. **Oxytocin** — This hormone stimulates the uterus to contract during childbirth and maintains labor during childbirth. Oxytocin is also secreted during suckling, and causes the production of milk from the mammary glands.

VIII. OVARIES

A. Location and Structure

The ovaries are two small glands located in the lower abdominal region of the female. The ovaries produce the female sex cell, the ovum, as well as hormones which are responsible for female sex characteristics and regulation of the menstrual cycle.

B. Function

The ovarian hormones are **estrogen** and **progesterone.** Estrogen is responsible for the development and maintenance of secondary sex characteristics, such as hair and breast development. Progesterone is responsible for the preparation and maintenance of the uterus in pregnancy.

IX. TESTES

A. Location and Structure

The testes are two small, ovoid glands suspended from the inguinal region of the male by the spermatic cord and surrounded by the scrotal sac. The testes produce the male sex cells, spermatozoa, as well as the male hormone called **testosterone**.

B. Function

Testosterone is an **androgen** (male steroid hormone) which stimulates and promotes the growth of secondary sex characteristics in the male (development of beard and pubic hair, deepening of voice, and distribution of fat).

Figure 18–7 reviews the major endocrine glands and the hormones they produce.

X. COMBINING FORMS

Combining Form	Definition	Terminology	Meaning
thyroid/o thyr/ð	thyroid gland	thyroidectomy _____	
		thyroiditis _____	
toxic/o	poison	thyrotoxicosis _____ *Caused by excessive thyroid secretion.*	
home/o	sameness, unchanging, constant	homeostasis _____	
calc/o	calcium	hypocalcemia _____	
		hypercalcemia _____	
		decalcification _____	
parathyroid/o	parathyroid glands	parathyroidectomy _____	
ster/o	solid structure	steroid _____ *Complex, solid, ring-shaped molecule.*	
adren/o	adrenal glands	adrenomegaly _____	

Endocrine Gland	Hormone	Action
Thyroid	Thyroxine	Regulates metabolism in body cells
Parathyroids	Parathyroid hormone	Regulates calcium in the blood
Adrenals:		
Cortex	Aldosterone (mineralocorticoid)	Regulates the amount of salts in the body
	Cortisol (glucocorticoid)	Regulates the quantities of sugars, fats, and proteins in cells
	Androgens, estrogens, and progestins	Maintain secondary sex characteristics
Medulla	Epinephrine (adrenaline)	Sympathomimetic
	Norepinephrine (noradrenaline)	Sympathomimetic
Pancreas:		
Islets of Langerhans	Insulin	Regulates the transport of glucose to the body cells
	Glucagon	Increases blood sugar by causing conversion of glycogen to glucose
Pituitary (hypophysis):		
Anterior lobe (adenohypophysis)	Pituitary growth hormone (GH; somatotropin, STH)	Increases bone growth
	Thyroid-stimulating hormone (TSH)	Stimulates production of thyroxine and growth of the thyroid gland
	Adrenocorticotropin (ACTH)	Stimulates secretion of hormones from the adrenal cortex, especially cortisol
	Gonadotropins:	
	Follicle-stimulating hormone (FSH)	Stimulates growth of eggs in the ovaries
	Luteinizing hormone (LH)	Important in sustaining pregnancy
	Prolactin (LTH)	Promotes growth of breast tissue and milk secretion
Posterior lobe (neurohyophysis)	Antidiuretic hormone (ADH; vasopressin)	Stimulates reabsorption of water by kidney tubules
	Oxytocin	Stimulates contraction of the uterus during labor and childbirth
Ovaries	Estrogen	Development and maintenance of secondary sex characteristics in the female
	Progesterone	Preparation and maintenance of the uterus in pregnancy
Testes	Testosterone	Growth and maintenance of secondary sex characteristics in the male

Figure 18–7   Major endocrine glands and the hormones they produce.

adrenal/o	adrenal glands	adrenalectomy _____
cortic/o	cortex, outer region of an organ	corticoid _____
kal/i	potassium	hypokalemia _____
natr/o	sodium	hypernatremia _____
gluc/o	sugar	glucocorticoids _____
		gluconeogenesis _____
glyc/o	sugar	hyperglycemia _____
		glycolysis _____
		glycogen _____
thym/o	thymus gland	thymectomy _____
somat/o	body	somatotropin _____

-tropin, like -trophy, means nourishment or development.

gonad/o	sex glands *(ovaries in the female, and testes in the male)*	hypogonadism _____ gonadotropin _____
lact/o	milk	lactogenic _____
		prolactin _____
andr/o	male	androgen _____
pancreat/o	pancreas	pancreatectomy _____
estr/o	female	estrogen _____
test/o	testes	testosterone _____
dips/o	thirst	polydipsia _____

Symptom associated with many disease conditions; for example, diabetes insipidus and diabetes mellitus.

ur/o	urine	antidiuretic _____
		polyuria _____
-physis	growth	adenohypophysis _____

Derived from glandular tissue in the embryo.

neurohypophysis _____

Derived from nervous tissue in the embryo.

cryohypophysectomy _____

_____

hypophyseal _____

-tocin	labor, delivery	oxytocin _____

XI. PATHOLOGICAL CONDITIONS

Thyroid

goiter   Enlargement of the thyroid gland.

Thyroid gland enlargement may be a symptom of many different conditions. Two of these conditions are:

endemic goiter This enlargement of the thyroid gland is due to deficiency of iodine in the diet. Because iodine is necessary to form thyroxine, too little thyroxine is produced and the thyroid enlarges in an effort to compensate for the deficiency.

exophthalmic goiter (also called **Graves' disease, toxic goiter, thyrotoxicosis,** or **hyperthyroidism**). This type of goiter is characterized by excessive thyroxine secretion leading to high oxygen consumption and a high metabolic rate. The etiology of the disorder is unclear, although it is currently thought to be an immunologic disorder. Tachycardia, exophthalmos (protrusion of the eyeballs), weight loss, and diaphoresis (sweating) are common symptoms. Treatment may include thyroidectomy or management with antithyroid drugs.

cretinism   Congenital hypothyroid condition.

This condition affects children and is the result of a congenital hypofunctioning of the thyroid gland. The children afflicted with cretinism are slow in both physical and mental development. They lack sufficient amounts of thyroxine for normal metabolic growth processes *in utero* and after birth. Treatment consists of administration of thyroid hormone which if continued for life can result in normal growth and development.

myxedema   Advanced hypothyroidism in adulthood.

This condition results when hypothyroidism occurs in adult life. The thyroid gland atrophies and little thyroxine is produced. The adult is obese, weak, and slow to action, and has low body temperature. The skin becomes dry and puffy because of collections of a mucus-like (myx/o = mucus) secretion under the skin. Recovery may be complete if thyroxine is administered soon after symptoms appear.

Parathyroid

osteitis fibrosa cystica   Bone inflammation with fibrous changes in bone and bone marrow.

This bone condition results from hyperparathyroidism. Excess of parathyroid hormone leads to increased amount of calcium in the blood (hypercalcemia). Because the hormone pulls calcium out of bones, it leaves the bones decalcified and susceptible to fracture and cysts (sacs of fluid or solid material). This condition is usually caused by a benign parathyroid tumor (adenoma). Treatment consists of surgical removal of the tumor.

hypoparathyroidism   Hypofunctioning of the parathyroid glands.

Decreased production of parathyroid hormone leads to hypocalcemia. As the calcium level in blood falls, the muscles and nerves of the body show weakness and display a condition called **tetany** (spasms and involuntary twitching of muscles). This condition is sometimes produced following accidental removal of or injury to the parathyroid glands. Treatment consists of administering calcium to raise its content in the blood.

Adrenal Cortex

Addison's disease   Hypofunctioning of the adrenal cortex.

This is a disease condition of hypoadrenalism caused by lack of sufficient adrenal cortex hormones (mineralocorticoids and glucocorticoids). Weakness, weight loss, yellow pigmentation of the skin, hypoglycemia (caused by lack of glucocorticoids), and large excretions of water and salts (caused by lack of mineralocorticoids) are all symptoms of Addison's disease. Treatment consists of administration of cortisone and adequate intake of salt.

Cushing's disease   Hyperfunctioning of the adrenal cortex (glucocorticoid secretion).

Overproduction of glucocorticoids leads to obesity, moonlike fullness of the face, elevated blood sugar, high blood pressure, and weakness. Cushing's disease may be caused by a benign or malignant adrenal cortex tumor or any abnormal growth of the adrenal glands. Treatment includes surgical removal of part of the adrenal glands or the tumor.

Adrenal Medulla

pheochromocytoma   Tumor occurring in the adrenal medulla.

The tumor cells (which stain dark or dusky color—phe/o = dusky) produce excess secretion of the catecholamines epinephrine and norepinephrine. The excess catecholamines produce hypertension, palpitations, severe headaches, sweating, flushing of face, and muscle spasms. Surgery to remove the tumor and administration of antihypertensive drugs are possible courses of treatment.

Pancreas

diabetes mellitus   Hypofunctioning of the pancreas.

This disease condition results from lack of insulin secretion by the pancreas (hypoinsulinism). Because deficiency of insulin prevents sugar from leaving the blood, sugar cannot enter the cells of the body. Hyperglycemia results, as well as glycosuria, polyuria (sugar in the blood acts as a diuretic), loss of weight (proteins and fats and all available foodstuffs, other than glucose, are burned), and ketonuria (fats are improperly burned, leading to ketosis, which is an accumulation of ketones in the body). Treatment depends on many factors, such as severity of the disease, age of the patient, and type of symptoms. Insulin is administered, and patients are restricted to a diet high in nutritive value and low in sugar.

hyperinsulinism   Excess of insulin.

This condition may be caused by a tumor of the pancreas (benign adenoma or carcinoma) or overdose of insulin. Excess insulin draws sugar out of the bloodstream, resulting in hypoglycemia. Fainting spells, convulsions, and loss of consciousness are common because a minimum level of blood sugar is necessary for proper mental functioning. If a tumor is the cause, it may be surgically resected and drugs administered to prevent hyperinsulin attacks.

Pituitary (Adenohypophysis)

gigantism   Hyperfunctioning of the pituitary gland before puberty, leading to abnormal overgrowth of the body.

Benign adenomas of the pituitary gland which occur before a child reaches puberty can produce this condition. Excessive pituitary growth hormone (somatotropin) is secreted before the growing ends of the long bones have closed and stopped their growth. Gigantism can be corrected by early diagnosis in childhood, followed by resection of the tumor or x-ray treatment.

acromegaly   Enlargement of the extremities caused by hyper-functioning of the pituitary gland after puberty.

Adenomas of the pituitary gland which occur during adulthood produce acromegaly. Hypersecretion of pituitary growth hormone causes the bones in the hands, feet, face, and jaw to grow abnormally large in size, producing a characteristic Frankenstein-type facial appearance.

dwarfism   Congenital hyposecretion of somatotropin.

The children affected are normal mentally but their bones remain small and underdeveloped. Treatment consists of administration of somatotropin. Achondroplastic dwarfs differ from hypopituitary dwarfs in that they suffer from a genetic defect in cartilage formation which adversely affects the growth of bones.

Simmonds' disease   Chronic pituitary gland insufficiency.

In this rare pathological condition, also called **pituitary cachexia** (wasting away), there is chronic pituitary insufficiency (caused by tumor, injury, surgery, or infection) which leaves the individual weak, debilitated, pale, and prematurely senile. Treatment consists of regular administration of hormones which are dependent upon normal pituitary functioning.

Pituitary (Neurohypophysis)

diabetes insipidus   Insufficient production of antidiuretic hormone from the neurohypophysis.

Deficient antidiuretic hormone causes the kidney tubules to fail to hold back (reabsorb) needed water and salts. Clinical symptoms include polyuria and polydipsia (excessive thirst).

inappropriate ADH   Excessive secretion of antidiuretic hormone.
  (IADH)

Excessive ADH secretion produces excess water retention in the body. Treatment consists of dietary water restriction. Tumor, drug reactions, and head injury are some of the possible etiological factors.

Figure 18–8 is a chart reviewing the various pathological conditions associated with hyposecretion and hypersecretion of the endocrine glands.

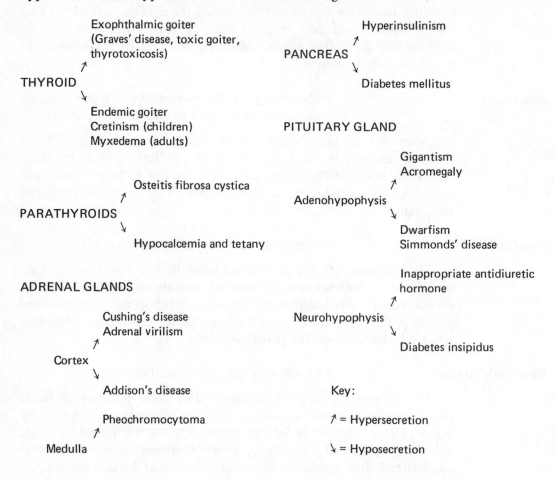

Figure 18–8   Review of pathological conditions related to endocrine organs.

XII. EXERCISES

A.   *Give the endocrine organs (including appropriate lobe or region) which produce the following hormones:*

    1.   follicle-stimulating hormone _____

    2.   vasopressin _____

    3.   aldosterone _____

    4.   insulin _____

    5.   thyroxine _____

6. cortisol _____

7. gonadotropic hormones _____

8. epinephrine _____

9. oxytocin _____

10. prolactin _____

11. somatotropin _____

12. glucagon _____

13. melatonin _____

14. estrogen _____

15. progesterone _____

16. testosterone _____

B. *Give the meaning of the following abbreviations:*

1. ADH _____

2. ACTH _____

3. GTT _____

4. LH _____

5. FSH _____

6. TSH _____

7. FBS _____

8. PTH _____

9. GH _____

10. LTH _____

C. *Indicate whether the following conditions are caused by hypersecretions or hyposecretions. Also, select from the list below the endocrine gland which is involved in each disease:*

thyroid	testes	anterior lobe of the pituitary
adrenal cortex	adrenal medulla	parathyroid gland
pancreas	posterior lobe of the pituitary	ovaries

Disease	Hypo or Hyper	Gland
1. Cushing's disease	_____	_____
2. tetany	_____	_____
3. Graves' disease	_____	_____
4. diabetes insipidus	_____	_____
5. acromegaly	_____	_____
6. myxedema	_____	_____
7. osteitis fibrosa cystica	_____	_____
8. diabetes mellitus	_____	_____
9. Addison's disease	_____	_____
10. gigantism	_____	_____
11. endemic goiter	_____	_____
12. cretinism	_____	_____
13. Simmonds' disease	_____	_____
14. pheochromocytoma	_____	_____
15. hypocalcemia	_____	_____
16. hyperinsulinism	_____	_____
17. dwarfism	_____	_____
18. inappropriate antidiuretic hormone	_____	_____

D. *Build medical terms:*

1. Abnormal condition (poison) of the thyroid gland _____

   _____

2. Removal of the thymus gland _____

3. Condition of deficiency or underdevelopment of the sex organs _____

   _____

4. Much thirst _____

5. Removal of the pituitary gland using cold temperatures _____

   _____

6. Sugar in the urine _____

7. Excessive calcium in the blood _____

8. Inflammation of the thyroid gland _____

9. Pertaining to producing milk _____

10. Enlargement of the adrenal gland _____

E. *Give the meaning of the following medical terms:*

1. steroids _____

2. catecholamines _____

3. adenohypophysis _____

4. tetany _____

5. exophthalmic goiter _____

6. mineralocorticoids _____

   _____

7. homeostasis _____

8. isthmus _____

9. glucocorticoids _____

_____

10. epinephrine _____

11. hypernatremia _____

12. hypokalemia _____

13. glycogenolysis _____

14. cachexia _____

ANSWERS

A. 1. Anterior lobe of the pituitary gland (adenohypophysis).
2. Posterior lobe of the pituitary gland (neurohypophysis).
3. Adrenal cortex.
4. Islets of Langerhans in the pancreas.
5. Thyroid gland.
6. Adrenal cortex.
7. Anterior lobe of the pituitary.
8. Adrenal medulla.
9. Posterior lobe of the pituitary.
10. Anterior lobe of the pituitary.
11. Anterior lobe of the pituitary.
12. Islets of Langerhans in the pancreas.
13. Pineal gland.
14. Ovaries.
15. Ovaries.
16. Testes.

B. 1. Antidiuretic hormone.
2. Adrenocorticotropin.
3. Glucose tolerance test.
4. Luteinizing hormone.
5. Follicle-stimulating hormone.
6. Thyroid-stimulating hormone.
7. Fasting blood sugar.
8. Parathyroid hormone.
9. Pituitary growth hormone.
10. Prolactin.

C. 1. Hypersecretion; adrenal cortex.
2. Hyposecretion; parathyroid gland.
3. Hypersecretion; thyroid gland.
4. Hyposecretion; posterior lobe of the pituitary gland.
5. Hypersecretion; anterior lobe of the pituitary gland.
6. Hyposecretion; thyroid gland.
7. Hypersecretion; parathyroid gland.
8. Hyposecretion; pancreas.
9. Hyposecretion; adrenal cortex.
10. Hypersecretion; anterior lobe of pituitary gland.
11. Hypersecretion; thyroid gland.
12. Hyposecretion; thyroid gland. A congenital condition.
13. Hyposecretion; anterior lobe of pituitary gland.
14. Hypersecretion; adrenal medulla.
15. Hyposecretion; parathyroid gland.

16. Hypersecretion; pancreas.
17. Hyposecretion; anterior lobe of pituitary gland.
18. Hypersecretion; posterior lobe of pituitary gland.

D.
1. Thyrotoxicosis.
2. Thymectomy.
3. Hypogonadism.
4. Polydipsia.
5. Cryohypophysectomy.
6. Glycosuria.
7. Hypercalcemia.
8. Thyroiditis.
9. Lactogenic.
10. Adrenomegaly.

E.
1. Complex substances derived from cholesterol; hormones from the adrenal cortex (corticoids) and sex hormones are steroids.
2. Complex substances derived from an amino acid; epinephrine (adrenaline) and norepinephrine (noradrenaline) are examples.
3. Anterior lobe of the pituitary gland.
4. Continuous contractions of muscles associated with low levels of parathyroid hormone.
5. Enlargement of the thyroid gland with eyeballs that bulge outward.
6. Steroid hormones from the adrenal cortex (outer region of the adrenal gland) which influence salt (minerals such as sodium and potassium) metabolism.
7. A state of equilibrium in the body with respect to functions, fluids, and times.
8. A narrow strip of tissue connecting two parts.
9. Steroid hormones from the adrenal cortex which influence sugar metabolism in the body.
10. Catecholamine hormone from the adrenal medulla.
11. Excessive sodium in the blood.
12. Deficient potassium in the blood.
13. Breakdown of glycogen to produce sugar.
14. Wasting away.

REVIEW SHEET 18

Combining Forms

adren/o	_____	lact/o	_____
adrenal/o	_____	natr/o	_____
andr/o	_____	pancreat/o	_____
calc/o	_____	parathyroid/o	_____
cortic/o	_____	somat/o	_____
dips/o	_____	ster/o	_____
estr/o	_____	test/o	_____
gluc/o	_____	thym/o	_____
glyc/o	_____	thyr/o	_____
gonad/o	_____	thyroid/o	_____
home/o	_____	toxic/o	_____
kal/i	_____	ur/o	_____

Suffixes

-ectomy	_____	-oid	_____
-emia	_____	-osis	_____
-genic	_____	-physis	_____
-lysis	_____	-stasis	_____
-megaly	_____	-tocin	_____

Additional Terms

acromegaly

Addison's disease

catecholamines

cortisone

cretinism

Cushing's disease

diabetes insipidus

diabetes mellitus

dwarfism

endemic goiter

exophthalmic goiter

fasting blood sugar (FBS)

gigantism

glucose tolerance test (GTT)

goiter

homeostasis

hyperinsulinism

hypoparathyroidism

hypothalamus

inappropriate ADH (IADH)

isthmus

myxedema

osteitis fibrosa cystica

pheochromocytoma   _____

Simmonds' disease   _____

steroids   _____

sympathomimetic   _____

tetany   _____

Give the locations of the following endocrine glands:

adenohypophysis   _____

adrenal cortex   _____

adrenal medulla   _____

hypophysis   _____

islets of Langerhans   _____

neurohypophysis   _____

ovaries   _____

parathyroid glands   _____

pineal gland   _____

suprarenal glands   _____

testes   _____

thymus gland   _____

thyroid gland   _____

Identify the actions of the following hormones and the glands from which they are produced:

adrenocorticotropic hormone (ACTH) _____

adrenaline   _____

aldosterone   _____

androgens _____

antidiuretic hormone (ADH) _____

cortisol _____

epinephrine _____

estrogen _____

follicle-stimulating hormone (FSH) _____

glucagon _____

glucocorticoids _____

gonadotropic hormones _____

hydrocortisone _____

insulin _____

luteinizing hormone (LH) _____

melatonin _____

mineralocorticoids _____

norepinephrine _____

oxytocin _____

parathyroid hormone (PTH) _____

pituitary growth hormone (GH) _____

progesterone _____

prolactin (LTH) _____

somatotropin _____

testosterone _____

thyroid-stimulating hormone (TSH) _____

thyroxine _____

vasopressin _____

CHAPTER 19

CANCER MEDICINE I: DEFINITIONS AND PATHOLOGICAL TERMS; CLASSIFICATION OF TUMORS

In this chapter you will:

Learn the medical terms related to the general characteristics of tumors;

Become familiar with terms used to describe the pathological appearance of tumors;

Understand the basis for classification, grading, and staging of cancer; and

Learn combining forms, prefixes, and suffixes related to the specialty of oncology.

This chapter is divided into the following sections:

I. INTRODUCTION

Cancer is a disease characterized by unrestrained and excessive division of body cells, occurring in any body tissue and at any age. Cancerous cells accumulate as large growths called **malignant tumors** which can penetrate, compress, and ultimately destroy the normal tissue of which they are a part. In addition to local growth, the cancerous cells may also invade adjacent tissues and may spread throughout the body by way of the blood and lymphatic vessels. It is this spreading of cancers from their site of origin to establish colonies in distant organs that is responsible for the lethality of malignant tumors if left untreated.

Deaths from cancer now make up almost one-fifth of all deaths in the United States. This chapter and the two that follow will explore the terminology related to this prevalent but poorly understood disease process. In this chapter, we will discuss the terms which describe the general characteristics of tumors, including abnormalities of growth and development. In addition, descriptions and examples of major categories of tumors, and systems for defining the size and extent of disease, will be examined.

In the next chapter (Chapter 20) we will learn about the process whereby a normal cell is transformed into a cancerous cell. Chapter 21 deals with terms pertaining to the causes and treatment of cancer.

II. VOCABULARY

anaplasia	Change in normal cells so that they revert to a more primitive, embryonic cell type.
benign	Not tending to become progressively worse or to recur; used to describe the growth of noncancerous tumors.
carcinoma	Cancerous tumor derived from epithelial tissues in the body (glandular, skin, linings of internal organs).
dedifferentiated	Lacking specialization in structure and function; undifferentiated.
differentiated	Specialized in structure and function.
encapsulated	Surrounded by a capsule.
grading	Evaluating the microscopic appearance of tumor cells to determine their degree of anaplasia.
hyperplasia	Increase in mass of a tissue or organ caused by new growth of cells.
infiltrative	Pertaining to the deposition or diffusion of a tissue onto or into another tissue; invasive.
invasive	Pertaining to extending beyond the boundaries of a specific type of tissue; infiltrative.
malignant	Tending to become progressively worse; used to describe the growth of cancerous tumors.

metastasis	Spreading of malignant tumor cells from the primary tumor site to distant regions of the body.
mixed tissue tumor	Tumor derived from different types of tissues (epithelial and connective tissues combined).
neoplasm	A mass of new, abnormal tissue; a tumor.
pedunculated	Possessing a stem or stalk (peduncle).
polyp	A growth extending outward from a mucous membrane. Polyps are usually benign, but may become malignant. Some polyps are pedunculated and others are sessile (having no stem).
sarcoma	Cancerous tumor derived from connective tissue in the body (blood, bone, muscle, fat, or cartilage).
sessile	Having no stem; describes a polyp attached directly to a membrane by a broad base.
solid tumor	A malignant growth consisting of a definite mass or lump.
staging	System of evaluating the spread of malignant tumors.
tumor	An enlargement or swelling due to a pathological overgrowth of tissue; tumors may be benign or malignant.

III. CHARACTERISTICS OF CANCEROUS TUMORS

Tumors (neoplasms) are masses or growths which arise from surrounding normal tissue. They may be either **malignant** (progressive and life-threatening) or **benign** (nonprogressive and not life-threatening). Benign tumors display slow growth and are **encapsulated** so that tumor cells cannot invade the surrounding tissue. Malignant tumors, in contrast, are rapidly growing and are not encapsulated. Malignant tumor growth is characteristically **invasive** and **infiltrative**, extending beyond the tissue of origin into adjacent organs.

In addition to the primary characteristics of increased numbers of cells (**hyperplasia**), a second feature of malignant neoplasms is **anaplasia**. Anaplasia is an abnormality in which cancerous cells resemble primitive, or embryonic, cells and lose the capacity for mature cellular functions. This means that cancerous cells are **dedifferentiated** (reverting to a less developed state) in contrast to the normal, healthy tissue of their origin. As opposed to malignant tumors, benign tumors are composed of more highly differentiated cells which are specialized in structure and function and more closely resemble mature tissue.

An example of anaplasia is seen in malignant white blood cells (leukocytes). Malignant leukocytes are unable to perform the function of normal, mature leukocytes, that is, to fight disease and infection. The anaplastic leukocyte is dedifferentiated and reverts back to a rapidly dividing, unspecialized, embryonic cell. Anaplastic cells in general lack orientation with respect to other tissues surrounding them; instead of an orderly arrangement, their distribution is often jumbled and disorganized.

A third characteristic of malignant neoplasms is the ability of the malignant cell to detach itself from the tumor site and establish a new tumor site at a remote region within the body. This ability reflects the lessened cohesiveness of hyperplastic and anaplastic tissue. In addition, it reflects the capacity of malignant cells to survive while floating freely in the blood and lymphatic vessels which transport the cells away from the original tumor site. The medical term used to describe this spreading of malignant tissue cells is **metastasis**. Benign tumors, as opposed to malignant tumors, display no metastasis.

IV. PATHOLOGICAL DESCRIPTIONS

The following terms are used to describe the appearance of a malignant tumor, either on gross (visual) inspection or by microscopic examination.

Gross Descriptions

cystic   Forming large open spaces filled with fluid. A cystic tumor is described as **mucinous** when the cystic spaces are filled with mucus (thick, sticky fluid secreted by mucous membranes). It is called **serous** when the fluid is thin or watery like serum. Cystic tumors are commonly found in the ovary.

polypoid   Growths which are like projections extending outward from a membrane base. **Sessile** polypoid tumors extend from a broad base, while **pedunculated** polypoid tumors extend from a stem or stalk. Polypoid tumors are commonly found in the colon.

ulcerating   Characterized by open, exposed surfaces resulting from death of overlying tissue. Ulcerating tumors may be found in the stomach, breast, and metastatic tumors of the skin.

inflammatory

Characterized by inflammation—that is, redness, swelling, and heat. Inflammatory tumors are found in the breast.

necrotic

Containing dead tissue. Any type of malignant tumor can display necrotic characteristics.

fungating

Mushrooming pattern of growth in which tumor cells pile one on top of another. Tumors of the colon are often fungating.

medullary

Large, soft, fleshy tumors. Thyroid and breast tumors are commonly medullary in consistency.

verrucous

Resembling a wartlike growth; circumscribed elevation of the skin. Commonly occurs in the gingiva (cheek).

Microscopic Descriptions

alveolar

Small, microscopic sacs within a malignant tumor. Alveolar-type tumors are commonly found in connective tissue, such as muscle, bone, fat, and cartilage.

follicular

Small, microscopic glandular sacs within a malignant tumor. This type of tumor is common in glandular malignancies such as thyroid cancers.

nodular

Forming multiple, microscopic nodules or tightly packed clusters of cells. The major type of tumors displaying nodularity are the malignant lymphomas.

diffuse

Not forming microscopic nodules; tumor cells are evenly spread throughout the tumor mass. Malignant lymphomas may be characterized by either diffuseness or nodularity.

carcinoma
in situ

Referring to localized tumor cells; those that have not invaded adjacent structures. Cancer of the cervix may begin as carcinoma *in situ*.

papillary

Forming microscopic, finger-like or nipple-like projections. Thyroid, bladder, and ovarian tumors are commonly described as papillary.

scirrhous	Hard, densely packed tumor, overgrown with fibrous tissue. Scirrhous-type tumors are commonly found in the breast and stomach.
pleomorphic	Tumors with a variety of types of cells present. Muscle, fat, and mixed-cell tumors are examples of pleomorphism.
epidermoid	Tumors of squamous epithelial cells (thin, platelike skin cells). These are found in the respiratory tract (trachea and lung).

V. CLASSIFICATION OF CANCEROUS TUMORS

Although about half of all cancer deaths are caused by malignancies of only three organs (lung, breast, and large intestine), more than 100 distinct varieties of cancer are recognized, each having a unique set of symptoms and requiring a specific course of therapy. It is possible to divide these 100 specific types of cancer into three broad groups on the basis of histogenesis—that is, by identifying the particular tissue from which the tumor cells have arisen. The major groups of malignant tumors are thus called **carcinomas**, **sarcomas**, and **mixed-tissue tumors**.

Carcinomas

Carcinomas, the largest group, are **solid tumors**, or masses, which are derived from epithelial tissue (external and internal tissue lining body surfaces, including skin, glands, digestive, urinary, and reproductive organs). Approximately 85 per cent of all malignant neoplasms are carcinomas.

The following list gives examples of specific carcinomas and the epithelial tissue from which they are derived. Benign tumors of epithelial origin are usually named by using the suffix -oma added to the type of tissue in which the tumor occurs. For example, a gastroma (also called gastric adenoma) is a benign tumor of the glandular cells lining the stomach. Malignant tumors of epithelial tissue origin are named by using the term -carcinoma added to the type of tissue in which the tumor occurs. For example, a gastric adenocarcinoma is a cancerous tumor of glandular cells lining the stomach.

Type of Epithelial Tissue	*Malignant Tumor*
Gastrointestinal tract:	
stomach	gastric adenocarcinoma
esophagus	esophageal adenocarcinoma
colon	carcinoma of the colon

Glandular tissue:

thyroid	carcinoma of the thyroid
adrenal glands	carcinoma of the adrenals
pancreas	carcinoma of the pancreas (pancreatic adenocarcinoma)
breast	carcinoma of the breast
prostate	carcinoma of the prostate

Skin:

squamous cell layer	squamous cell carcinoma
basal cell layer	basal cell carcinoma
melanocyte	malignant melanoma

Lung	adenocarcinoma of the lung; oat cell (small cell) carcinoma; epidermoid carcinoma

Kidney	hypernephroma (renal cell carcinoma)

Reproductive organs	cystadenocarcinoma of the ovaries; adenocarcinoma of the uterus; squamous cell (epidermoid) carcinoma of the vagina and cervix; carcinoma of the penis; seminoma (carcinoma of the testes); choriocarcinoma of the uterus or testes

Sarcomas

Sarcomas, a rarer type of cancer than carcinomas, are derived from supportive and connective tissue, such as bone, fat, muscle, cartilage, bone marrow, and lymphatic tissue, or from blood cells. Sarcomas account for approximately 10 per cent of all malignant neoplasms.

The following list gives examples of specific types of sarcomas and the connective tissue from which they are derived. Benign tumors of connective tissue origin are named using the suffix -oma added to the type of tissue in which the tumor occurs. For example, a benign tumor of bone is called an osteoma. Malignant tumors of connective tissue origin are often named by using the term -sarcoma added to the type of tissue in which the tumor occurs. For example, an osteosarcoma is a malignant tumor of bone derived from flesh (sarc/o = flesh) or connective tissue.

Type of Connective Tissue	*Malignant Tumor*
Bone	osteosarcoma (osteogenic sarcoma)
Muscle:	
smooth (visceral) muscle	leiomyosarcoma
striated (skeletal) muscle	rhabdomyosarcoma
Cartilage	chondrosarcoma
Fat	liposarcoma
Fibrous tissue	fibrosarcoma
Blood vessel tissue	hemangiosarcoma
Hematopoietic tissue:	
leukocytes	leukemia
bone marrow cells	multiple myeloma
lymphocytes	lymphosarcoma or lymphoma; reticulum cell sarcoma; Hodgkin's disease
Nerve tissue:	
embryonic nerve tissue	neuroblastoma
neuroglial tissue	astrocytoma (tumor of neuroglial cells called astrocytes)
meningeal tissue	meningeal sarcoma

Mixed-Tissue Tumors

Mixed-tissue tumors are derived from tissue which is capable of differentiating into epithelial as well as connective tissue. The tumors are thus composed of several different types of cells. Examples of mixed-tissue tumors can be found in the kidney, ovaries, and testes.

Type of Tissue	*Malignant Tumor*
Kidney	Wilms' tumor (embryonal adenosarcoma)
Ovaries and testes	teratoma (tumor composed of bone, muscle, skin, gland cells, cartilage, etc.)

VI. GRADING AND STAGING SYSTEMS

Two methods of categorizing malignant tumors are called **grading** and **staging**. They are based on different aspects of tumor growth and appearance.

When grading a tumor, the pathologist is concerned with the microscopic appearance of the tumor cells, specifically with their degree of anaplasia. In most cases, four grades are used. Grade I tumors are very well differentiated so that they closely resemble the normal parent tissue of their origin. Grade IV tumors are so anaplastic (dedifferentiated) that recognition of the tumor's cells of origin may even be difficult. Grades II and III are intermediate in appearance, moderately or poorly differentiated, as opposed to well differentiated (Grade I) and dedifferentiated (Grade IV).

Grading is of value in prognosis of certain types of cancers, such as cancer of the urinary bladder, melanomas, and brain tumors (astrocytomas). Patients with Grade I tumors have a high survival rate, while patients with Grade II, III, and IV tumors have a poorer survival rate.

Grading is also used in evaluating the cytology (cell appearance) of cells obtained from normal body fluids in preventive screening tests, such as Pap smears of the uterine cervix, tracheal secretions, or stomach secretions. Examination of free cells from tissue and fluids allows the pathologist to rule out the presence of malignant neoplasms in these organs. For example, a Grade I Pap smear contains only normal-appearing cervical epithelial cells, while a Grade IV smear contains highly anaplastic malignant cells. Intermediate grades necessitate repeat smears at frequent intervals to detect early malignant transformations.

The staging of cancerous tumors is based on the extent of spread of the tumor rather than on its microscopic appearance. A **TNM** staging system is in use and has been applied to breast, head, neck, and other cancers. T (tumor) refers to the size and degree of local extension of the tumor; N (regional lymph nodes) refers to the number of regional lymph nodes which have been invaded by tumor; M (distant metastasis) refers to the presence or absence of metastases of the tumor cells.

VII. COMBINING FORMS, SUFFIXES, AND PREFIXES

Combining Form	Definition	Terminology	Meaning
onc/o	tumor	oncology	_____
carcin/o	cancer	carcinoma	_____
		carcinolytic	_____
sarc/o	flesh, connective tissue	sarcoma	_____
aden/o	gland	adenocarcinoma	_____

leiomy/o	smooth muscle	leiomyosarcoma _____
rhabdomy/o	striated muscle	rhabdomyosarcoma _____
lip/o	fat	liposarcoma _____
oste/o	bone	osteosarcoma _____
scirrh/o	hard	scirrhous _____
medull/o	middle, soft	medullary _____
papill/o	nipple-like, finger-like	papillary _____
polyp/o	small growths on a stalk *(polyps)*	polyposis _____
cyst/o	sac of fluid, cyst	cystic _____
alveol/o	small sac	alveolar _____
follicul/o	small sac	follicular _____
ple/o	more	pleomorphic _____
terat/o	monster	teratoma _____
-plasia	formation, growth	dysplasia _____
		hyperplasia _____
-plasm	formation, growth	neoplasm _____
-oid	resembling	polypoid _____
-oma	tumor	hypernephroma _____
ana	up, backward, again	anaplasia _____
epi	upon	epidermoid _____
		epithelial _____

meta   beyond, change,   <u>meta</u>stasis _____
                             near

                                           <u>meta</u>plasia _____

VIII. EXERCISES

A. *Build medical terms:*

1. New growth or formation _____

2. Excessive growth (in numbers of cells) _____

3. Pertaining to sacs filled with fluid _____

4. Tumor of striated muscle derived from flesh (connective) tissue _____

    _____

5. (Benign) tumor of a gland _____

6. Beyond control (spreading of a malignant neoplasm) _____

    _____

7. Cancerous tumor of gland tissue _____

8. Cancerous tumor of melanocytes _____

9. Tumor of fat derived from flesh (connective) tissue _____

    _____

10. Pertaining to finger-like projections _____

B. *Give the meaning of the following:*

1. carcinoma *in situ* _____

2. teratoma _____

3. dedifferentiation _____

4. infiltration _____

5. TNM system _____

6. grading of malignant tumors _____

7. anaplasia _____

8. epithelial _____

9. encapsulated _____

10. mucinous _____

11. epidermoid _____

12. verrucous _____

C. *Match the following gross and microscopic descriptions of tumors with their meanings:*

scirrhous _____

medullary _____

nodular _____

diffuse _____

alveolar _____

cystic _____

follicular _____

polypoid _____

papillary _____

necrotic _____

fungating _____

inflammatory _____

ulcerating _____

pleomorphic _____

1. Microscopic nipple-like projections.

2. Forming microscopic, tightly packed clusters of cells.

3. Small glandular sacs within carcinomas.

4. Microscopic sacs within sarcomatous tumors.

5. Hard, overgrown with fibrous tissue.

6. Resembling a growth on a stalk.

7. Even spreading out of tumor cells (microscopic appearance).

8. Forming large open spaces filled with fluid.

9. Large, soft, fleshy tumors.

10. Mushrooming pattern of growth with tumor cells piling one on top of another.

11. Open, exposed surfaces upon the tumor.

12. Microscopic appearance of many types of tumor cells present.

13. Characterized by redness, swelling, and heat.

14. Containing dead tissue.

D.   *What is the difference between a* carcinoma *and a* sarcoma? _____

_____

_____

_____

ANSWERS

A.   1.   neoplasm
    2.   hyperplasia
    3.   cystic
    4.   rhabdomyosarcoma
    5.   adenoma

    6.   metastasis
    7.   adenocarcinoma
    8.   malignant melanoma
    9.   liposarcoma
    10.   papillary

B.   1.   Malignant growths which are noninvasive (localized).
    2.   Malignant neoplasm composed of cells derived from different types of tissue (mixed-tissue tumor).
    3.   A reversion of cells from a more complex form to a simpler, more embryonic state, anaplasia.
    4.   Abnormal growth of malignant cells into tissue surrounding it.
    5.   Staging system to describe the extent of spread of a malignant tumor (T = tumor size; N = lymph nodes; M = metastasis).
    6.   System to describe the microscopic appearances of tumors according to their degrees of anaplasia.
    7.   Reversion of adult cells to more primitive, embryonic cell types.
    8.   Pertaining to cells which cover the outer and inner surfaces of the body and give rise to glandular tissue.
    9.   Within a capsule.
    10.   Full of mucus.
    11.   Describing tumors composed of squamous epithelial cells (skin cells).
    12.   Describing tumors resembling wartlike growths.

C.

5	8	10
9	3	13
2	6	11
7	1	12
4	14	

D.   A carcinoma is a cancerous tumor composed of cells of epithelial tissue (skin lining the outside and inside of the body). Examples are glandular tumors, skin cancers, and cancers of the linings of internal organs.

A sarcoma is a cancerous tumor composed of cells of connective tissue or flesh tissue (bone, fat, blood, muscle, cartilage). Examples are tumors of bone (osteosarcoma), fat (liposarcoma), and cartilage (chondrosarcoma).

REVIEW SHEET 19

Combining Forms

aden/o	_____	onc/o	_____
alveol/o	_____	oste/o	_____
carcin/o	_____	papill/o	_____
cyst/o	_____	ple/o	_____
follicul/o	_____	polyp/o	_____
leiomy/o	_____	rhabdomy/o	_____
lip/o	_____	scirrh/o	_____
medull/o	_____	terat/o	_____

Prefixes and Suffixes

ana	_____	-oma	_____
epi	_____	-plasm	_____
-meta	_____	-plasia	_____
-oid	_____		

Additional Terms

alveolar _____

anaplasia _____

benign _____

carcinoma *in situ* _____

cystic _____

dedifferentiated _____

differentiated _____

diffuse _____

encapsulated _____

epidermoid _____

follicular _____

fungating _____

grading _____

hyperplasia _____

infiltrative _____

inflammatory _____

invasive _____

malignant _____

medullary _____

metastasis _____

mixed-tissue tumor _____

mucinous _____

necrotic _____

neoplasm _____

nodular _____

papillary _____

pedunculated _____

pleomorphic _____

polypoid _____

sarcoma _____

scirrhous

serous

sessile

solid tumor

staging

tumor

ulcerating

verrucous

CHAPTER 20

CANCER MEDICINE II: CELLULAR ASPECTS

In this chapter you will:

Learn concepts and terminology related to the transformation of a normal cell into a cancerous cell;

Review the major structures and functions of a cell;

Identify terms which pertain to the structure of DNA and how it functions in a cell;

Learn about the genetic code and its relationship to protein syntheses and cellular differentiation; and

Differentiate between the stages in the growth cycle of a cell.

The chapter is divided into the following sections:

I. INTRODUCTION

In the previous chapter we discussed the general characteristics of cancers, including the terminology which describes the various abnormalities displayed by malignant tissue. In this chapter, we will concentrate at the level of the individual cell and discuss the process of transformation of a normal cell into a cancerous one. We will focus on the characteristics of DNA, the genetic material within the cell which controls the cell's multiplication and differentiation.

At the cellular level, cancer is primarily a disease of excessive and uncontrolled cell multiplication. While normal cells will cease to divide once they come in contact with adjacent cells (a process known as **contact inhibition**), cancerous cells are not affected by contact and continue to divide relentlessly.

Another important characteristic of malignant cells is their **anaplastic** appearance; that is, the cells are undifferentiated, primitive, and immature. Differentiation is a normal process in cell development whereby unspecialized, immature body cells undergo a change to assume the capabilities of more specialized cells. For example, in bone marrow, immature cells during a period of days normally undergo change in their structure and become functionally mature blood cells known as erythrocytes, leukocytes, and thrombocytes. It is this normal change, or differentiation, which allows a particular blood cell to carry on its specialized functions in the body—such as carrying gases, engulfing bacteria to fight disease, and aiding in the clotting of blood.

However, when a cell becomes cancerous, these normal processes of cellular differentiation are thwarted. For example, in the blood cancer known as leukemia, the normal bone marrow progression from immature cell to mature leukocyte does not occur. Undifferentiated, immature cells, poorly equipped structurally to carry on the important disease-fighting functions of the normal leukocyte, replace mature leukocytes in the circulating blood and bone marrow.

The transformation of a normal cell into a cancerous one (displaying unrestrained, anaplastic, as well as metastatic, growth) is only partially understood at present. However, even though basic scientific answers are beyond reach, we will attempt in this chapter to become familiar with some of the general ideas and terminology related to malignant transformation and ongoing cancer research.

II. VOCABULARY

adenine	One of four bases in the DNA molecule.
amino acids	Molecules which form the building blocks of proteins. There are 20 different kinds of amino acids found in proteins.
anabolism	Building up of new molecules in the cytoplasm of the cell. Larger molecules are formed from the combination of smaller molecules. Protein synthesis from amino acids is an example of anabolism.
bases	Special chemical compounds which form DNA.
catabolism	Breaking-down process in cells. Energy-containing molecules (foods) are broken down in the presence of oxygen to release energy for activities or storage in the cell.

chromosomes	Located in the nucleus, these small, rod-shaped bodies contain the genetic material (DNA) which determines heredity.
cytoplasm	Contents of the cell exclusive of the nucleus.
cytosine	One of four bases which are part of the DNA molecule.
deoxyribose	The sugar found in deoxyribonucleic acid (DNA).
differentiation	Process of specialization of cells. Skin cells, bone cells, muscle cells, and so forth, have characteristic sets of proteins which make them differentiated for their functions in the body.
DNA (deoxyribonucleic acid)	A large molecule composed of sugar, phosphate, and bases. It is found in the cell nucleus, within chromosomes, and its function is to control the activities and reproduction of the cell. Regions in the DNA molecules are called genes.
endoplasmic reticulum	Tiny membrane network in the cytoplasm which is the site of protein synthesis.
enzyme	Protein made in the endoplasmic reticulum of a cell. Enzymes promote and control all chemical processes within the cell but remain unchanged themselves.
G-1 period	Part of the growth cycle of a cell. Period of time which extends from completion of previous cell division to the synthesis of new DNA in the nucleus.
G-2 period	Part of the growth cycle of a cell. Period of time which follows DNA synthesis and ends with the actual division of the cell.
generation time	Time it takes for a cell to complete a full growth cycle from one cell division to the next.
genes	Basic units of heredity which are located within chromosomes. Genes are regions on a DNA molecule which control the synthesis of specific enzymes and other proteins.

genetic code

The system by which genetic information is passed from the DNA molecule in the nucleus to the protein-making machinery in the cytoplasm of a cell. The specific sequence of bases on the DNA molecule is thought to determine the sequence of amino acids in a protein molecule.

growth cycle

The sequence of changes in the life of a cell which extends from one cell division to the next.

guanine

One of the four bases which are part of the DNA molecule.

helical

Pertaining to being shaped like a helix, or spiral.

M-period

Part of the growth cycle of a cell. Period of time during which the cell divides. M stands for mitosis.

messenger RNA
  (mRNA)

Molecule which is formed from DNA and transfers the genetic code to the cytoplasm where protein synthesis occurs.

metabolism

The sum total of the activities of the cell (anabolism and catabolism).

mitochondria
  (singular: mitochondrion)

Structures in the cytoplasm which are the site of the chemical breakdown of molecules and subsequent release of energy.

mitosis

Process of cell division involving the production of two identical daughter cells from a parent cell.

mutation

Change in the genetic material (DNA) of a cell. It can be caused by chemicals, viruses, or radiation, or may occur spontaneously.

nucleic acids

DNA and RNA; large molecules containing phosphate, carbon, hydrogen, oxygen, and nitrogen, and built up from smaller compounds called nucleotides.

nucleolus

Large RNA-containing structure in the cell nucleus.

nucleotide

Chemical compound composed of a base with an attached sugar and phosphate. This is the building block of a nucleic acid.

nucleus

Portion of the cell which contains hereditary material (DNA).

phosphate	Compound which is part of a nucleotide of DNA and RNA.
proteins	Large molecules containing carbon, nitrogen, and oxygen, and which are built up from amino acids. Proteins are necessary for growth and tissue repair and are important constituents of blood.
protein synthesis	The putting together of amino acids to form large molecules called proteins.
purine	One of the two types of bases found in DNA and RNA, and contained in foods like meat, fish, spinach, and poultry. The two important purine bases in DNA are adenine and guanine.
pyrimidine	The second type of base found in nucleic acids. Two important pyrimidine bases found in DNA are thymine and cytosine. RNA contains the pyrimidine called uracil, as well as cytosine.
replication	The process of cell division whereby an exact copy of the parent cell is formed; mitosis.
ribose	Sugar which is found in ribonucleic acid (RNA).
ribosomes	Particles on the endoplasmic reticulum. They contain RNA and are the site of protein synthesis.
RNA (ribonucleic acid)	A nucleic acid which closely resembles DNA. It is found in the cell nucleus **and** cytoplasm and plays an important role in the synthesis of proteins.
S-period	Part of the growth cycle of the cell. Period of time during which synthesis of new DNA takes place.
template	A mold or form used as a guide in reproducing a shape or structure. DNA is a template for its own reproduction and the reproduction of RNA as well.
thymine	One of four bases which are part of the DNA molecule.
transfer RNA (tRNA)	A ribonucleic acid molecule which transfers amino acids from cytoplasm onto the ribosomes to form protein chains.
uracil	One of the bases which are formed in the RNA molecule.

III. BASIC CELL STRUCTURE

In order to understand how a cancerous change can occur in a cell, we will first review and examine further the major parts of a cell. Consult Figure 3–1 (in Chapter 3) as you read the following.

All human body cells, whether they be bone, muscle, blood, nerve, or skin, have specific structures in common. Each cell is divided into two major compartments. The large area of the cell is called the **cytoplasm**, and the smaller central region surrounded by the cytoplasm is called the **nucleus**.

Cytoplasm

The cytoplasm, protected by the cell membrane, contains structures which carry on the complicated **metabolism** of the cell. Metabolism includes all enzyme-mediated chemical processes that go on in the cell. It consists of **anabolism**, which is the building up of complex molecules, such as proteins, and **catabolism**, which is the breaking down or breaking apart of larger molecules to release energy. This energy can be used then to carry on the work of the cell.

Some of the structures within the cytoplasm which carry on these metabolic functions are:

Mitochondria. These are small, threadlike bodies which contain enzymes to help break down food molecules and release energy. In the presence of oxygen, food is catabolized and energy is released to support the activities of the cell or to be put into storage for later use.

Endoplasmic Reticula. These are structures in the cell which are composed of a network of membranes so small that they are visible only with an electron microscope. There are two types of endoplasmic reticula: a rough-surfaced, granular type and a smooth-surfaced agranular type. The granular endoplasmic reticulum contains numerous particles called **ribosomes**. Ribosomes are composed of a substance called ribonucleic acid (RNA). The RNA within the ribosomes directs the synthesis of proteins in the cell. **Enzymes** are examples of large protein molecules which are made within the granular endoplasmic reticula of the cell.

Nucleus

While the cytoplasm carries on the important work of the cell, building up and breaking down molecules, the nucleus contains structures and substances which direct this cytoplasmic work. Some of these structures are:

Nuclear Membrane. This membrane surrounds the nucleus and contains many pores which allow molecules to pass back and forth between the nucleus and the cytoplasm.

Nucleolus. This large body in the nucleus contains RNA and protein and is the site of the manufacture of ribosomes in the cell. All of the ribosomes found in the cytoplasm are manufactured in the nucleolus and transported to the granular endoplasmic reticulum where they participate in the formation of proteins.

Chromosomes. These are threads of genetic material which condense during the process of cell division into 46 small rod-shaped bodies. Each chromosome is made up of a long series of hereditary units known as **genes.** These units are segments of a large molecule called **deoxyribonucleic acid,** or **DNA,** which is located in each chromosome.

DNA is found in the nucleus of a cell, and it plays an essential role in both the replication (division) of a cell and the cell's ability to grow by making new proteins (protein synthesis). When a cell reproduces itself, the DNA material in each chromosome is copied so that exactly the same genetic information is passed to the next generation of cells. This process is called self-replication. In addition, within the nucleus DNA is able to copy its genetic information onto a ribonucleic acid (RNA) molecule. The RNA molecule can then leave the nucleus, carrying information from DNA, enter the cytoplasm, and direct the protein synthesis within the granular endoplasmic reticulum of the cell.

The kinds of proteins that a cell can make determine the specific characteristics (differentiation) of the cell (fat, nerve, bone, or blood cell). Characteristics such as eye color, skin color, hair color, height, capacity for intelligence, and thousands of other characteristics are determined by the nature of the protein synthesized within the cell.

In summary, the two major roles of DNA are self-replication and control of cell protein synthesis. Figure 20–1 illustrates these two functions of DNA.

If DNA molecule is responsible for the normal processes of cell reproduction and differentiation, and cancer is a disorder of cell reproduction and differentiation, it follows that cancer researchers are interested in analyzing the nature of this important molecule, how it operates within a cell, and how it may be changed in an abnormal or cancerous cell.

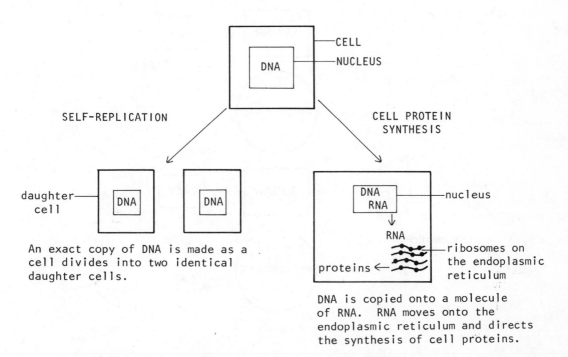

Figure 20–1   The two functions of DNA.

IV. STRUCTURE OF DNA

DNA is a large, complex molecule composed of a single chain of individual units called **nucleotides**. Each nucleotide consists of three basic elements: (1) a sugar called **deoxyribose**; (2) a chemical substance called **phosphate**; and (3) a chemical compound called a **base**.

The nucleotide chains of DNA are arranged in two long strands twisted around each other. There are hundreds and thousands of nucleotides linked chemically on each double-stranded DNA molecule.

Figure 20–2 shows how three nucleotide units are arranged on one strand of DNA.

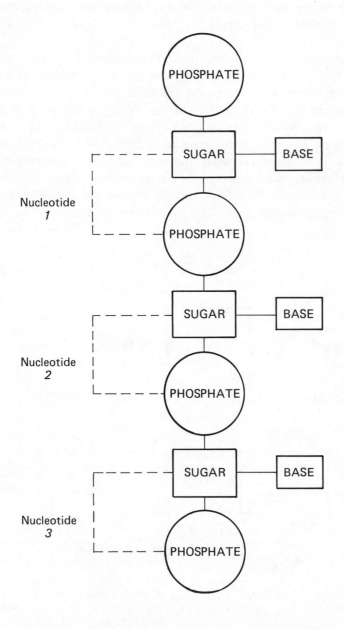

Figure 20–2   Three nucleotide units are arranged on one strand of DNA.

There are four different kinds of bases on the double-stranded DNA molecule. All the bases contain the element nitrogen, but each is different because of the individual arrangement of elements within the base. Two of the bases are compounds called **purines**. The names of the purines in DNA are **adenine** (A) and **guanine** (G). The other bases are compounds known as **pyrimidines**, and they are called **cytosine** (C) and **thymine** (T).

On the DNA double strand the bases serve as connections between the two opposing (complementary) strands. Like rungs of a ladder, they link one DNA strand to its complementary strand through chemical bonds. This linkage is accomplished in a specific manner. An **adenine** base on one DNA strand links only with a **thymine** base on the opposing DNA strand. Similarly, a **cytosine** base links only with a **guanine** base on the opposite DNA strand.

ADENINE pairs with THYMINE

CYTOSINE pairs with GUANINE

To summarize, then, each DNA molecule within a chromosome is composed of thousands of nucleotides (combinations of deoxyribose, phosphate, and a base). The nucleotides are arranged in two complementary strands in a **helical** (spiral) fashion (something like a twisted ladder). If we could untwist the DNA ladder, the nucleotides would be arranged in a pattern which is represented in Figure 20–3.

The specific kind of genetic information that a cell possesses is determined by the sequence of base pairs (A-T and C-G) on DNA molecules in the cell nucleus. Thus, a base sequence on a two-stranded DNA molecule which reads $\frac{\text{GATAGTC}}{\text{CTATCAG}}$ would be different genetic information than a base pair sequence of $\frac{\text{TCGACTCA}}{\text{AGCTGAGT}}$. Each different type of cell in the body, whether it be muscle, bone, skin, or nerve, has the same basic set of genetic information. It is reasonable to assume that if a cell becomes diseased or abnormal and the abnormality continues in the descendants of that cell (as in cancerous growths), there may have been a change in the genetic information, such as the sequence of bases, in that particular cell and that change is passed on from generation to generation of those cells.

In the transformation of a normal cell into a cancerous cell, a crucial change is thought to take place in the structure of DNA, either by addition of extra material, faulty copying (replication) of DNA, or loss of genetic material. Such changes in the genetic material of the cell may cause **mutations**, which are permanent, heritable alterations in cell structure or function and may lead to cancerous growths.

V. THE GENETIC CODE

The **genetic code** is the specific sequence of base pairs on the molecules of DNA in the nucleus of a cell. In the English language, words are created by the specific order and arrangement of the 26 letters of the alphabet. The language of the genetic code has only four letters (A, T, C, and G), which stand for the bases adenine, thymine, cytosine, and guanine. The order in which these bases are arranged on the DNA molecules determines the kinds of **proteins** the cell can make.

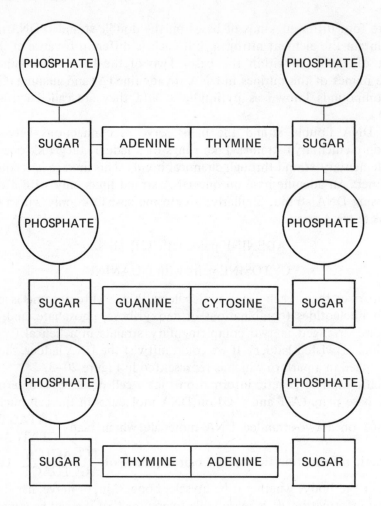

Figure 20-3 General pattern of nucleotide arrangement in a DNA molecule.

Since so many cellular activities are carried on by proteins, it is the specific protein molecules in a cell which reflect the cell's particular kind of differentiation. Thus, for example, in addition to the basic proteins common to all cells, muscle cells contain certain muscle proteins, skin cells contain skin proteins, and nerve cells possess their own particular type of proteins.

The relationship between the genetic code in the DNA molecule and the differentiation of a cell can be illustrated by the following sequence:

$$\text{genetic code in DNA} \xrightarrow{\textit{directs}} \text{protein synthesis} \xrightarrow[\textit{leads to}]{\textit{which}} \text{CELL DIFFERENTIATION}$$

How, then, can the genetic code which is in the nucleus of the cell dictate the order and kinds of proteins which are synthesized in the cytoplasm of the cell?

The answer to this question is that there is a special molecule which can travel from the nucleus of the cell into the cytoplasm to carry the genetic code information for protein synthesis. This is an RNA molecule appropriately called **messenger RNA (mRNA)**. The mRNA molecule, like DNA, is composed of nucleotides and is actually formed from DNA within the nucleus of the cell.

When the DNA molecule in the nucleus makes an mRNA molecule, the DNA molecule serves as a **template** (model) for the construction of mRNA. The sequence of bases on the new mRNA molecule is the pattern set by the parent DNA strand. This copying is accomplished even though mRNA is not identical to DNA (mRNA contains the base **uracil** instead of the base **thymine** on DNA, and mRNA contains ribose sugar instead of deoxyribose).

An mRNA molecule, containing a base sequence (such as A, U, G, C, A, C . . .) determined by the DNA molecule it was created from, thus carries the genetic code. This code is transferred to the ribosomes on the endoplasmic reticulum of the cell by the mRNA molecule as it passes from the nucleus into the cytoplasm. The specific sequence of bases in mRNA calls for the attachment of specific **amino acids** (subunits of protein) to form a large protein chain on the ribosomes. In other words, the particular amino acid sequence in a protein is determined by the order of bases on the mRNA molecule which in turn has been copied from DNA in the nucleus of the cell.

In addition, another cytoplasmic RNA molecule, called **transfer RNA (tRNA)**, is responsible for helping to bring and attach the specific amino acids together on the ribosomes to form a protein chain.

Scientists now know that a sequence of three bases (triplet) contains the necessary message to call for the attachment of a specific amino acid in the protein chain. For example, the mRNA base code sequence GUC (guanine, uracil, cytosine) on mRNA calls for the attachment of the amino acid **valine**, while the mRNA base code sequence AUG (adenine, uracil, guanine) calls for the attachment of the amino acid **methionine**. It is the particular sequence of amino acids on a protein chain which determines the types of proteins and **enzymes** (proteins necessary for proper cellular functioning) that a cell can produce.

The following sequence summarizes the process whereby the genetic code in the DNA molecule can determine the specific proteins and enzymes made by a cell and, therefore, the differentiation of a cell:

$$\text{genetic code in DNA} \xrightarrow[\text{onto}]{\text{copied}} \text{mRNA} \xrightarrow[\text{sequence of}]{\text{directs}} \text{amino acids} \xrightarrow[\text{build up}]{\text{which}} \text{proteins (such as enzymes)} \xrightarrow[\text{to}]{\text{leading}} \text{CELLULAR DIFFERENTIATION}$$

One of the disorders of a cancer cell is its lack of differentiation (anaplasia). It is conceivable that the etiology of cancer may be related to some factor which causes a change in the specific amino acids and proteins that a cell makes, thus leading to improper differentiation, or **dedifferentiation**. Changes in the DNA molecule or in the mRNA molecule could thus result in improper amino acid sequence for protein synthesis and produce cellular abnormalities. As noted earlier in this chapter, the term used to describe such a change in genetic material leading to differences or abnormalities in cell structure and function is **mutation**. In the next chapter we will discuss some of the possible factors which may lead to mutation and malignant changes in cells. Some of these etiologic agents are radiation, chemicals and drugs, and viruses.

VI. GROWTH CYCLE OF CELLS

Some scientists approach the problem of the change in a cell from normal to cancerous by examining the sequence of events as the cell undergoes growth and division. The process of cell division, which is the production of identical daughter cells from a parent cell, is called **mitosis**. During mitosis, the genetic material (DNA) in chromosomes duplicates itself so that each daughter cell receives an exact copy of the DNA in the parent cell.

Once the parent cell has divided and the daughter cells are produced, those daughter cells grow and differentiate until **they** begin to divide and reproduce themselves. This cycle of division to growth and differentiation and back to division is called the **growth cycle**. The growth cycle of a cell can be represented by the following:

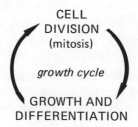

The growth cycles of different cells in the body are variable. Skin cells and the cells lining the digestive tract replace themselves daily. Nerve cells in the brain and spinal cord never undergo cell division. Bone marrow cells divide every two or three days to form new blood cells. And, depending on the individual type, the growth cycle of the cancer cell is greatly changed from that of the normal cell from which it originated.

In order to study the growth cycles of normal and cancerous cells, scientists have divided the growth cycle into several specific time periods.

The **G-1 period** (G stands for gap) extends from the completion of the previous cell division to the beginning of DNA duplication prior to the next division. During the G-1 period the cell grows and synthesizes new proteins (differentiation).

The **S period** (S stands for synthesis) follows and covers the time in which new DNA synthesis occurs.

The **G-2 period** extends from the end of DNA synthesis to the beginning of actual cell division.

The **M period** (M stands for mitosis) is the time of actual cell division whereby two identical daughter cells are produced.

Figure 20–4 shows the periods in the cell cycle and the approximate lengths of time of each period in a hypothetical 24-hour growth cycle. The time it takes for a cell to complete its growth cycle is called the **generation time**.

G-1	=	9.5 hours
S	=	10.5 hours
G-2	=	3. hours
M	=	1. hour
		24 hours

Figure 20-4   Periods in a 24-hour growth cycle of a cell.

Is there a difference in the growth cycle of a cancer cell and that of a normal cell of one particular type of tissue? Scientists have found that there is often a shortening of the G-1 time in a cancerous cell in relation to the G-1 time of its normal cell type. Thus, normal hepatocytes have a longer G-1 time than their malignant counterparts. It has been shown that the length of time that a cell remains in the G-1 period prior to DNA replication determines the frequency of cell division. Longer G-1 periods (giving the cell time to grow and properly differentiate) mean slower reproductive rates; and shorter G-1 periods diminish the time for growth and differentiation and increase the reproductive rate.

Cancer cells, which have short G-1 periods, are thus produced at a faster rate than they are lost, and the cells that are produced lack the functions of the normally differentiated cells of their type.

VII. COMBINING FORMS AND TERMINOLOGY

Combining Form	Definition	Terminology	Meaning
kary/o	nucleus	karyotype _____	
nucle/o	nucleus	nucleoprotein _____	
		nucleotide _____	
mut/a	mutation, genetic change	mutagenesis _____	
bol/o	to cast or throw	anabolism _____	
		catabolism _____	
		metabolism _____	
som/o	body	somatic cells _____	
rib/o	sugar	ribosome _____	

		deoxyribose _____
chrom/o	color	hyperchromatic _____
		chromosome _____
mit/o	thread	mitochondria _____
		mitosis _____
prote/o	first, protein	proteolysis _____
		protein _____
zym/o	leavening agent, catalyst	enzyme _____
		zymolysis _____

VIII. EXERCISES

A. *Match the following cellular structures with their function in the cell:*

1. chromosomes

2. granular endoplasmic reticulum

3. nuclear membrane

4. mitochondria

5. nucleolus

_____ structures in cytoplasm where molecules are broken down to produce energy.

_____ site of ribosome synthesis within the nucleus.

_____ contains genes which are segments on a DNA molecule.

_____ site of protein synthesis in cell.

_____ surrounds nucleus and allows materials to pass in and out of the nucleus.

B. *Match each term in Column I with an appropriate definition in Column II:*

Column I

1. self-replication

2. differentiation

Column II

_____ tiny granules on an endoplasmic reticulum.

_____ large protein molecules which aid in chemical reactions.

3. anabolism

4. metabolism

_____ duplication of DNA material within the nucleus of a cell.

5. catabolism

_____ process of cell division whereby two identical daughter cells are produced from a single parent cell.

6. enzymes

7. ribosomes

_____ specialization.

8. amino acids

_____ sum total of all chemical reactions in the cell.

9. helical

_____ spiral-shaped.

10. mitosis

_____ breaking-down and energy-releasing process in the cell.

_____ simple molecules which are the building blocks of proteins.

_____ building-up or synthesizing process in the cell.

C. *Give the meaning of the following medical terms:*

1. mRNA _____

_____

2. DNA _____

_____

3. purine _____

4. pyrimidine _____

5. template _____

6. genetic code _____

_____

7. generation time _____

_____

8. karyotype _____

D. *Name the bases in DNA and explain how they pair up in the double-stranded molecule of DNA:*

_____

_____

_____

E. *Give two important functions of DNA in the cell:*

_____

_____

_____

_____

F. *What is a mutation, and how might it cause a cell to become cancerous?*

_____

_____

_____

_____

_____

G. *Name the bases in RNA. How is mRNA formed, and what is its function?*

_____

_____

_____

_____

_____

_____

H. *Name the phases in the growth cycle of a cell and explain what occurs during each phase:*

_____

_____

_____

_____

_____

_____

I. *Does a cancerous cell of a specific type have a longer or shorter G-1 period? How does this explain its abnormal characteristics of dedifferentiation and fast rate of reproduction?*

_____

_____

_____

_____

_____

_____

ANSWERS

A. 4
5
1
2
3

B. 7   4
6   9
1   5
10   8
2   3

C. 1. Messenger RNA. This molecule is formed or copied from a molecule of DNA in the nucleus of the cell. It carries hereditary information to the protein-making region of the cell where it dictates the type of proteins manufactured by the cell.
2. Deoxyribonucleic acid. This large molecule is found in the nucleus and contains the hereditary information which controls the activities of the cell.
3. Compound which is part of nucleic acid. Purine bases in DNA are adenine and guanine.
4. Compound which is part of nucleic acid. Pyrimidines in DNA are thymine and cytosine.
5. A mold or form from which another substance is copied.

6. The information which is transferred from the DNA molecules in the nucleus to the protein-making machinery in the cytoplasm. The information determines the sequence of amino acids needed for protein synthesis.
7. The time it takes a cell to divide, grow, and differentiate before dividing again; the time it takes a cell to complete its growth cycle.
8. The configuration of chromosomes in the nucleus of the cell.

D. DNA bases are: adenine, guanine, cytosine, thymine. Adenine always pairs with thymine, and guanine always pairs with cytosine.

E. DNA can replicate itself exactly so that copies of the hereditary material within a parent cell are passed on to daughter cells. Also, DNA can direct the synthesis of amino acids in the cytoplasm, thereby controlling the differentiation and protein-making process in the cell.

F. A mutation is any change in the genetic material of the cell. If, for instance, the base sequence in DNA is altered in any way (by viruses, chemicals, or radiation, or spontaneously), the genetic information that the cell needs to make proteins or replicate itself would obviously be different from the normal, and might lead to a cancerous growth of cells.

G. RNA bases are: adenine, cytosine, guanine, uracil. mRNA is formed or copied from a strand of DNA according to the specific base sequence in DNA. mRNA carries the base sequence (genetic code) to the endoplasmic reticulum (protein-making machinery) in the cytoplasm and specific amino acids arrange to form proteins according to the base sequence on the mRNA.

H. G-1 = period between the end of the last cell division and the beginning of new DNA synthesis in preparation for the next cell division. Time of cell growth and differentiation.
S = period of DNA synthesis.
G-2 = period between DNA synthesis and beginning of actual cell division.
M = period of cell division or mitosis.

I. A cancerous cell has a shorter G-1 period in its growth cycle. A shorter G-1 period means less time for growth and differentiation (cancerous cells are usually poorly differentiated) and also faster reproductive rate since the cell division period would occur more frequently.

REVIEW SHEET 20

Combining Forms

bol/o _____   nucle/o _____

chrom/o _____   prote/o _____

kary/o _____   rib/o _____

mit/o _____   som/o _____

mut/a _____   zym/o _____

Additional Terminology

adenine _____

amino acids _____

anabolism _____

bases _____

catabolism _____

chromosomes _____

contact inhibition _____

cytoplasm _____

cytosine _____

DNA _____

differentiation _____

endoplasmic reticulum _____

enzyme _____

G-1 period _____

G-2 period _____

generation time _____

genes _____

genetic code _____

growth cycle _____

guanine _____

helical _____

M period _____

mRNA _____

metabolism _____

mitochondria _____

mitosis _____

mutation _____

nucleic acids _____

nucleolus _____

nucleotide _____

nucleus _____

proteins _____

purine _____

pyrimidine _____

replication _____

RNA _____

ribosomes _____

S period _____

template   _____

thymine   _____

tRNA   _____

uracil   _____

CHAPTER 21

CANCER MEDICINE III: ETIOLOGY AND TREATMENT OF CANCER

In this chapter you will:

Recognize the terms which apply to the various etiological theories of cancer: heredity, radiation, chemicals, and viruses;

Investigate medical terms which relate to current methods of cancer treatment: surgery, radiotherapy, and chemotherapy; and

Become familiar with combining forms which apply to carcinogenesis and cancer therapy.

This chapter is divided into the following sections:

I. INTRODUCTION

The investigations into the etiology of cancer (**carcinogenesis**) represent one of the most perplexing areas of research for the modern scientist. As we have discussed in the previous chapter, in all probability the answers to the mystery of carcinogenesis lie in the functioning of molecules of DNA and RNA within the nuclei of normal and cancerous cells. However, it is likely that agents from the environment, such as radiation, chemicals and drugs, and different types of viruses, may produce cancer by initiating changes in the hereditary material (DNA) in a cell. While the mechanism of this process is at present unclear, it is hoped that in the future better understanding of neoplastic transformations will lead to the development of vaccines or other measures which will prevent the carcinogenic process. Section II of this chapter explores the terminology related to some of the possible etiological factors contributing to cancerous growths.

In the absence of specific information regarding the etiology of human cancer, present medical efforts are directed primarily at treating established cancer disease. The object of treatment is to remove or kill as many cancerous cells as possible without harmful or toxic effects to normal cells. It is an irony, perhaps, that the same type of agents, such as radiation and certain chemicals and drugs, which may be responsible for malignant transformations are also useful in the treatment of cancer. Section III investigates terminology related to the various types of cancer treatment.

II. ETIOLOGY OF CANCER

A. Vocabulary

alkylating agents	Chemical compounds which add an alkyl (CH_3CH_2Cl) group to other molecules. They are highly reactive and are carcinogenic.
aromatic amines	Carcinogenic chemicals which contain a nitrogen molecule attached to a ring of carbon atoms. Aromatic amines are found as by-products of industrial and natural chemical processes.
aromatic hydrocarbons	Chemicals which contain hydrogen and carbon. These compounds, which are often carcinogenic, are found as a by-product of coal combustion, cigarette smoking, and other chemical reactions.
arsenicals	Carcinogenic compounds containing arsenic (a poisonous element).
asbestos	A carcinogen which is found in pipe insulation and shipbuilding equipment.
benzpyrene	A compound which comes from tobacco smoke and is believed to be an agent causing lung cancer.

Burkitt's lymphoma	A malignant cancer of the lymph glands found predominantly in tropical Africa. This tumor is thought to be caused by a specific virus.
carcinoembryonic antigen (CEA)	A unique protein antigen found in the patient's bloodstream in a wide variety of cancers.
culture	Growing microorganisms or cells in a growth medium (food) in the laboratory.
diethylstilbestrol (DES)	An estrogen compound which was formerly used to prevent miscarriage during pregnancy, but which is now known to cause cancer in female offspring exposed to the drug during their mothers' pregnancy.
host cell	A living cell which is invaded by a parasite such as a virus.
inert	Not active.
in vitro	In glass; refers to an experiment performed in a laboratory with isolated biological materials or chemicals.
in vivo	In life; refers to an experiment performed in a whole, living animal.
ionizing radiation	Energy given off by radioactive atoms and x-rays. This type of radiation can be carcinogenic.
latent	Hidden, concealed, dormant.
mutation	Change in genetic material which is potentially capable of being transmitted to offspring and which can produce changes in structure and function of cells and tissue.
nonionizing radiation	Energy given off by the sun (ultraviolet rays). This type of radiation may be carcinogenic.
oncogenic DNA and RNA viruses	Those viruses composed of DNA and protein or RNA and protein which produce cancer in laboratory animals.
Pap test	Cytological examination of the lining of the cervix to diagnose cervical carcinoma (named for a man named Papanicolaou).

parasite

An organism that lives within or at the expense of another organism (host). Viruses are parasites of host cells.

polyposis coli syndrome

Hereditary malignant neoplasms in the colon and rectum.

retinoblastoma

Tumor of the retina which is thought to be caused by mutation (genetic change) in the egg and sperm cells which produce the embryo.

RNA reverse transcriptase

An enzyme which is found in oncogenic RNA viruses. This enzyme is thought to help in translating the genetic code information in reverse fashion from viral RNA to the DNA of the host cell. The enzyme is also called RNA-dependent DNA polymerase.

vinyl chloride

A carcinogen found in industrial sprays and chemicals.

virion

Virus; a minute microorganism which is parasitic and dependent on nutrients from host cells for growth and reproduction.

xeroderma pigmentosum

Hereditary malignant skin neoplasm caused by inability of DNA in skin cells to repair itself after damage by ultraviolet radiation.

B. Heredity

Some forms of cancer are transmitted from parents to offspring through defects in the DNA of germinal cells (egg and sperm cells). If the genetic apparatus (DNA) of an egg or sperm cell carries a carcinogenic change, or cancerous **mutation**, the mutation can be transmitted through the mutated germinal (germ) cell to the resulting offspring, who would be predisposed to cancer. The mutation is usually the result of the loss of genetic information for making a specific protein needed to maintain the structure and function of DNA itself.

This theory of carcinogenesis is supported by work with experimental animals and by knowledge of certain inherited cancers in man. Examples of known inherited cancers in man are retinoblastoma, polyposis coli syndrome, and xeroderma pigmentosum.

Retinoblastoma is a tumor of the retina of the eye. It is frequently an inherited disorder, and most of its victims are very young children. In most cases, the removal of the affected eye is indicated to prevent spread of tumor cells. It is known that individuals who survive the cancerous lesion in childhood have an almost 50 per cent chance of passing it on to their offspring.

Xeroderma pigmentosum is an inherited condition which causes extreme sensitivity to sunlight and predisposes the individual to the development of many cutaneous neoplasms early in life. The genetic mutation in this disorder appears to prevent the repair of DNA which becomes damaged by the ultraviolet rays of the sun.

Polyposis coli syndrome is a neoplastic condition consisting of the growth of numerous polyps in the colon and rectum. Its occurrence is definitely inherited in families and has a frequency of about 1 in 8000 live births, or approximately 500 cases per year. The polyps become cancerous with advancing age.

C. Chemicals and Drugs

A large, rapidly growing list of chemical carcinogens is known. It is thought that the chemical carcinogens act on normal cells in a **mutagenic** manner. The chemical or drug might alter the structure of a gene (DNA) in such a way that the normal control mechanisms for cell growth are disrupted and cells begin to grow in a cancerous or uncontrolled manner. In one type of cancer—leukemia—animal studies have shown that a chemical carcinogen can activate a **dormant**, or **latent**, virus in the cell. The virus might then cause changes in the DNA of the cell, which would lead to a malignant cellular transformation.

A partial list of chemicals and drugs known to be inducers of cancer follows:

Chemicals or Drugs	Examples	Carcinogenic Effect
aromatic hydrocarbons (chemicals containing hydrogen and carbon in a ring or circular configuration)	soots, pitch, coat tar, **benzpyrene** (found in cigarette, cigar, and pipe smoke, and automobile exhaust)	produce cancer of the lung, skin cancer, leukemia, and scrotal carcinoma in laboratory animals and man
alkylating agents (compounds which add an alkyl group to DNA)	mustard gas, melphalan, busulfan	produce leukemia in laboratory animals
aromatic amines (aromatic compounds containing nitrogen and hydrocarbons)	naphthylamine, nitrous amines, butter yellow (previously used to color margarine)	produce liver cancer in rodents and bladder cancer in dogs
vinyl chloride, asbestos, and **arsenicals**	sprays, metals, industrial chemicals, and their products	produce epithelial tumors and lung tumors in man
diethylstilbestrol (DES)	estrogen compound	produces vaginal carcinoma in female offspring of women who have taken the drug during that pregnancy

D. Radiation

The term **radiation** refers to the energy given off by the atoms of specific substances. Cells can become cancerous when they are exposed to the effects of either ionizing radiation or nonionizing radiation.

Ionizing radiation consists of small particles, or fragments, given off by radioactive atoms and x-rays. The radiation causes the production of **ions**, or charged atoms, which can lead to the conversion of a normal cell into a cancerous one by affecting the DNA in the cell nucleus. There are many examples of the damaging effect of ionizing radiation. Leukemia is an occupational hazard of radiologists who are exposed to x-rays routinely. There is also a high incidence of leukemia among the survivors of the atomic bomb destructions in Nagasaki and Hiroshima. Partial body irradiation may also be leukemogenic when a large area of hematopoietic tissue is irradiated. Examples of this are observed in adults irradiated for spondylitis (inflammation of the vertebrae) and in children who are irradiated for enlarged glands in the mediastinum (region within the thoracic cavity).

Nonionizing radiation refers to the invisible, ultraviolet rays given off by the sun. These rays may be carcinogenic, especially to persons with lightly pigmented, or fair, skin.

While we do not know the mechanism by which radiation exerts its carcinogenic effect, several hypotheses have been suggested. One is that the radiation may cause changes in the structure of chromosomes, which impair the normal functioning of the cell. This is illustrated in a form of leukemia in which part of a chromosome is characteristically missing in all tumor cells. Another hypothesis is that the radiation produces a mutation in a part of a gene which regulates only the cell division process for the cell, transforming the cell into a cancerous one. A third hypothesis centers around the theory that radiation weakens the resistance of a cell to invasion by a cancer-producing virus, or activates a **latent** (concealed) cellular virus which may cause the cellular transformation.

E. Viruses

Investigations into the understanding of the etiological role (if any) of viruses in human carcinogenesis represent one of the most challenging aspects of current cancer research. Although viruses have been shown to cause cancer in many laboratory animals, there is at present no conclusive evidence that they cause human cancer. Also, it is important to remember that viruses are **not** thought to transmit cancers in the typical pattern seen with infectious diseases such as measles, chickenpox, mumps, and upper respiratory illness.

A **virus**, also called a **virion**, is a minute, electronmicroscopic particle consisting of one or more molecules of either DNA or RNA and covered by a protein coat. The viruses which contain DNA are known as DNA viruses, and those which contain only RNA are called RNA viruses. Figure 21–1 illustrates the structure of a virus.

A virus particle possesses no cytoplasm or structures, such as mitochondria and ribosomes. It cannot carry on essential life functions, such as anabolism and catabolism, on its own. Thus, when floating in the air and in the environment, it exists in an **inert, dormant** (inactive) state.

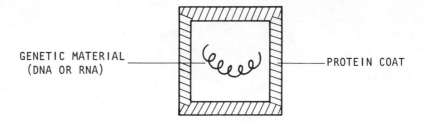

GENETIC MATERIAL
(DNA OR RNA) ———————————— PROTEIN COAT

Figure 21-1 Structure of a virus.

Viruses grow and multiply themselves only when they have invaded living cells. They are cell **parasites**. Figure 21–2 shows the interaction between a **DNA virus** (1) and a **host cell** (2) which it has invaded. As the virus invades the host cell it loses its **protein coat** (3) and injects its **genetic material (DNA)** (4) into the nucleus of the host cell. This viral DNA material can then be replicated (5) within the host cell by using the raw materials of the host cell. In addition, the viral DNA can make **mRNA** (messenger RNA) (6), which is capable of entering the cytoplasm of the host cell and directing the production of **new protein coats** (7) for newly replicated DNA viral material (8). It is possible, as well, for the viral DNA to be integrated into the **host cell DNA** (9) and make **new protein antigens** (10) which can influence the metabolism and functioning of the host cell so that it is transformed into an abnormal cell type.

Various techniques can be used to identify viruses. An electron microscope (EM) can visualize suspected oncogenic viruses. *In vitro* cell culture experiments (growing colonies of tumor cells on laboratory plates or in test tubes) provide another method of watching the growth of viral tumors. In cell culture, the presence of an oncogenic virus can be detected by the formation of small tumors and multilayered cells.

Immunologic and biochemical tests are also used to detect viruses, as well as any antiviral antibodies which may be formed when they invade host cells. Some cells when they become cancerous produce a specific protein antigen whose presence can be detected in the bloodstream; one of these antigens is called **carcinoembryonic antigen**, or **CEA**.

In vitro and *in vivo* (within living organisms) experiments with laboratory animals have shown that certain DNA and RNA viruses can cause cancer in mammals (warm-blooded animals with backbones). Some **oncogenic DNA viruses** which have been investigated are listed below:

Polyoma virus

Occurs naturally in adult mice, and when injected into newborn rodents (mice or rats) produces tumors.

SV-40
 (simian vacuolating virus)

Isolated from Rhesus monkey kidney cells. When injected into newborn hamsters it produces sarcomas.

Adenoviruses

These are human viruses which cause cancer in other mammals. They can cause acute respiratory disease, but are not oncogenic, in man.

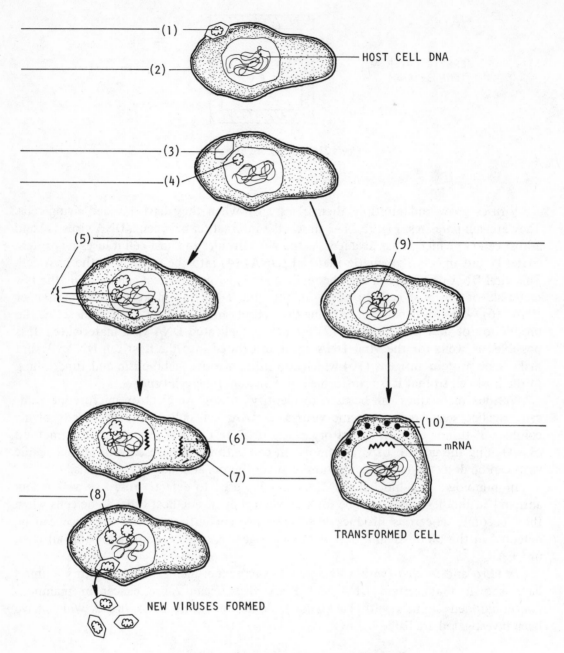

HOST CELL DNA

TRANSFORMED CELL

NEW VIRUSES FORMED

Figure 21-2 Interaction of virus with a host cell.

Herpes virus

These viruses have been isolated from renal carcinoma cells of leopard frogs and are oncogenic when injected into tadpoles. They can produce leukemia in owl monkeys and marmosets.

Epstein-Barr virus
(EBV)

This virus is found in **Burkitt's lymphoma** cells that are grown in **culture** (on a glass plate or test tube in the laboratory). Burkitt's lymphoma is a type of lymphatic cancer found predominantly in children (ages 2 to 14), with high incidence of occurrence in tropical West Africa, New Guinea, and Papua.

The oncogenic **RNA viruses** have RNA genetic material within their nuclei instead of DNA. Recently, an enzyme called **RNA reverse transcriptase**, also called **RNA-dependent DNA polymerase**, has been found in all oncogenic RNA viruses but not in most nononcogenic RNA viruses. It is thought that the enzyme enables viral RNA to serve as a model for making new DNA strands in a host cell which has been invaded by an RNA virus. These new DNA strands, whose production was directed by the viral RNA and its enzyme RNA reverse transcriptase, can then produce proteins in the host cell which may lead to abnormal cell tumor growth.

Figure 21–3 summarizes the various etiological factors in carcinogenesis.

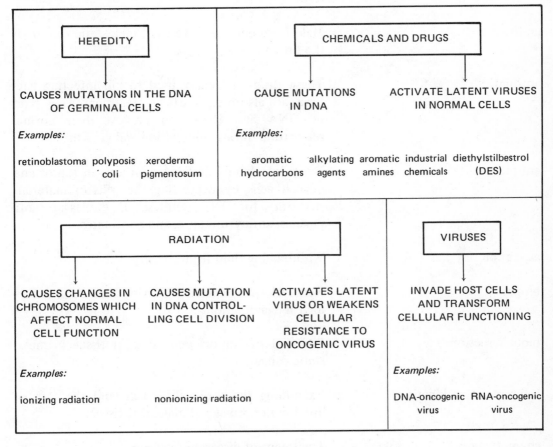

Figure 21-3 Etiological factors in carcinogenesis.

III. TREATMENT OF CANCER

The three major approaches to cancer treatment are **surgery**, **radiotherapy**, and **chemotherapy**. Each method may be used alone but often they are coordinated in the total treatment of the cancer patient. The specific medical terms relating to each of these treatment areas will be discussed in the sections following the vocabulary list.

A. Vocabulary

alkylating agents	Compounds which add an alkyl chemical group to other molecules. They are highly reactive chemicals and are used in cancer chemotherapy. Examples are melphalan, chlorambucil, and nitrogen mustard.
androgens	Male hormones used to treat metastatic cancer of the breast.
antibiotics	These drugs, normally used to kill infecting bacteria, are also used in cancer treatment. They bind to DNA and RNA and prevent their normal replication during cell division and growth.
antimetabolites	Drugs which inhibit DNA synthesis in tumor and normal cells by depressing the cells of materials necessary for DNA synthesis. Examples are antipurines, antipyrimidines, and antifolates.
aspiration	Withdrawing fluid from a cavity.
biopsy	Removal of a segment of living tissue for pathological examination.
block resection	Removal of tumors and adjacent tissue in metastatic cancer.
cell population kinetics	Examining the way cells divide and the rate of division in normal and malignant tissue.
chemotherapy	Treatment of disease using drugs.
combination chemotherapy	Use of two or more drugs in combination as antitumor treatment.
corticoids	Hormones from the adrenal cortex. Used to treat lymphomas and leukemia.

cryosurgery	Operative procedure using extremely cold temperatures to freeze tissue.
electrocautery	Use of an electric probe to burn tissue.
estrogens	Female hormones used to treat cancer of the prostate gland in males and breast cancer in females over 65.
excisional biopsy	Diagnostic surgery to remove a tumor.
exfoliative cytology	Scraping cells from tissue to examine them for diagnosis of cancer.
fractionation	Giving radiotherapy in short, fractional doses.
germinal cells	Egg cells or sperm cells.
growth fraction	Percentage of cells in a tissue which are going through cell division.
lethal	Producing death.
local excision	Surgical procedure to remove a small area of tumor.
modality	A method of cancer treatment, such as surgery or radiation.
myelosuppression	Decreasing bone marrow function by means of chemicals or radiation.
needle biopsy	Insertion of a needle into a tumor or organ to remove a core of tissue or fluid for diagnosis.
nonresponsive tumor	A tumor which is not severely damaged by drug therapy. These tumors often have a low growth rate.
pharmacokinetics	The study of the distribution and removal of drugs in the body over an extended period of time.
radiocurable tumor	A tumor which can be completely eradicated by radiation therapy.
radioresistant tumor	A tumor which requires very large doses of radiation to produce death of cells.

radiosensitive tumor	A tumor which is easily killed by radiation with little effect on surrounding normal tissue.
radiotherapy	Treatment of disease using radiation.
responsive tumor	A tumor which will be killed by drug therapy. These tumors often have a high growth rate.
surgery	Branch of medicine dealing with manual operative procedures (excision, incision, and so forth).

B. Surgery

In potentially curable cancer patients, when the tumor is localized and has not spread beyond the regional lymph nodes, surgical excision may offer an effective means of cure. The tumor, plus a margin of normal tissue, is removed.

Some common cancers in which surgery may be curative are those of the stomach, lower esophagus, large and small bowel, bone, breast, and endometrium.

The following is a list of terms used in describing surgical procedures in diagnosis as well as treatment of malignant diseases:

1. **Excisional Biopsy.** With very small tumors, removal of the tumor and a margin of normal tissue provides both a specimen for diagnosis and cure at the same time. This procedure is used for small tumors of the skin or subcutaneous tissue.

2. `Incisional Biopsy. In this procedure the tumor is cut into, and a piece of it is removed for examination to establish the diagnosis. The procedure is used if excisional biopsy would create an unnecessary major defect (cosmetic, emotional, or social), or if x-ray therapy is to be used to treat the tumor.

3. **Needle Biopsy.** This procedure involves plunging a needle through the skin into the cancerous tissue or organ to obtain a sample for biopsy. It is frequently used for patients who have incurable malignant lesions. Liver nodules and bone marrow are the most common sites for needle biopsy, although it is also used in lymph nodes, lung, and breast. Inserting a needle to withdraw (aspirate) free cells from a fluid-filled cavity is another form of needle biopsy.

4. **Exfoliative Cytology.** This procedure involves scraping cells from the region of suspected disease and examining the cells under a microscope. The **Pap test**, to detect carcinoma of the cervix, is an example of how this procedure is applied.

5. **Local Excision.** Cancers of low-grade malignancy can be managed by local excision if metastases to lymph nodes occur rarely (basal cell carcinoma and squamous cell carcinoma are examples).

6. **Block Resection.** Tumors which metastasize to regional lymph nodes generally require dissection of a large area of tumor and surrounding tissues containing affected lymph nodes. The surgeon usually starts with the nodes farthest from the tumor and dissects toward the primary tumor. Radical mastectomy, gastrectomy, and colectomy are examples of this procedure.

7. **Special Surgical Techniques.** **Cryosurgery** in the nervous system and urogenital tract is effective in freezing malignant tissue. **Electrocautery** is used to burn the malignant tissue in carcinomas of the rectum.

C. Radiotherapy

The goal of radiotherapy is to delivery a maximal dose of ionizing radiation to the tumor tissue and a minimal dose to normal tissue in the region of the tumor. In reality, this goal is difficult to obtain and usually one accepts a degree of residual normal cell damage as a sequel to destruction of the **lethal** (fatal) tumor. The effect of the high-dose radiation to cells is to break up the DNA molecules and stop the functioning of the cell.

Some terms used in the medical field of radiation therapy for cancer are listed below:

1. **Radiosensitive Tumor.** A tumor in which irradiation can cause acute loss of cells or hypoplasia without damage to surrounding vascular or interstitial tissue. Hematopoietic and lymphopoietic tissues are the most radiosensitive tumor tissues.

2. **Radioresistant Tumor.** A tumor which requires large doses of radiation to produce acute loss or atrophy of tumor cells and in which the results of radiation are usually associated with its effect on surrounding structures (vessels and interstitial cells) rather than with its direct effects on the tumor tissue. Connective tissues are the most radioresistant tumor tissues.

3. **Radiocurable Tumor.** A tumor that can be completely eradicated by radiation therapy. Radiocurable tumors are usually localized tumors with no metastases. Examples are Hodgkin's disease and lymphomas.

4. **Fractionation.** The method of giving radiotherapy in short, fractional doses. This procedure allows larger doses to be given to tumor tissue without damaging normal tissue.

D. Cancer Chemotherapy

Cancer chemotherapy is the treatment of cancer using drugs. It is probably the most important factor responsible for long-term survival in several types of cancer (Burkitt's lymphoma, choriocarcinoma, acute lymphocytic leukemia, Hodgkin's disease, and others). Chemotherapy may be used alone or in conjunction with the other methods, or **modalities**, of cancer treatment, such as radiation and surgery.

Studies of **cell population kinetics** (what happens to a cell during cell division and how fast groups of cells are dividing in a total tissue mass) are important in understanding how to use drugs to treat cancer. These studies provide information on the rate of cell division in normal and cancerous tissue.

The term used to describe the percentage of cells in a tissue which are progressing through the process of **mitosis** (cell division) is **growth fraction**. A high tumor growth fraction means that a large percentage of tumor cells are in the process of dividing. A large growth fraction also means that the cells which are proliferating are going through active DNA synthesis as a prelude to mitosis. Because most antitumor drugs have their major killing effect during and against DNA synthesis, a tumor with a large growth fraction (more cell division and more DNA synthesis) will be more seriously damaged by these drugs than will a low growth fraction tumor. A highly **responsive tumor** is one which will be killed by drugs, while a **nonresponsive tumor** is not significantly affected by drug treatment.

The field of **pharmacokinetics** represents the study of drugs and their effect on cell division of normal and tumor tissue. Obviously, the ideal is to develop drugs which kill large numbers of tumor cells without harming normal cells. Because some normal tissue cells, such as bone marrow and gastrointestinal lining cells, have large growth fractions, they will suffer a great deal from antitumor drugs. Scientists working in the field of pharmacokinetics of cancer chemotherapy are interested in the proper design of drug dosages, concentrations, and schedules of administration, so that they can achieve the greatest tumor kill with the least toxicity to normal cells.

Combination chemotherapy refers to the use of two or more antitumor drugs together to kill a specific type of malignant growth. In chemotherapy, drugs are given according to a written **protocol**, or plan which details exactly how the drugs will be given. Usually drug therapy is continued until the patient achieves a complete **remission**, which is the absence of all signs of disease. At times, chemotherapy is given as an **adjuvant** to surgery. This means that the drugs are used to kill possible hidden disease in patients who are otherwise free of any evidence of malignancy.

The list below gives the general categories of cancer chemotherapeutic agents, how they are thought to act to kill tumor cells, toxic side effects which may accompany their use, names of specific antitumor drugs, and the type of cancer against which the drug is effective:

1. **Alkylating Agents.** These are man-made compounds containing two or more chemical groups called alkyl groups ($CH_2 CH_2 Cl$). Alkylating agents interfere directly with the process of DNA synthesis by preventing new DNA molecules from forming properly. Side effects include nausea and vomiting, diarrhea, bone marrow depression (myelosuppression), which leads to lack of production of blood cells, and alopecia (baldness). These are common side effects because the cells in the gastrointestinal tract, bone marrow, and scalp are rapidly dividing cells (high growth fraction) which, along with tumor cells, are susceptible to the lethal effects of chemotherapeutic drugs. The side effects disappear after treatment is suspended.

Drug	*Type of Cancer It Is Used to Treat*
Nitrogen mustard	lymphomas
Chlorambucil (Leukeran)	myeloma and chronic lymphocytic leukemia
Cyclophosphamide (Cytoxan)	Burkitt's lymphoma, neuroblastoma
Phenylalanine mustard (PAM, melphalan)	myeloma and breast cancer

2. **Antimetabolites.** These drugs inhibit the synthesis of substances which are necessary for the replication of DNA. Substances necessary for the synthesis of DNA are **folic acid, purines,** and **pyrimidines.** Thus, the antimetabolite drugs which are effective in stopping cell division in this manner are called **antifolates, antipurines,** and **antipyrimidines.** Side effects are myelosuppression, with leukopenia, thrombocytopenia, and bleeding; and oral and digestive tract toxicity, including stomatitis, nausea, and vomiting.

Drug	*Type of Cancer It Is Used to Treat*
Methotrexate (MTX)	acute leukemia and choriocarcinoma (malignancy of embryonic tissue in the uterus)
6-Mercaptopurine (6-MP)	acute leukemia
5-Fluorouracil (5-FU)	breast cancer and colon cancer
Cytosine arabinoside (Ara-C)	leukemia

3. **Hormones.** It is known that the growth of some tumors (breast and prostate) is accelerated or depressed by specific hormones. By changing the body hormonal status, it is possible to ·inhibit tumor growth. Fluid retention, masculinization, feminization, nausea, and vomiting are some possible side effects of the hormonal drug use.

Drug	*Type of Cancer It Is Used to Treat*
Estrogens (female hormones)—diethylstilbestrol (DES)	prostate cancer, and breast cancer in women over 65
Androgens (male hormones)—testosterone propionate (TP)	metastatic breast cancer
Progestins (female hormone)—hydroxyprogesterone (Delalutin)	adenocarcinoma of the endometrium
Corticoids (adrenal cortex hormone)—prednisone	acute lymphocytic leukemia and lymphoma

4. **Antibiotics.** These drugs bind to DNA and RNA in the cell and prevent their replication, leading to decreased cell division and death of tumor cells. Toxic effects from their use include alopecia, stomatitis, myelosuppression, and gastrointestinal disturbances.

Drug	*Type of Cancer It Is Used to Treat*
Adriamycin, daunomycin	
Bleomycin	childhood tumors,
	leukemia, sarcomas,
Actinomycin D	and solid tumors
Mithramycin	

5. **Miscellaneous Drugs.** Most of these drugs cause myelosuppression as well as nausea and vomiting.

Drug	Type of Cancer It Is Used to Treat
L-Asparaginase	acute lymphoblastic leukemia
Bischloroethylnitrosourea (BCNU)	brain tumors, Hodgkin's disease, lymphomas
Procarbazine (Matulane)	Hodgkin's disease and ovarian cancer
Vinblastine (Velban)	Hodgkin's disease, choriocarcinoma, and breast cancer
Vincristine (Oncovin)	Hodgkin's disease, acute lymphocytic leukemia, breast cancer, lymphomas, and Wilms' tumor

6. **Drug Combinations**

Abbreviation	Drugs	Type of Cancer It Is Used to Treat
MOPP	Nitrogen mustard, Oncovin, prednisone, procarbazine.	Hodgkin's disease
POMP	Prednisone, Oncovin, methotrexate, 6-mercaptopurine	acute leukemia
CVP or COP	Cytoxin, Oncovin (vincristine), prednisone	lymphoma
CMF	Cytoxin, methotrexate, 5-fluorouracil	breast cancer

Figure 21–4 reviews the major methods of cancer treatment.

IV. COMBINING FORMS

Combining Form	Definition	Terminology	Meaning
mut/a	change, mutation	mutagen _____	
retin/o	retina of the eye	retinoblastoma _____	
germ/o	sprout, seed	germinal cell _____	
carcin/o	cancer	carcinogenesis _____	
onc/o	tumor, mass	oncogenesis _____	

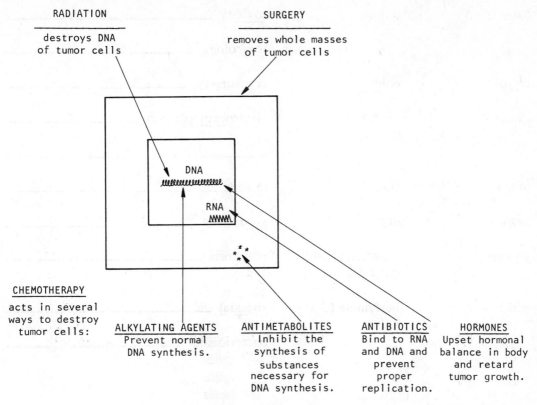

Figure 21-4 Treatment of cancer.

ion/o	charged particles, ions	ionic _____
		ionizing _____
radi/o	rays, x-rays	radiotherapy _____
		radioresistant _____
		radiosensitive _____
vir/o	virus, poison	virology _____
		virion _____
		viremia _____
chem/o	drug, chemical	chemotherapy _____
pharmac/o	drugs, chemicals	pharmacology _____
tox/o	poison	toxemia _____

toxic/o	poison	toxicity _____
		toxicology _____
cry/o	cold	cryosurgery _____
cauter/o	heat, burn	electrocauterization _____
		_____
mit/o	thread	mitosis _____
xer/o	dry	xeroderma _____
polyp/o	growths, usually on stalks	polyposis _____
-cidal	pertaining to killing	viricidal _____
		bacteriocidal _____

V. EXERCISES

A. *Give the meanings of the following medical terms:*

1. germinal _____

2. retinoblastoma _____

3. latent _____

4. lethal _____

5. culture _____

6. mitosis _____

7. antibiotics _____

8. parasite _____

9. *in vitro* _____

10. host cell _____

B. *Match the CARCINOGENS in Column I with an associated term in Column II:*

Column I	*Column II*
1. ionizing radiation	_____ estrogen compound; diethylstilbestrol.
2. alkylating agents	_____ virus from rhesus monkey kidney cells; produces sarcomas in baby hamsters.
3. spontaneous genetic mutation	_____ benzpyrene (found in cigarette, cigar, and pipe smoke).
4. DES	_____ ultraviolet light from the sun.
5. aromatic hydrocarbons	_____ carcinogenic compounds containing nitrogen attached to a carbon ring.
6. nonionizing radiation	
7. aromatic amines	_____ change in DNA molecule in sex cells.
8. SV-40	_____ x-rays and radioactive substances.
	_____ highly reactive carcinogenic compound which adds an alkyl group to DNA. Mustard gas is an example.

C. *Build medical terms:*

1. The originating of tumors _____

2. Abnormal condition of polyps _____

3. The study of poisons _____

4. Viruses in the blood _____

5. Pertaining to killing bacteria _____

6. Pertaining to treatment with drugs _____

D. *Give the meaning of the following medical terms:*

1. virion _____

2. RNA reverse transcriptase _____

_____

3. xeroderma pigmentosum _____

_____

4. arsenical _____

5. Burkitt's lymphoma _____

_____

6. aspiration _____

7. pharmacokinetics _____

8. growth fraction _____

9. combination chemotherapy _____

10. antimetabolite _____

_____

E. *Match the abbreviation in Column I with an associated term in Column II:*

Column I   *Column II*

1. CEA   _____   deoxyribonucleic acid

2. EBV   _____   5-fluorouracil

3. DNA   _____   cytosine arabinoside

4. 5-FU   _____   carcinoembryonic antigen

5. RNA   _____   6-mercaptopurine

6. ARA-C   _____   Epstein-Barr virus

7. 6-MP   _____   bischloroethylnitrosourea

8. BCNU   _____   ribonucleic acid

F. *Give the meanings for the following terms:*

1. radiocurable tumor _____

2. radiosensitive tumor _____

3. fractionation _____

4. radioresistant tumor _____

G. *Match the surgical procedure for cancer diagnosis and treatment in Column I with a closely associated term in Column II:*

Column I	Column II
1. needle biopsy	_____ removal of tumor and a margin of normal tissue for diagnosis.
2. block dissection	_____ burning lesion to kill cells.
3. incisional biopsy	_____ scraping of cells to examine for cancerous changes.
4. excisional biopsy	
5. exfoliative cytology	_____ removal of entire tumor and regional lymph nodes.
6. cryosurgery	_____ freezing lesion to kill cells.
7. electrocautery	_____ aspiration of fluid from tumor.
	_____ cutting into tumor to remove section for diagnosis.

H. *Tell whether the following chemotherapeutic drugs are:*

(A) Alkylating agents (C) Hormones (E) Other types of drugs
(B) Antimetabolites (D) Antibiotics

1. Vincristine _____

2. Prednisone _____

3. Bleomycin _____

4. L-Asparaginase _____

5. ARA-C _____

6. DES _____

7. Adriamycin _____

8. Chlorambucil _____

9. Methotrexate _____

10. Phenylalamine mustard _____

11. Vinblastine _____

12. 5-Fluorouracil _____

13. Cytoxin _____

14. Nitrogen mustard _____

15. 6-Mercaptopurine _____

I. Provide the answers called for:

1. Name some of the toxic side effects of cancer chemotherapy:

2. What are antifolates, antipyrimidines, and antipurines?

3. Name some hormones used as cancer chemotherapeutic agents:

4. Name some antibiotics which are used in cancer chemotherapy:

ANSWERS

A.
1. Pertaining to reproductive cells; egg and sperm cells.
2. Malignant tumor of the eye; it is hereditary.
3. Hidden.
4. Pertaining to producing death; fatal.
5. To grow substances on growth medium (food) in the laboratory.
6. Cell division.
7. Drugs to combat bacterial infection; also used in cancer treatment.
8. Organism which needs another living organism for growth and reproduction of itself.
9. Experiment in glass tube or plate in the laboratory.
10. Cell which is invaded by a parasitic cell.

B. 4
8
5
6
7
3
1
2

C.
1. oncogenesis
2. polyposis
3. toxicology
4. viremia
5. bacteriocidal
6. chemotherapy

D.
1. Virus.
2. Enzyme in oncogenic RNA viruses which is able to help transfer the genetic information on an RNA virus onto a molecule of new DNA made in a host cell.
3. Malignant neoplastic skin condition which occurs when DNA of skin cells is unable to repair itself after ultraviolet radiation damage. The inability to repair itself is thought to be inherited.

4. Carcinogenic metal (arsenic).
5. Malignant lymphatic neoplasm occurring predominantly in tropical Africa.
6. To withdraw fluid with a needle.
7. The effect of drugs on cell division.
8. That portion in a mass of tumor or normal cells which is actively undergoing cell division.
9. Use of two or more antitumor agents to treat cancer.
10. A chemotherapeutic agent which inhibits DNA synthesis by depriving cells of raw materials necessary to make more DNA.

E. 3
   4
   6
   1
   7
   2
   8
   5

F. 1. Tumor which can be completely eradicated by radiotherapy.
2. Tumor in which radiation can cause loss of tumor cells without damage to normal cells in the surrounding region.
3. Giving radiotherapy in short doses.
4. Tumor which requires large doses of radiation, which damages normal tissue surrounding the tumor.

G. 4
   7
   5
   2
   6
   1
   3

H.

1. E	6. C	11. E
2. C	7. D	12. B
3. D	8. A	13. A
4. E	9. B	14. A
5. B	10. A	15. B

I. 1. Myelosuppression, nausea and vomiting, and alopecia.
2. These are antimetabolites which can be used as chemotherapeutic agents to deprive a cell of material necessary for DNA synthesis and thereby stop its division.
3. Prednisone, estrogens (DES), androgens (testosterone propionate), progestins (Delalutin).
4. Adriamycin, bleomycin, actinomycin D, mithramycin.

REVIEW SHEET 21

Combining Forms

carcin/o	_____	pharmac/o	_____
cauter/o	_____	polyp/o	_____
chem/o	_____	radi/o	_____
cry/o	_____	retin/o	_____
germ/o	_____	tox/o	_____
ion/o	_____	toxic/o	_____
mit/o	_____	vir/o	_____
mut/a	_____	xer/o	_____
onc/o	_____		

Suffixes

-blast	_____	-genesis	_____
-cidal	_____	-therapy	_____
-emia	_____	-osis	_____

Additional Terms for Etiology of Cancer

alkylating agents _____

aromatic amines _____

aromatic hydrocarbons _____

arsenicals _____

asbestos _____

benzpyrene _____

Burkitt's lymphoma _____

carcinoembryonic antigen (CEA) _____

culture _____

diethylstilbestrol (DES) _____

host cell _____

inert _____

in vitro _____

in vivo _____

ionizing radiation _____

latent _____

mutation _____

nonionizing radiation _____

oncogenic DNA and RNA viruses _____

Pap test _____

parasite _____

polyposis coli syndrome _____

retinoblastoma _____

RNA reverse transcriptase _____

vinyl chloride _____

virion _____

xeroderma pigmentosum _____

Additional Terms for Cancer Treatment

alkylating agents _____

androgens _____

antibiotics _____

antimetabolites _____

aspiration _____

biopsy _____

block resection _____

cell population kinetics _____

combination chemotherapy _____

corticoids _____

cryosurgery _____

electrocautery _____

estrogens _____

exfoliative cytology _____

fractionation _____

germinal cells _____

growth fraction _____

lethal _____

modality _____

myelosuppression _____

needle biopsy _____

nonresponsive tumor _____

pharmacokinetics _____

radiocurable tumor _____

radioresistant tumor _____

responsive tumor _____

CHAPTER 22

RADIOLOGY AND NUCLEAR MEDICINE

In this chapter you will:

Investigate the terms which apply to x-rays, how they are produced, and what they can do;

Compare and distinguish the different techniques used by radiologists in diagnosis and treatment of disease;

Identify the various x-ray views and patient positions used in x-ray examinations;

Investigate basic terms relating to the nature of radioactivity and radioactive substances;

Recognize the terms which apply to the role of radioactivity in the diagnosis and treatment of disease; and

Become familiar with combining forms pertaining to the medical specialties of radiology and nuclear medicine.

This chapter is divided into the following sections:

I. INTRODUCTION

Radiology (also called **roentgenology** after the discoverer, Wilhelm Roentgen) is the medical specialty concerned with the study of x-rays. **X-rays** are invisible waves of energy which are produced by a machine and, when focused on an organism, can aid in diagnosis as well as in treatment of disease. Section II of this chapter explores the terms which apply to the characteristics and uses of x-rays in medicine.

Nuclear medicine is the medical specialty which studies the characteristics and uses of **radioactive substances** in the diagnosis and treatment of disease processes. Radioactive substances are those materials which emit high-speed particles and energy-containing rays from the interior (nucleus) of their matter. The particles and rays which are emitted are called **radioactivity**, and can be of three types: **alpha particles**, **beta particles**, and **gamma rays**. Gamma rays are similar to x-rays and are used effectively as a diagnostic label to trace the path and uptake of chemical substances in the body. Radioactivity in high-intensity doses can also be used therapeutically to destroy tissues and stop the growth of malignant cells. Section III of this chapter explores the terminology of radioactive substances and their use in nuclear medicine.

II. RADIOLOGY

A. Vocabulary

barium enema	Rectal instillation of a dense substance, barium sulfate, to outline the large bowel (colon) for a clearer view of it in x-ray studies.
barium swallow	Oral ingestion of barium sulfate used to outline the upper gastrointestinal tract for x-ray study.
Bucky grid	Series of lead strips placed near the x-ray film to absorb scattered radiation before it can strike the x-ray film.
catheterization	Process of inserting or withdrawing fluids using a tube.
cineradiography	Use of motion picture techniques to record a series of x-ray images.
computerized axial tomography (CAT)	Specialized radiological diagnostic technique in which a series of x-rays is taken from several points around a single plane or level of the body. From these x-rays a single, composite picture (scan) is developed by a computer. The scan represents a horizontal cross-section of the various tissues present at that level of the body. The machine used

for this procedure is called an **ACTA scanner**. Another similar type instrument for reconstructing cross-sectional planes of the body is an **EMI scanner**.

contrast techniques

Materials or gases (called contrast media) are injected into a cavity, vessel, or fluid to obtain contrast with surrounding tissue when shown on the x-ray film.

film badge

Radiation detection device worn by technicians and radiologists to record the amount of radiation to which they are exposed.

fluorescence

The emission of a type of radiation, glowing light, which is a result of exposure to absorption of radiation from another source (i.e., x-rays).

fluoroscopy

The process of using x-rays to produce a visible (fluorescent) image on a screen after the x-rays pass through the body.

iodine compounds

Used as a radiopaque contrast medium in x-ray and fluoroscopy studies of body cavities, blood vessels, and body fluids.

ionization

The separation of stable substances into charged particles called ions.

laminagraphy

Tomography.

megavoltage

High-energy radiation generated by a machine and used in curative x-ray radiation therapy for cancer.

myelogram

X-ray record of the spinal cord made by injecting radiopaque dye or air into the cerebrospinal fluid to provide contrast.

nuclear medicine

Study of radioactive substances and radioactivity in the diagnosis and treatment of disease.

orthovoltage

Low-energy radiation used in palliative (symptom-relieving but not curative) radiotherapy.

oscilloscope

Instrument used in ultrasound scanning to visualize the sound waves coming back as echoes from tissues in the body.

photon	Unit of energy; an x-ray or other form of energy, such as a light ray.
rad	*R*adiation *a*bsorbed *d*ose—a unit of absorbed radiation in the body.
radiology	The study of x-rays and their use in the treatment and diagnosis of disease.
radiolucent	Permitting the passage of x-rays. Radiolucent structures appear black on the x-ray film.
radiopaque	Obstructing the passage of x-rays. Radiopaque structures appear white on the x-ray film.
roentgenology	The study of roentgen rays as they are used for diagnostic and therapeutic purposes.
scattered radiation	The deviation, or spreading out, of x-rays as they pass through a material or medium.
stereoscopy	Process of visualizing depth in an x-ray image by taking two successive radiograms and viewing both simultaneously with a special viewer.
thermography	Special diagnostic technique which detects regions of heat and cold in the body; useful in diagnosis of malignant lesions (hot areas) in soft tissue, especially in the breast.
tomography	A special radiographic technique in which a series of x-rays are taken at different depths in order to define images not clearly seen on usual x-ray films; also called laminagraphy.
ultrasonography	Special diagnostic technique which projects ultrasound (high-frequency sound waves) through the body. Echoes formed by differences in density of tissues are recorded by special instruments, providing a map, or scan, of underlying tissues.
xeroradiography	A technique substituting Xerox paper for x-ray film as a substance upon which x-rays are recorded.
x-rays	High-energy waves emitted from an x-ray machine.

B. X-Rays: Characteristics and Production

Characteristics.   There are several characteristics of x-rays which make them useful to physicians in the diagnosis of disease. The most important of these characteristics is that x-rays are waves of energy which can **cause exposure of a photographic plate**. Thus, if a photographic plate were placed alone in front of a beam of x-rays, the x-rays, traveling unimpeded through the air, would expose the plate and cause it to blacken.

Another characteristic of x-rays is that they **penetrate different substances in varying degrees**. Suppose, then, that a human form is placed between the x-ray beam and the photographic plate. The x-rays now have to pass through the different media (densities) of the body, such as air (in lungs and respiratory tubes), water (in blood vessels and tissue fluid), fat (surrounding muscles and organs), and metal (calcium in bones). X-rays are able to penetrate the different densities of the body in varying degrees. Air, being the least dense substance, is penetrated easily, while water, fat, and metal (most dense) are penetrated with increasing difficulty. If the x-ray beams focused on the body are stopped (absorbed) by the high density of a body substance (e.g., calcium in bones), the x-ray beams will not reach the photographic plate, and white areas will be left unexposed on the x-ray film. The fact that some x-rays are partially or totally absorbed by the different densities of the body organs and tissues before reaching the photographic film accounts for the varying degrees of whiteness of images created on the film. Figure 22–1 is an example of an x-ray photograph.

The thickness, or density, of the part of the body through which the x-rays travel thus determines in large part the degree of penetration of the rays. Lung tissue, which contains a great deal of air, transmits x-rays readily and appears blackish on the photographic plate, while the bony tissue of the ribs contains calcium (metal) and does not transmit x-rays well, leaving white shadows on the photographic plate.

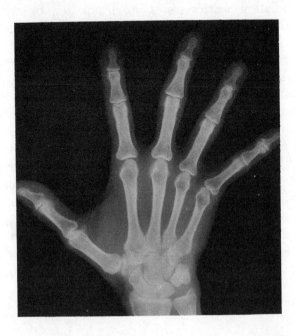

Figure 22–1 X-ray photograph of the hand. (From Poznanski, A. K.: The Hand in Radiologic Diagnosis. Philadelphia, W. B. Saunders Co., 1974.)

A substance is said to be **radiolucent** if it permits some passage of x-rays. Lung tissue is an example of a radiolucent substance in the body. **Radiopaque** substances are those which are impenetrable to the passage of x-rays. Bones are radiopaque substances.

Other characteristics of x-rays, in addition to their ability to expose a photographic plate and penetrate different tissues of the body, are their **invisibility, ability to travel in straight lines**, and **ability to be scattered by the materials they traverse**. The fact that x-rays are invisible and not detectable by man's other senses is important from the point of view of radiation safety. Although exposure to x-rays in low intensities may be safe for patient diagnostic purposes, radiation workers exposed to x-rays occupationally do not receive any sensory warning indicating their daily exposure to x-rays. Most technicians and radiologists wear a **film badge** which is like a Geiger counter that constantly detects and records the amount of radiation to which a person is exposed.

The ability of x-rays to travel in straight lines is important in diagnosis of disease because it makes possible the formation of accurate shadow images on the photographic plate behind the object which is x-rayed. The ability of x-rays to travel in straight lines also permits the x-ray beam to be directed accurately at a tumor site in the body in x-ray therapy.

Scattering of radiation occurs when x-rays come into contact with radiopaque objects. Thus, a person standing near an **irradiated** patient (patient receiving radiation) does receive a small amount of radiation scatter, which is a potentially serious occupational hazard to those working in the x-ray field. Scatter can also blur images on the photographic plate and expose areas of the film which would otherwise be in shadow. In taking diagnostic x-ray pictures, a grid, which contains a large number of thin lead strips arranged parallel to the x-ray beams, is placed in front of the film to absorb scattered radiation before it can strike the x-ray film. This is called a **Bucky grid**. In therapy, radiation scatter can cause irradiation of areas not in the direct treatment field, so that adjacent healthy tissues are inevitably irradiated along with the tumor being treated.

A final characteristic of x-rays is an ability to ionize substances through which they pass. **Ionization** means that the x-rays interact with the neutral **atoms** (minute particles) of the substances which they impinge upon so that **electrons** (negatively charged particles) are gained or released from the previously neutral atoms. The x-ray beam thus converts a neutral atom into an **ion** (charged particle).

Once x-rays cause ionization of neutral atoms of matter by releasing negatively charged particles called electrons, those electrons can then strike other atoms and ionize them as well. The ionizing effect of x-rays is most important in living organisms. Because of its ability to rearrange and disrupt atoms, ionizing radiation can cause chemical changes in the cells through which it passes, and is able to affect the functioning of those cells. This change is noted when normal cells become cancerous after exposure to x-rays. Ironically, in x-ray therapy the strongly ionizing ability of x-rays is made use of to kill malignant cells and thereby stop the growth of the cancerous lesions.

Some of the many characteristics of x-rays are summarized in the following list:

1. Invisible.
2. Travel in straight lines.

3. Expose a photographic plate.
4. Penetrate different substances to varying degrees casting shadows on photographic film.
5. Scattered by the substances through which they pass.
6. Ionize atoms of the material through which they pass.

Production. Follow Figure 22–2 as you read the following simplified description of how x-rays are produced.

X-rays (also called **photons**) are produced by an electric current (1) which sets up a stream of rapidly moving **electrons** (2) within a **vacuum tube** (3) (tube without air). The high-speed electrons moving within the vacuum tube strike the atoms of a **target structure** (4), usually made of a metal called **tungsten**. This tungsten target structure, within the vacuum tube, is designed to withstand the collision of fast electrons and even slows down the high-speed electrons. The result of the electrons colliding with the atoms of the target structure is that x-rays, or **photons** (5), are produced.

The following sequence summarizes the major events in the production of x-rays:

electric current $\longrightarrow$ stream of electrons (within vacuum tube) $\xrightarrow{\text{strike}}$ target structure (tungsten) $\xrightarrow{\text{producing}}$ x-rays (photons)

C. Diagnostic Techniques

Fluoroscopy. This x-ray procedure uses a fluorescent screen instead of a photographic plate to derive a visual image from the x-rays which emerge from the patient. The fact that ionizing radiation such as x-rays can produce **fluorescence** (rays of light energy emitted as a result of exposure to and absorption of radiation from another source) is the basis for fluoroscopy. The x-rays from the x-ray tube, after passing in varying degrees through the densities of the human body, cast shadows on the fluorescent screen. The fluorescent screen glows when struck by the x-rays.

A major advantage of fluoroscopy over normal radiography is the almost instantaneous picture which is presented of the x-ray transmission on the fluorescent screen. Internal organs, such as the heart, can be observed in motion, and the patient's position can be changed to provide the right view at the right time so that the most useful diagnostic information can be obtained.

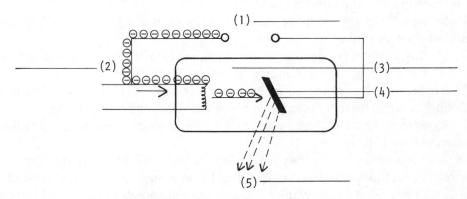

Figure 22–2 Production of x-rays.

Several disadvantages of fluoroscopy should be noted as well. The image projected on the fluorescent screen is fleeting and cannot always be compared with those observed at previous examinations. Also, higher doses of x-rays are necessary to produce fluorescence than would normally be needed to produce an x-ray picture, and detail is much poorer on the fluorescent screen than on the x-ray film.

Image-intensifier systems for fluoroscopy can brighten fluoroscopic images and can be combined with still and movie cameras to obtain a permanent record of the fluoroscopic examination (**cineradiography**).

Contrast Techniques. In a normal x-ray film and in fluoroscopy, the natural differences in the density of body tissues (e.g., air in lung, calcium in bone) allow for contrasting shadow images projected on the x-ray film and fluorescent screen. However, when ionizing x-rays pass through two adjacent substances of body parts of the same density, their images cannot be distinguished on the film or on the screen. Thus, two substances of water density, like the heart and blood tissues, cannot be differentiated because they are of the same density. It is necessary, then, to inject a **contrast medium** into the structure or fluid to be visualized so that the specific part, organ, tube, or liquid can be contrasted with its adjacent structures.

Some artificial contrast material used in diagnostic radiological and fluoroscopic studies are:

Barium Sulfate. Barium sulfate is a metallic paste contrast medium which is mixed in water and is used for upper and lower GI (gastrointestinal) examinations. A **barium swallow** is oral ingestion of barium sulfate for radiological and fluoroscopic examination of the esophagus, stomach, duodenum, and small intestine. A **barium enema** opacifies the lumen (passageway) of the colon by use of an enema containing barium sulfate.

Iodine Compounds. These radiopaque compounds contain up to 50 per cent iodine and are used predominantly in the following tests:

1. **Intravenous pyelogram (IVP)** — x-ray record of the renal pelvis and urinary tract after injecting contrast medium (dye) into a vein.

2. **Retrograde pyelogram (RP)** — x-ray record of the renal pelvis and urinary tract after injecting dye directly into the urethra, bladder, and ureters. The dye flows back up to the kidneys through the ureters.

3. **Salpingogram** — x-ray record of the fallopian tubes after injecting dye directly into the fallopian tubes via the vagina and uterus.

4. **Bronchogram** — x-ray record of the bronchial tubes after injecting radiopaque contrast medium into the bronchi via the trachea.

5. **Sialogram** — x-ray record of the salivary ducts after injection of radiopaque dye directly into the salivary ducts.

6. **Myelogram** — x-ray record of the spinal cord after injecting radiopaque dye into the subarachnoid space surrounding the spinal cord.

7. **Angiogram** — x-ray record of blood vessels and heart chambers after injecting dye through a catheter (tube) into the appropriate vessel or heart chamber.

8. **Lymphangiogram** — x-ray record of lymphatic vessels after injecting radiopaque dye into the lymphatic system.

Air and Other Gases. Air, oxygen, carbon dioxide, and nitrous oxide may be used as contrast media after fluid is removed from organs such as the brain ventricles and spinal cord. **Pneumoencephalography** and **myelography** are examples of this technique.

Stereoscopy. Stereoscopy is a special radiographic technique in which an illusion of depth of an object is obtained. Two successive radiographs of the part of the body to be viewed are taken from different angles while the patient is immobilized. The resulting films are then examined simultaneously using a stereoscopic viewing device which merges the images, giving the appearance of depth to the picture. This technique is used in studies of the skull, as well as of other anatomical areas.

Tomography. Tomography (also called **laminagraphy**) is a technique for taking x-ray pictures in sections so that radiographs of a desired layer of the body are obtained, while at the same time structures in front of and behind that layer are blurred out. A laminagraph, or tomograph, consists of an apparatus in which the x-ray tube and x-ray film rotate at the same time but in opposite directions while the patient remains stationary and x-ray pictures are taken. Everything is displaced or blurred except in the plane of the structure which is to be studied. Multiple pictures are taken which are like x-ray slices at different depths through the patient. The tomogram obliterates all extraneous material and focuses on the one small segment which is to be viewed. Calcifications and lesions which are missed on conventional radiographs can be picked up with tomography.

Computerized Axial Tomography. Computerized axial tomography (CAT) is a revolutionary techniq... ...ines called **ACTA** (*a*utomated *c*omputerized *t*ransverse *a*xial) s... ...EMI, Ltd., a company in England which first built the ... s of ionizing x-rays through a patient while rotating ... n of the body. The absorption rates of the x-ray... ...etected and relayed to a computer device whic... the absorption capacities of the different b... computer then synthesizes all the information... x-ray views and projects a single composite p...

The AC... ...more sensitive in detecting disease in soft body... hage of a horizontal slice of the human body... ordinary x-ray technique. This scanning tech... umors and hematomas, abnormal spinal cord l... kidneys, and pancreas. It has also been helpful ... ms in blood vessels. (Figure 22–3 shows an EMI ...

Xeroradiogra... ...chnique uses the technology of the Xerox office copier... Xerox paper instead of on an x-ray film. Ionizing radiation passes ... dy and is detected on a dry paper without chemical solutions. Within 90 seconds, an image of the soft tissues of the body can be obtained on specially treated Xerox paper and then observed under ordinary light. Because of the ability to visualize more detail in soft tissues of the body, such as the breast, xeroradiography is thought to enhance the diagnosis of nonpalpable (unable to be felt) lesions and minute calcifications of the breast. (Figure 22–4 shows examples of xeroradiographs.)

Thermography. Unlike x-ray diagnosis, thermography requires no physical agent applied to the body. It is the body's own heat energy which produces the diagnostic record. Warm areas of the body appear light; cool areas of the body appear dark; and intermediate temperature regions are recorded as a gray color on the thermogram. The

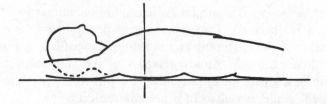

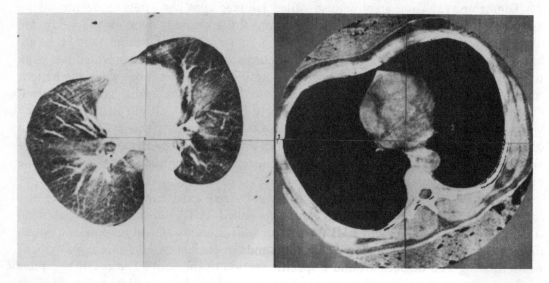

Figure 22-3 EMI body scan photographs. On the left are the lungs, showing their blood vessels. On the right is the heart, spinal column, and rib cage. The diagram above shows the point on the human body where the images were taken. (Courtesy of EMI Medical Inc. X-Ray Systems, Northbrook, Illinois.)

technique has been particularly useful in aiding the diagnosis of breast tumors, because breast tumors produce more heat than the normal tissue surrounding it. (Figure 22–5 is an example of a breast thermogram.)

Ultrasonography.   Ultrasonography is not a technique which uses the transmission of ionizing radiation to diagnose or treat disease. Ultrasound employs very high frequency, inaudible sound waves which bounce off body tissues and then are recorded to give information about the anatomy of an internal organ. Sound waves are emitted in short, repetitive pulses from a special instrument. The instrument is placed near or on the skin, which is covered with water, oil, or a thick jelly to assure good transmission of sound waves from the air into the body. As the instrument is moved over the skin, sound waves pass through the skin and strike the different body tissues which are of varying density and elasticity (stiffness). Ultrasound waves move with different speeds in tissues which differ in density and elasticity. An echo reflection of the sound wave as it hits the various body tissues passes back to the special instrument.

Ultrasonic echoes are then recorded on an **oscilloscope** (instrument for visualizing sound waves), which is part of the instrument which emits the sound waves. A pictorial representation of the "slice" of the body over which the instrument passes is reproduced by a series of dots on the oscilloscope. The position of each dot reflects the location of an echo within the body, and the brightness of each dot reflects the relative strength of each individual echo. The record produced by ultrasonography is appropriately called an **echogram**.

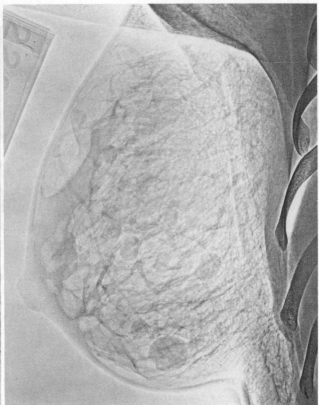

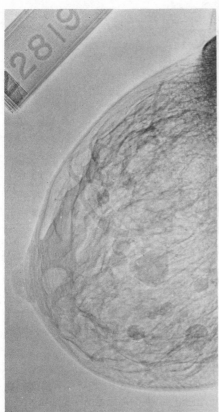

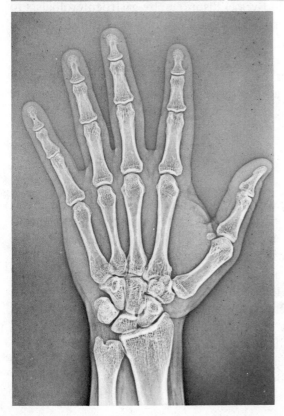

Figure 22-4 Xeroradiographs. Photographs above reveal multiple fibroadenomas with palpable masses in both breasts. Xeroradiograph of the hand shows bony structure detail and soft tissue as well. (Top, from Wolfe, J. N.: Mammography. Radiologic Clinics of North America, *12*:189, 1974; left, from Poznanski, A. K.: The Hand in Radiologic Diagnosis. Philadelphia, W. B. Saunders Co., 1974.)

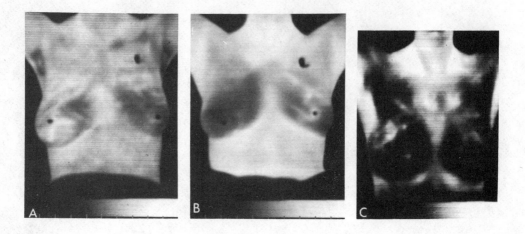

Figure 22–5   Breast thermograms. *A*, Warm diffuse heat area (light area indicates heat) in the right breast. *B*, Periareolar heat, left breast. *C*, Focal heat, upper right breast. (From Isard, H. J., and Ostrum, B. J.: Breast thermography — the mammatherm. Radiologic Clinics of North America, *12*:167, 1974.)

Ultrasonography is used as a diagnostic tool not only by radiologists but also by neurosurgeons and ophthalmologists to detect intracranial and ophthalmic lesions, by cardiologists to detect heart valve and blood vessel disorders, by gastroenterologists to locate abdominal masses outside the digestive tubes, by obstetricians to differentiate single and multiple pregnancies, and by gynecologists to locate tumors, cysts, and breast lesions.

The technique has several advantages in that the sound waves are nonpainful, nonionizing, and noninjurious to tissues at the energy ranges utilized for diagnostic purposes. (Figure 22–6 is an example of an echogram, or ultrasonogram.)

D. X-Ray Therapy

Not only are x-rays helpful in detecting disease, but they can be used as therapy as well. Large doses of ionizing radiation to body tissues can be lethal (fatal) to the cells which are **irradiated**. X-ray therapy has been particularly helpful as a lethal agent in the treatment of malignant neoplasms, as discussed in Chapter 21.

The machines used for x-ray therapy are different from those used for diagnostic x-ray. Therapy machines deliver rays of many times higher intensity and are of two general types: **Orthovoltage** machines deliver low-energy radiation which is used in palliative treatment (relieving symptoms but not curing) of cancer patients; **megavoltage** machines generate high-energy radiation and are used to treat deeper tissues of the body in curative radiotherapy for cancer. The dose unit of radiation absorbed by body tissue is called a **rad** (*r*adiation *a*bsorbed *d*ose).

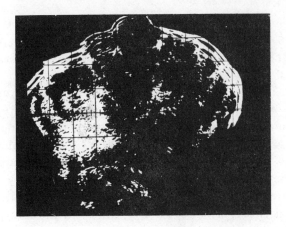

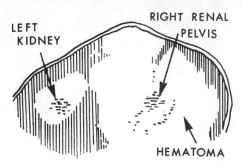

Figure 22–6 Echogram of the kidneys showing a retroperitoneal hematoma surrounding the right kidney. (From Saunders, R. C.: Renal ultrasound. Radiologic Clinics of North America, *13*:417, 1975.)

E. X-Ray Positioning

In order to take the best possible view of the part of the body being radiographed, the patient, film, and x-ray tube must be positioned in the most favorable alignment possible. There are special terms used by radiologists to designate the position or direction of the x-ray beam, the patient's position, and the motion and position of the part of the body to be viewed. The following is only a partial list of the many positions which are used in getting the best possible x-ray film of the part of the body to be viewed:

1. **PA view** (*p*ostero*a*nterior). In this view, the patient is upright with his back to the x-ray machine and the x-ray tube is aimed horizontally at a distance of about 6 feet from the film. The reason the tube is 6 feet from the film is that this distance enhances the sharpness and reduces the magnification of the object to be viewed. To test this yourself, place your finger above a piece of paper under a table lamp and adjust the lamp back and forth farther from and closer to your finger. When the lamp

is farther away, the shadow of your finger appears smaller and in sharper focus. You should also notice that the closer your finger moves to the paper, the sharper and smaller your finger's shadow becomes. It is obvious, then, that the closer a patient is to the x-ray film plate, the clearer the x-ray picture will be.

2. **AP view** (*antero*posterior). In this view, the patient may be **supine** (lying on the back) and the x-ray tube aimed from above at the anterior of the body with the beam passing from anterior to posterior. Because of low ceilings, AP views are usually taken at 3 feet, meaning that there is less sharpness and greater magnification of the image. The AP view may also be taken with the patient in the upright position.

3. **Lateral view** (from the side). In this view, the x-ray beam passes from one side of the body toward the opposite side. In taking a right lateral view, the right side of the body is held closely against the x-ray film and the x-ray beam passes from the left to the right through the body.

4. **Oblique view.** In this view, the x-ray tube is positioned on an angle. Oblique views are used to show regions that would be hidden and superimposed in routine AP and PA views.

5. **Lordotic view.** This view is taken by elevating and angling the x-ray tube downward so that the collarbones are projected out of the view of the x-ray picture.

The following terms are used to describe the position of the patient or part of body in the x-ray examination:

6. **Supine.** Lying on the back.

7. **Prone.** Lying on the belly (face down).

8. **Decubitus.** Lying down (usually on the side with the x-ray beam horizontally positioned); sometimes called a **cross-table lateral.**

9. **Recumbent.** Lying down (may be prone or supine).

10. **Adduction.** Moving the part of the body toward the midline of the body, toward the body.

11. **Abduction.** Moving the part of the body away from the midline or away from the body.

12. **Eversion.** Turning outward.

13. **Inversion.** Turning inward.

14. **Extension.** Lengthening or straightening a flexed limb.

15. **Pronation.** Turning downward; lying on one's abdomen.

16. **Supination.** Turning the part upward; lying on one's back.

17. **Flexion.** Bending a part.

III. NUCLEAR MEDICINE

A. Vocabulary

alpha particle	High-energy particle produced by the disintegration of radioactive substances.
atom	The smallest particle of an element having the same properties of that element.

atomic number	Number of protons (positively charged particles) in an atom. A sodium atom has 11 protons and its atomic number is 11.
atomic weight	Number of heavy particles (neutrons plus protons) in an atom. A sodium atom has 11 protons and 12 neutrons and its atomic weight is 23.
beta particle	A common type of charged particle produced and emitted from disintegrating radioactive substances.
cold nodule	Area on a scan, as in a thyroid scan, showing less than normal cellular activity. Used to identify a malignant lesion.
electron	Negatively charged particle within an atom. Electrons circulate in orbits surrounding the central nucleus of an atom.
element	A basic type of matter, composed of like atoms, which cannot be broken down into dissimilar parts by ordinary chemical means.
gamma rays	High-energy rays emitted from disintegrating radioactive substances. They are similar to x-rays.
Geiger counter	An instrument used to measure radioactive rays and particles (alpha, beta, and gamma rays) emitted from radioactive substances.
half-life	Time required for half the atoms of a radioactive substance to lose their radioactivity by undergoing disintegration.
ion	A charged particle; a particle carrying an electric charge.
ionization	The separation of stable substances (atoms) into charged particles, or ions.
isotopes	Atoms of the same element having the same atomic number (number of protons) but different atomic weights (number of neutrons and protons).
neutrons	Neutral particles located in the nucleus of an atom.
nuclear medicine	The study of radioactivity and its application in medical diagnosis and treatment.

nucleus
In chemistry, the central core of an atom, containing the heavy particles called neutrons and protons.

nuclide
The combination of protons, neutrons, and electrons in an atom of an element.

protons
Positively charged particles within the nucleus of an atom.

radioactive isotopes
Atoms of an element which emit particles, or energy. Also called radioisotopes.

radioactivity
The ability of an atom to emit high-energy alpha, beta, or gamma rays from its nucleus.

radionuclides
Atoms of an element which emit particles or waves of energy.

radiopharmaceuticals
Compounds which incorporate radionuclides. They are used for diagnostic tracer studies or in therapy.

scan
A composite picture of the distribution of a radioactive substance in the body.

scintillation counter
Instrument used to detect radioactivity from radiopharmaceuticals used in tracer studies.

tagging
Attaching a radionuclide to a body chemical to follow its course throughout the body.

tracer studies
Studies in which radionuclides are used as tags, or labels, attached to body chemicals and followed as they migrate throughout the body.

B. The Atom and Basic Concepts of Radioactivity

The emission of energy as particles or rays from the nucleus of an atom is called **radioactivity**. In order to understand such a definition, as well as the role of radioactivity in medicine, it is essential to understand some of the terminology of the **atom**.

Atoms are small particles of which all elements are made. An **element** is an aggregation, or collection, of only a single type of atom. Examples of elements are oxygen, hydrogen, sodium, nitrogen, calcium, and over 100 other substances in the living and nonliving world. Atoms are the smallest particles within these elements.

Atoms are so small that they are undetectable by even the most powerful microscope known to man. Without being able to see atoms, scientists have performed experiments which prove that atoms have electrical properties and consist of charged particles. The central core of an atom is called the **nucleus**, and the nucleus contains positively charged particles called **protons**. Neutral particles called **neutrons** are also located in the nucleus of an atom. Protons and neutrons thus compose the nucleus of the atom. Negatively charged particles called **electrons** are found circulating in orbits, or clouds, of energy surrounding the central nucleus core of the atom. The number of protons (positively charged particles) always equals the number of electrons (negatively charged particles) which are circulating around the nucleus. For example, the element sodium has 11 protons and 11 electrons; hydrogen has one proton and one electron; and oxygen has eight protons and eight electrons.

Figure 22–7 illustrates the composition of an atom of the element sodium (chemical symbol: Na). Na has 11 protons, 11 electrons, and 12 neutrons. The specific composition and configuration of protons, electrons, and neutrons in an atom is referred to as a **nuclide**.

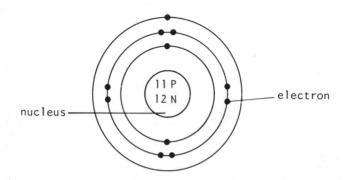

Figure 22-7   Sodium atom containing 11 protons, 11 electrons, and 12 neutrons.

The number of protons in an atom of an element is equal to the **atomic number** of that element. Hydrogen has one proton, and its atomic number is 1; sodium has 11 protons, and its atomic number is 11. The number of protons **plus** the number of neutrons equals the **atomic weight** of an atom. The atomic weight of sodium is, then, 11 protons plus 12 neutrons, or 23. It is common practice to indicate the atomic weight of an element as a number to the left and slightly above the chemical symbol of the element. For example, an atom of sodium is written ^{23}Na.

While the atomic number (number of protons) of an element never changes, its atomic weight may change with the addition or subtraction of neutrons. More neutrons increase the atomic weight, while fewer neutrons decrease the atomic weight. **Isotopes** are atoms of the same element having the same atomic number (number of protons) but different atomic weights (number of neutrons). For example, Figure 22–8 shows the three isotopes of hydrogen (^{1}H, ^{2}H, ^{3}H) and three isotopes of sodium (^{22}Na, ^{23}Na, ^{24}Na). All the isotopes of hydrogen have one proton and the atomic number of 1, but their atomic weights are 1, 2, and 3, depending on the number of neutrons in the atom. All the isotopes of sodium have 11 protons and the atomic number of 11, while their atomic weights are 22, 23, and 24, depending on the number of neutrons in each atom.

Most atoms in nature exist in a nuclide form with a stable, specific number of protons and neutrons and electrons. ^{1}H and ^{23}Na are stable nuclide forms of the elements hydrogen and sodium. Atoms that have unstable nuclei (more or fewer neutrons than the stable form) are said to be **radioactive isotopes** (radioisotopes) or

radionuclides. The term radioactive comes from the fact that the instability of the nucleus causes the emission of energy in particles and rays (radiation) from the nucleus of the atom. Thus, while the nuclide ^{23}Na is the stable form of the element sodium and is nonradioactive, ^{22}Na and ^{24}Na are both unstable, radioactive forms with either too few or too many neutrons in their nuclei. When atoms of an element are or become radioactive, they are called **radionuclides**.

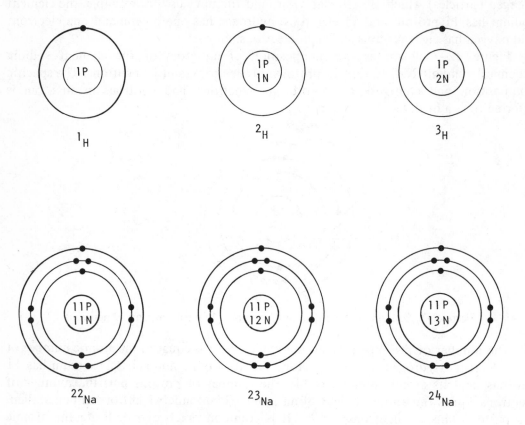

Figure 22–8 Isotopes of hydrogen and sodium.

Some elements, such as radium and uranium, never exist in a stable state and are normally radioactive (radionuclides). In a continuous attempt to reach a stable state, they spontaneously disintegrate and emit radiation. Other, normally stable, elements, such as hydrogen, iodine, and sodium, can be transformed into radionuclides so that the radiation they emit may be used in medicine and science. Man-made radionuclides are produced when high-energy particles are used to bombard stable forms of elements (hydrogen, iodine, mercury). When these elements are bombarded, the number of neutrons in their nuclei changes, and a process of nuclear disintegration is initiated which causes the emission of radiation. Once an element has become radioactive, it continues to emit energy particles and rays spontaneously. Figure 22–9 illustrates in diagram form the change from stable atom to radionuclide and its resultant production of radioactivity.

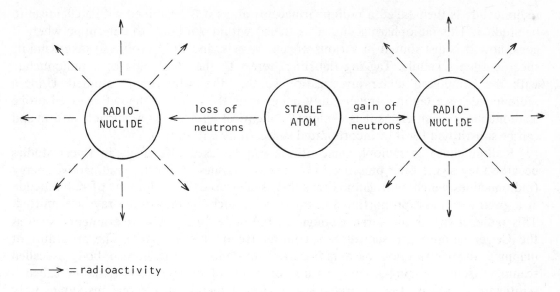

— —→ = radioactivity

Figure 22–9 Production of radioactivity.

Each radionuclide has a characteristic rate at which it disintegrates. The term **half-life** refers to the time required for a radioactive substance to lose half of its atoms and thus half of its radioactivity by disintegration. For example, any quantity of ^{131}I (iodine-131) is radioactive and has a half-life of 8 days. This means that no matter when ^{131}I is measured, 8 days later half the radioactive material will have disappeared. The difference in half-life of various materials is very great. Radium-226 (^{226}Ra) has a half-life of 1622 years, while ^{138}I has a half-life of 8 seconds.

Radionuclides (radioactive isotopes) emit three types of radiation: **alpha**, **beta**, and **gamma** rays. Alpha rays are actually composed of charged particles (protons) and neutrons, which are much heavier than electrons. Because of their large mass, they collide very easily with any atoms they encounter and, thus, they penetrate matter very poorly. They are dangerous rays because of their strong ability to **ionize** atoms, that is, to disrupt or excite neutral atoms by detaching an electron from the atom and making it a charged particle.

Beta rays are streams of electron particles which are lighter than alpha rays and can penetrate matter to a greater distance. They have less ionizing power than alpha rays and are less dangerous.

Gamma rays are similar to high-energy x-rays. They are not particles with charge and mass as are alpha and beta rays, but are waves of electromagnetic energy. This means that they have greater penetrating ability than alpha or beta rays and even greater ionizing power because they can more easily detach electrons from the atoms they collide with in the material through which they pass.

C. Diagnosis of Disease Using Radioactivity

Radionuclides (radioisotopes) have been used with success as diagnostic aids in medicine. In **tracer studies**, a specific radionuclide is incorporated into a chemical substance whose course of action and path in the body is to be analyzed. The radionuclide is then called a **radiopharmaceutical**, as it is combined with a chemical to be studied. This radiopharmaceutical is traced within the body to determine where it goes; how it is distributed in various organs, vessels, and fluids; routes it takes; and its specific time schedule. **Tagging** (labeling) refers to the combining of a radionuclide with the compound under investigation so that the latter can be studied. Using a radionuclide as a tag in a tracer study depends on the fact that the radioactive isotope (radionuclide) of an element is chemically identical with the nonradioactive form and can be substituted for it or incorporated successfully within it.

Radionuclides as radiopharmaceuticals can be used effectively in tracer studies because they signal their presence in organs and tissues by emitting radioactive energy (radionuclides which emit gamma rays are usually used). The amount of radionuclide at a given location is proportional to the rate at which the radioactive rays are emitted. This radioactivity is measured throughout the body by sensitive instruments, such as the **Geiger counter** and **scintillation counter** (scint/i means spark). The procedure of mapping the distribution of a radioactive substance in the human body is called **scanning** (scintiscanning). The picture, or map, of an organ or tissue is called a **scintigram** or a **scan**. Devices called scintillation cameras can respond instantaneously to radioactivity from all areas and incorporate the information from the scan with a total image. **Uptake** refers to the rate of absorption of the radionuclide into an organ or tissue. The radionuclide may be administered intravenously, orally, intracutaneously, or intramuscularly. A **cold nodule**, or **cold spot**, is detected on a scan as an area of less than normal activity. A cold spot may contain a malignant lesion. (Figure 22–10 shows an example of a total-body bone scan and a lung scan.)

The following is a partial list of some types of scanning studies used in the diagnosis of disease. Also listed is the radionuclide tracer agent and the disease it is used to detect.

Scan	*Radionuclide*	*Disease*
Thyroid scan	Iodine-125 (^{125}I) Iodine-131 (^{131}I) *Iodine is the main constituent of thyroid hormone, and radioiodine accumulates in the thyroid.*	Thyroid disease (hyperthyroidism)
Liver (hepatic) scan	Gold-198 (^{198}Au) *Gold is ingested by the phagocytes of the liver.*	Hepatomas, liver damage
Kidney (renal) scan	Mercury-197 (^{197}Hg) Mercury-203 (^{203}Hg)	Kidney disease and lesions
Brain scan	Technetium-99m (^{99m}Tc) Mercury-197 (^{197}Hg) Mercury-203 (^{203}Hg)	Benign or malignant brain lesions

Bone marrow scan	Iron-52 or iron-59 (^{52}Fe, ^{59}Fe) *Iron is metabolized in bone marrow.*	Iron deficiency and hemolytic anemia, hematopoietic disorders
Spleen scan and red cell survival studies	Chromium-51 (^{51}Cr) Technetium-99m (^{99m}Tc)	Hemolytic anemia
Bone scan	Strontium-85 (^{85}Sr)	Primary and metastatic bone neoplasms
Gallium scan	Gallium-6 (^{6}Ga)	Localizes in malignancy

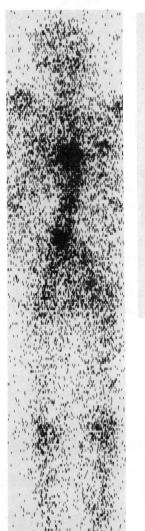

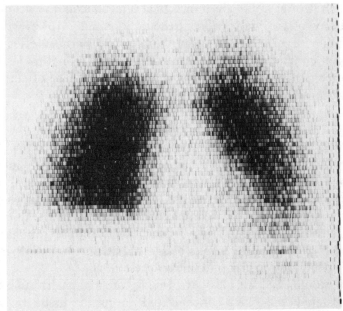

Figure 22–10   Total-body bone scan on the left shows darkened areas of increased radiopharmaceutical uptake in the thoracic and lumbar spine. Scan above shows lungs (anterior view) and was taken following intravenous injection of an appropriate radiopharmaceutical. (Left, from James, A. E., Jr., and Squire, L. F.: Nuclear Medicine. Philadelphia, W. B. Saunders Co., 1973; above, from DeLand, F. H., and Wagner, H. N., Jr.: Atlas of Nuclear Medicine: Lung and Heart. Philadelphia, W. B. Saunders Co., 1970.)

D. Treatment of Disease Using Radioactivity

The basic principle in the use of radionuclides for disease therapy is that, given in regulated doses, radionuclides are capable of suppressing or destroying the activity of diseased tissue, especially malignant neoplastic growth. Since normal tissue can be destroyed during the treatment, methods of dosage must be geared toward producing the greatest tumor kill without damaging normal tissue. Destruction of tissue is accomplished by the strongly ionizing effect of the radioactive rays (beta and gamma rays are used most frequently) from radionuclides. Radionuclides in lower doses are used as palliative agents when destruction of the tumor growth is impossible.

Radionuclides are administered internally, in liquid or solid form, or externally. In external administration, the radionuclide is housed in a shielded unit located at a distance from the patient, and a beam of radiation is aimed at a designated part of the patient's body.

There are important criteria which must be satisfied before a radionuclide can be safely used as a therapeutic agent. One such criterion is that the half-life of the radionuclide must be neither too short nor too long. Radionuclides with half-lives of less than several hours are impractical and uneconomical unless the user lives close to the source of the production of the radionuclide. However, if the half-life is very long, irradiation of healthy tissue may result, with harmful effects on the patient. Thus, it has been concluded that half-lives of about 12 hours to 12 days are suitable to allow the effect on the patient to be evaluated and to be effective while not exposing the patient to undue irradiation damage.

Some radioisotopes of especially long half-life, such as cobalt-60 and cesium-137, are used as external sources of gamma radiation so that the detrimental effect of their long half-life is avoided. **Teletherapy** (tele = distant) is the process of using cobalt-60 (^{60}Co), or other ionizing radiation, as an external source of radiation in a manner similar to x-rays. However, the gamma rays from the cobalt teletherapy sources are of higher energy than the x-rays. Shielded (protected) units which emit ^{60}Co gamma rays from a distance are the teletherapy sources. This treatment is especially useful for tumors which lie deep in the body, because the gamma rays are so penetrating. Machines which deliver supervoltage radiation for radiotherapy are called betatrons, cobalt teletherapy units, and linear accelerators.

It would be an ideal treatment of malignant disease if radionuclides were administered and then concentrated in tumor tissue by normal processes, finally destroying the tumor by local irradiation. However, in only a few cases has this ideal been achieved. One example is radioactive phosphorus (^{32}P) and its use in leukemia and polycythemia vera. When ^{32}P is administered intravenously, it disappears from circulation, later to be found incorporated into bone marrow cells, liver, spleen, and lymph nodes. In these organs, ^{32}P is effective in suppressing erythrocyte production as therapy for polycythemia and in suppressing leukocyte production as therapy for leukemia.

Radionuclides used in therapy may be injected intravenously to migrate selectively to body tissues. In addition, they may be enclosed in removable containers or needles for insertion into malignant tissues. Also, intracavitary administration is used, especially to irradiate tumors of the urinary bladder.

The following list names some important radionuclides, their use as therapeutic agents, and their method of administration in the body:

Radionuclide	Use	Method of Administration
Cobalt-60 (^{60}Co)	Cancers of breast, uterus, larynx, and bladder.	Intracavitary with radio-cobalt rods, pellets, or beads (larynx, uterus, and bladder).
		Interstitial with needles and wires into breast.
		Teletherapy with a tele-cobalt unit (all deep-lying tumors).
Phosphorus-32 (^{32}P)	Leukemia, polycythemia vera, Hodgkin's disease.	Intravenous injection in liquid form.
Gold-198 (^{198}Au)	Palliative treatment, or management of ascites and pleural effusion associated with metastasis. Prevents dissemination of tumor cells after surgery.	Intracavitary or inter-stitial injection in liquid form.
Iodine-131 (^{131}I)	Hyperthyroidism, thyroid carcinoma, heart failure (reduction in thyroid acitivity puts less strain on the function of the heart).	Oral administration of radioiodine.
Cesium-137 (^{137}Cs)	Cancerous tumor.	Teletherapy unit.

Radiotherapy, although it is a palliative and curative agent, can produce uncomfortable side effects. Most of these side effects are due to administering doses which are above the limit of tolerance of the target tissue. Physicians are restricted in the amount of radiotherapy which they can administer because of this factor. Some of the side effects or complications of radiotherapy are:

(1) Irritation of mucous membranes (mucositis); for example, in the mouth, pharynx, vagina, or bladder.
(2) Diarrhea.
(3) Nausea and dysphagia as a reaction to radiotherapy of the mouth and throat.
(4) Nephritis, pericarditis, pneumonitis, hepatitis, myelitis, and fibrosis of the skin.
(5) Bone marrow suppression.
(6) Alopecia (baldness).

IV. COMBINING FORMS

Combining Form	Definition	Terminology	Meaning
radi/o	rays, radioactivity	radiologist _____	
		radiotherapy _____	
		radionuclides _____	
		radioiodine _____	
roentgen/o	x-rays	roentgenology _____	
		roentgenotherapy _____	
		roentgenography _____	
tele/o	distant, far	teletherapy _____	
		teleradiography _____	
is/o	equal, same	isotope _____	
		radioisotope _____	
ion/o	wander, going	ion _____	
		ionization _____	
		ionizing radiation _____	
therm/o	heat	thermography _____	
xer/o	dry	xeroradiography _____	
son/o	sound	ultrasonography _____	
ech/o	sound	echocardiography _____	
luc/o	light, transparent	radiolucent _____	
opaq/o opac/o	dark, impervious to light rays	radiopaque _____	
		opacification _____	

fluor/o	luminous	fluoroscopy _____
cine/o	movement	cineradiography _____
stere/o	solid, three-dimensional	stereoscopy _____
tom/o	to cut	tomography _____
		intravenous tomogram _____
		_____
scint/i	spark	scintiscanner _____
		scintillation counter _____
		_____
-graphy	process of recording	roentgenography _____
-graph	instrument to record	radiograph _____
-gram	record	cholescintigram _____
intra-	within	intracavitary _____
		intravenous _____
inter-	between	interstitial _____

V. EXERCISES

A. *List six characteristics of x-rays:*

1. _____

2. _____

3. _____

4. _____

5. _____

6. _____

B. *Give the meaning of the following:*

1. Bucky grid _____

2. roentgenology _____

3. nuclear medicine _____

   _____

4. radiolucent _____

5. radiopaque _____

6. film badge _____

7. scattered radiation _____

8. irradiation _____

9. radioactivity _____

10. ionization _____

C. *Match the terms in Column I with their meanings in Column II:*

Column I		Column II
1. electron _____		a. Positively charged particle in nucleus of an atom.
2. proton _____		
3. ion _____		b. Unit of energy, as an x-ray, with no electrical charge.
4. neutron _____		c. Smallest particle of an element having the same properties of that element.
5. photon _____		
		d. Particle in nucleus of atom, has no charge.

6. atom _____

        e. Negatively charged particles normally circulating around the nucleus of an atom.

        f. Charged particle, can be positive or negative.

D. *Give the name of the special diagnostic technique which fits the following definitions:*

1. Radiopaque substances are introduced into the body and x-rays are taken to follow their distribution in organs, tubes, vessels, and fluids:

   _____

2. Use of motion picture techniques to help record x-ray images: _____

   _____

3. X-ray technique of blurring out all planes except the one that is to be seen in detail; successive x-ray "cuts" or "slices" of a region of the body: _____

   _____

4. Use of the echoes of inaudible sound waves to diagnose disease: _____

   _____

5. X-ray beams are focused from the body onto a special screen which almost instantaneously glows as a result of the ionizing effect of x-rays: _____

   _____

6. Three-dimensional x-ray views are produced by taking two successive radiographs and viewing both simultaneously with a three-dimensional viewer:

   _____

7. Natural body heat used as a clue to malignant lesions as an instrument detects hot and cold regions of the body: _____

   _____

8. X-ray images are projected on dry Xerox paper instead of x-ray photographic

   film: _____

9. Horizontal slice pictures of the body are made by means of technique which takes hundreds of successive x-ray pictures all around the body; information about density of tissues is released to a computer which synthesizes the data and presents a composite picture of the part of the body on a screen:

   _____

E. Give the meaning of the following x-ray diagnostic studies:

1. ventriculography (cerebral pneumography) _____

   _____

2. barium swallow _____

   _____

3. retrograde pyelography _____

   _____

4. sialogram _____

5. angiogram _____

6. cholecystography _____

7. intravenous pyelography _____

   _____

8. myelogram _____

9. barium enema _____

   _____

10. lymphangiography _____

    _____

11. bronchogram _____

12. hysterosalpingography _____

_____

13. heart catheterization _____

_____

14. venogram _____

F. *Match the following x-ray positions in Column I with their meanings in Column II:*

Column I	Column II
1. PA _____	a. On the side.
2. supine _____	b. Turned inward.
3. prone _____	c. Movement away from the midline.
4. AP _____	d. Lying on belly.
5. lordotic _____	e. On an angle downward so that collarbone is projected out of view.
6. lateral _____	f. Bending a part.
7. oblique _____	g. Lengthening a part.
8. decubitus _____	h. Lying on the back.
9. adduction _____	i. Lying down (prone or supine).
10. inversion _____	j. On an angle.
11. abduction _____	k. Lying down (on side, cross-table lateral).
12. recumbent _____	l. Anterior to posterior view.
13. eversion _____	m. Turning outward.
14. flexion _____	n. Posterior to anterior view (from 6 feet).
15. extension _____	o. Movement toward the midline.

G. *Give the meaning of the following terms:*

1. nuclide _____

2. atomic number _____

3. atomic weight _____

4. isotopes _____

5. radioisotopes _____

6. radionuclide _____

7. alpha particles _____

8. beta particles _____

9. gamma rays _____

10. half-life _____

H. *Match the terms in Column I with their definitions in Column II:*

Column I		Column II
1. tagging	_____	a. Instrument to detect radioactivity.
2. scintillation counter	_____	b. Radiation absorbed dose.
3. radioisotope	_____	c. Treatment from distant or external radioactive source.
4. scintigram	_____	d. Relieving pain without curing.
5. cold nodule (spot)	_____	e. Low-energy radiation used in palliative radiotherapy.
6. orthovoltage	_____	f. Record of radioactivity used in tracer studies.
7. rad	_____	g. Radioactive treatment wherein the source of radiation is placed directly within the body tissue.
8. teletherapy	_____	
9. interstitial implantation	_____	h. Radioactive labeling of a chemical compound and tracing its path in the body.

10. palliative _____   i.   Atomic form of an element which emits radioactivity.

j.   Region of less than normal activity revealed by radioactive scanning.

I. Give the meanings of the following combining forms:

1. therm/o _____   7. ion/o _____

2. xer/o _____   8. fluor/o _____

3. ech/o _____   9. stere/o _____

4. roentgen/o _____ 10. tom/o _____

5. son/o _____   11. scint/i _____

6. cine/o _____

ANSWERS

A. 1. Invisible.
2. Travel in straight line.
3. Expose a photographic plate.
4. Ionize atoms.
5. Scattered by the material through which they pass.
6. Penetrate different densities in varying degrees.

B. 1. Series of lead strips used near x-ray films to absorb scattered radiation.
2. Process of the study of x-rays.
3. Medical specialty involving the study of radioactivity and its application in diagnosis and treatment of disease.
4. Permitting the passage of energy rays yet offering some resistance to them.
5. Impenetrable by energy rays.
6. Radiation detection device worn by radiologists and x-ray technicians and others working in the x-ray field.
7. The spreading out of x-rays as they penetrate matter.
8. The penetration of energy rays through an object or substance.
9. The ability of a substance to emit high-energy particles and rays.
10. The dissociation of stable substances into charged particles.

C. 1. e
2. a
3. f
4. d
5. b
6. c

D. 1. contrast techniques.
2. cineradiography.
3. tomography (laminagraphy).
4. ultrasonography.
5. fluoroscopy.
6. stereoscopy.
7. thermography.
8. xeroradiography.
9. ACTA or EMI scanning (computerized axial tomography).

E.
1. Process of x-ray recording the ventricles of the brain using air as a contrast medium.
2. Oral ingestion of barium sulfate, a metallic contrast medium used for studies of the upper gastrointestinal tract, after which x-rays are taken.
3. Process of x-ray recording the renal pelvis and other urinary tract organs by injecting contrast dye back up through the urethra and into the urinary bladder.
4. X-ray record of the salivary gland and saliva.
5. X-ray of blood vessels using an iodine compound as a contrast medium.
6. Process of x-ray recording of the gallbladder using contrast media.
7. Process of x-ray recording of the urinary system by injecting contrast dye or medium through veins.
8. X-ray record of the spinal cord.
9. Rectal administration of barium sulfate as a contrast medium in x-ray studies of the lower gastrointestinal tract.
10. Process of x-ray recording of the lymph vessels by injecting a contrast medium into lymph fluid.
11. X-ray record of the bronchial tubes using a contrast medium.
12. Process of x-ray recording of the uterus and fallopian tubes using contrast medium.
13. Injecting contrast medium through tubes into the heart and blood vessels surrounding the heart and then taking x-ray pictures.
14. X-ray record of veins; contrast medium is injected.

F.
1. n	6. a	11. c
2. h	7. j	12. i
3. d	8. k	13. m
4. l	9. o	14. f
5. e	10. b	15. g

G.
1. Combination of proton, neutron, and electron in the atom of an element.
2. Number of protons in the nucleus of an atom.
3. Number of protons and neutrons in the nucleus of an atom.
4. Forms of an atom which have the same atomic number but differ in atomic weight.
5. Forms of an atom which are radioactive; they emit radioactive rays.
6. Radioisotope; form of an atom which is radioactive.
7. High-energy radioactive particles produced by the disintegration of radioactive atoms.
8. High-energy charged particles produced from radioactive atoms.
9. High-energy radioactive rays, emitted from radioactive atoms.
10. The time it takes for radioactive atoms to lose half their radioactivity.

H.
1. h	6. e
2. a	7. b
3. i	8. c
4: f	9. g
5. j	10. d

I.
1. heat	7. wandering, going
2. dry	8. luminous, light
3. sound	9. three-dimensional, solid
4. x-rays	10. cut
5. sound	11. spark
6. motion, moving pictures	

REVIEW SHEET 22

Combining Forms

cine/o	_____	radi/o	_____
ech/o	_____	roentgen/o	_____
fluor/o	_____	scint/i	_____
ion/o	_____	son/o	_____
is/o	_____	stere/o	_____
luc/o	_____	tele/o	_____
myel/o	_____	therm/o	_____
opac/o	_____	tom/o	_____
opaq/o	_____	xer/o	_____

Suffixes and Prefixes

-graph	_____	intra-	_____
-graphy	_____	-scope	_____
-gram	_____	-scopy	_____
inter-	_____	-therapy	_____

Additional Terms in Radiology

abduction _____

adduction _____

angiogram _____

AP view _____

barium enema _____

barium swallow _____

bronchogram _____

Bucky grid _____

catheterization _____

cineradiography _____

computerized axial tomography _____

contrast techniques _____

decubitus _____

EMI scanner _____

eversion _____

extension _____

film badge _____

flexion _____

fluorescence _____

fluoroscopy _____

intravenous pyelogram (IVP) _____

inversion _____

laminagraphy _____

lateral view _____

lordotic view _____

lymphangiogram _____

megavoltage _____

oblique view _____

orthovoltage _____

oscilloscope   _____

PA view   _____

photon   _____

prone   _____

rad   _____

radiology   _____

radiolucent   _____

radiopaque   _____

recumbent   _____

retrograde pyelogram (RP)   _____

roentgenology   _____

salpingogram   _____

scattered radiation   _____

sialogram   _____

stereoscopy   _____

supine   _____

thermography   _____

tomography   _____

ultrasonography   _____

xeroradiography   _____

x-rays   _____

Additional Terms for Nuclear Medicine

alpha particle   _____

atom   _____

atomic number _____

atomic weight _____

beta particle _____

cold nodule _____

electron _____

element _____

gamma rays _____

Geiger counter _____

half-life _____

ion _____

ionization _____

isotope _____

neutron _____

nuclear medicine _____

nuclide _____

proton _____

radioactive isotope _____

radioactivity _____

radionuclide _____

radiopharmaceutical _____

scan _____

scintillation counter _____

tagging _____

teletherapy _____

tracer studies _____

CHAPTER 23

PHARMACOLOGY I

In this chapter you will:

Differentiate between various subdivisions in the field of pharmacology;

Learn about drug names, drug standards, and reference information related to drugs;

Identify the various routes of drug administration;

Recognize the terms which describe different types of drug actions and drug toxicities; and

Build medical terms related to pharmacology using new combining forms, prefixes, and suffixes.

This chapter is divided into the following sections:

I. INTRODUCTION

Drugs are chemical substances used in medicine in the treatment of disease. These chemical substances can come from many different sources. Drugs are obtained from various parts of **plants**, such as the roots, leaves, and fruit. Examples of such drugs are digitalis (from the foxglove plant), and antibiotics such as penicillin and streptomycin (from plants called molds). Drugs can also be obtained from **animals**; for example, hormones are secretions from the glands of animals. Drugs can be made from chemical substances which are **synthesized** in the laboratory. Anticancer drugs, such as methotrexate and prednisone, are examples of laboratory-synthesized drugs. Some drugs are contained in food substances; these drugs are called **vitamins**. Drugs are dispensed and stored in an area known as a **pharmacy**.

The field of medicine which studies drugs, their nature, origin, and effect in the body is called **pharmacology**. Pharmacology is a large medical specialty and contains many subdivisions of study, including pharmacodynamics, molecular pharmacology, chemotherapy, and toxicology.

Pharmacodynamics involves the study of how drugs exert their effects in the body. Scientists interested in pharmacodynamics study the processes of drug **absorption** (how drugs pass into the bloodstream), **metabolism** (changes drugs undergo within the body), and **excretion** (removal of the drug from the body).

Molecular pharmacology concerns the study of the interaction of drugs and cells or subcellular entities, such as DNA, RNA, or enzymes. These studies provide important information about the mechanism of action of the drug.

Chemotherapy is the subdivision of pharmacology which studies drugs that are capable of destroying microorganisms, parasites, and cells within the body without destroying the body itself. Chemotherapy includes treatment of infectious diseases, mental illness, and cancer.

Toxicology is the study of harmful chemicals and their dangerous effects on the body. Toxicology includes the study of the potentially harmful effects of any drug on the body; any drug, if given in high enough doses, can have harmful actions on the body. Toxicological studies in animals are required by law before new drugs can be tested in individuals. A toxicologist is also interested in finding proper **antidotes** to these harmful effects. Antidotes are substances given to neutralize unwanted effects of drugs.

In this first of two pharmacology chapters, we will discuss some of the general concepts and terms which describe the actions, toxicities, and administration of drugs. In the next chapter, we will explore specific classes of drugs and their effects on the body.

II. VOCABULARY

additive	Drug action in which the combination of two similar drugs is equal to the sum of the effects of each.
anaphylaxis	Hypersensitive reaction of the body to a drug or foreign organism. Symptoms may include hives, asthma, rhinitis, and so forth.
antidote	An agent that is given to counteract an unwanted effect of a drug.
brand name (trade name)	Commerical name for a drug, normally the property of the drug manufacturer.
chemical name	Chemical formula for a drug.

chemotherapy	Treatment of illness using chemicals; usually refers to treatment of infectious disease, cancer disease, or mental illness.
contraindications	Factors in the patient's condition which prevent the use of a particular drug or treatment.
cumulation	Drug action resulting from the administration of small repeated doses of a drug that are not eliminated from the body quickly enough, so that the drug builds up, or accumulates; this may be produced intentionally, or it may be unintentional and have harmful effects.
drugs	Chemical substances used as medicines in the treatment of disease.
drug toxicity	Harmful and dangerous complications which may arise from the use of drugs. Examples of common toxic effects of drugs are blood dyscrasias, such as aplastic anemia and leukopenia; cataracts; neuropathy; collagen disorders; and photosensitivity.
Food and Drug Administration (FDA)	Governmental agency having the legal responsibility for enforcing proper drug manufacture and clinical use.
generic name	The legal, noncommercial name for a drug.
Hospital Formulary	Reference listing of drugs and their appropriate clinical usage found in most hospitals and libraries; published by the American Society of Hospital Pharmacies.
idiosyncrasy	A rare type of toxic effect produced in a peculiarly sensitive individual but not seen in most patients.
molecular pharmacology	Study of the interaction of drugs and cells or subcellular entities such as DNA, RNA, or enzymes.
National Formulary (N.F.)	Large, up-to-date list of drugs and official standards for their manufacture; issued by the American Pharmaceutical Association.
parenteral administration	Administration of drugs by injection into skin, muscle, or veins (places other than the digestive tract).

pharmacodynamics

Study of how drugs achieve their effects in living organisms, including their absorption, metabolism, and excretion from living systems.

pharmacology

The study of drugs, their nature, origin, and effect on living organisms.

Physicians' Desk Reference
  (PDR)

Reference book listing drug products; published privately.

potentiation

A type of drug action in which the combined effect of using two drugs together is greater than the sum of the effects of using each one alone; also called synergism.

side effect

A toxic (harmful) effect which routinely results from the use of a drug.

suppositories

Cone-shaped objects containing medication which are inserted into the rectum, vagina, or urethra, from which the medication is absorbed into the bloodstream.

synergism

Type of drug action in which the effect of two drugs acting together is greater than the sum of each acting alone; potentiation.

tolerance

Condition of becoming resistant to the action of a drug as treatment progresses so that larger and larger doses must be given to maintain the desired effect.

toxicology

Study of harmful substances and their effect on living organisms.

United States Pharmacopeia
  (U.S.P.)

An authoritative list of drugs, formulas, and preparations which sets a standard for drug manufacturing and dispensing.

III. DRUG NAMES, STANDARDS, AND REFERENCES

Names

A drug can have three different names. The **chemical name** is the chemical formula for the drug. This name is often long and complicated.

The **generic** or **official name** is a shorter, less complicated name which is recognized as identifying the drug for legal and scientific purpose. The generic name is public property and any drug manufacturer may use it. There is only one generic name for each drug.

The **brand name** or **trade name** is the private property of the individual drug manufacturer and no competitor may use it. Brand names often have the superscript ® after or before the name. Most drugs have several brand names because each manufacturer producing the drug gives it a different name. When a specific brand name is ordered on a prescription by a physician, it must be dispensed by the pharmacist; no other brand name may be substituted. It is common practice to capitalize the first letter of a brand name.

The following lists give the chemical, generic, and brand names of the well known antibiotic drug, ampicillin. Note that the drug can have several brand names but only one generic, or official, name.

Chemical Name	*Generic Name*	*Brand Name*
alpha-aminobenzyl P	ampicillin	Amcill capsules
		Omnipen
		Penbritin
		Polycillin
		Principen/N

Standards

While the **Food and Drug Administration** (FDA) has the legal responsibility for deciding whether a drug may be distributed and sold, there are definite standards for drugs set by an independent committee of physicians, pharmacologists, pharmacists, and manufacturers. This committee is called the **United States Pharmacopeia** (U.S.P.). Two important standards of the U.S.P. are that the drug must be clinically useful (useful for patients) and available in pure form (made by good manufacturing methods). If a drug has U.S.P. after its name, it has met with the standards of the Pharmacopeia. A list of drugs is published by the U.S.P. every 5 years, but not all drugs are listed in it. The **National Formulary** (N.F.) is a larger list of drugs which meet purity standards. The letters U.S.P. and N.F. after a drug indicate that the manufacturer claims his product conforms to U.S.P. or N.F. standards. It is up to the FDA to inspect and enforce the claims of drug manufacturers.

References

Libraries and hospitals have two large reference listings of drugs which give important information about drugs. The most complete and up-to-date is the **Hospital Formulary**, published by the American Society of Hospital Pharmacists. This listing gives information about the characteristics of drugs and their clinical usage (application to patient care).

The **Physicians' Desk Reference** (PDR) is published by a private firm, and drug manufacturers pay to have their products listed. The PDR is a useful reference with several different indexes to identify drugs (generic and chemical name index, product identification index, manufacturers' index, drug classification index) and full descriptions, precautions and warnings, and information about recommended dosage and administration for each drug.

IV. ADMINISTRATION OF DRUGS

The route of administration of a drug (how it is introduced into the body) is very important in determining the rate and completeness of its absorption into the bloodstream and the speed and duration of the drug's action in the body.

The many different methods used by physicians and allied health personnel to administer drugs are listed below, with a brief discussion of each method:

Oral Administration. This route of administration is by mouth. Drugs given orally must pass into the stomach and be absorbed into the bloodstream through the intestinal wall. Although this method is probably most acceptable to patients from the standpoint of convenience, it may have several disadvantages. If the drug is destroyed in the digestive tract by digestive juices or if the drug cannot pass through the intestinal mucosa, it will be ineffective. Also, oral administration is slower than other methods and disadvantageous if time is a factor in therapy.

Sublingual Administration. In this route of administration, drugs are not swallowed but are placed under the tongue and allowed to dissolve in the saliva. Absorption may be rapid for some agents. Nitroglycerin tablets are taken this way to treat attacks of chest pain (angina pectoris). The nitroglycerin is rapidly absorbed into the bloodstream and opens coronary arteries to increase blood flow to the heart muscle.

Rectal Administration. **Suppositories** (cone-shaped objects containing drugs) and aqueous (water) solutions are inserted into the rectum (distal end of the digestive tract). At times, drugs are given by rectum when oral administration presents difficulties, such as when the patient is nauseated and vomiting.

Parenteral Administration. This type of administration is accomplished by injection through a **syringe** (syring/o = tube) under the skin, into muscle, into a vein, or into a body cavity. There are several types of parenteral injections:

Subcutaneous Injection. This injection is sometimes called a **hypodermic injection**, and is given just under the several layers of the skin. The outer surface of the arm and the anterior surface of the skin are usual locations for subcutaneous injections.

Intradermal Injection. This shallow injection is made into the upper layers of the skin. It is used chiefly in skin testing for allergic reactions. Short needles are used, and an elevation appears on the skin when an intradermal injection is given properly.

Intramuscular Injection (I.M.). This injection is given into the muscle, usually into the buttocks. When drugs are irritating to the skin or when a large volume of a long-acting drug is to be given, I.M. injections are advisable.

Intravenous Injection (I.V.). This injection is given directly into the veins. It is given when an immediate effect from the drug is desired or when the drug cannot be given into other tissues. Good technical skill is needed in administering this injection, since leakage of drugs into surrounding tissues may result in damage to tissues.

Intrathecal Injection. This injection is made into the sheath of membranes (meninges) which surround the spinal cord and brain. The effects of the drug so administered are usually limited to the central nervous system, and intrathecal injections are often used to produce anesthesia.

Intracavitary Injection. This injection is made into a body cavity, as, for example, into the peritoneal or pleural cavity.

Inhalation. In this method of administration, vapors, or gases, are taken into the nose or mouth and are absorbed into the bloodstream through the thin walls of the air sacs in the lungs. **Aerosols** (particles of the drug suspended in air) are administered by inhalation.

Topical Application. This is the local external application of drugs on skin or mucous membranes of the mouth or other surface. It is commonly used to accelerate the healing of abrasions, for **antiseptic** treatment of a wound, and as an **antipruritic** (against itching). Topical application may also include administration of drugs into the eyes, ears, nose, and vagina. Lotions are used most often when the skin is moist, or "weeping," and ointments and creams are used when the lesions are dry.

Figure 23–1 is a chart summarizing the various routes of drug administration.

Oral	Sublingual	Rectal	Parenteral	Inhalation	Topical
Tablets	Tablets	Suppositories	Injections: Subcutaneous Intradermal Intramuscular Intravenous Intrathecal Intracavitary	Aerosols	Lotions Creams Ointments

Figure 23–1   Routes of drug administration.

V. TERMINOLOGY OF DRUG ACTION

There are certain terms which describe the action and interaction of drugs in the body once they are administered and have been absorbed into the bloodstream. These terms are listed below with explanations of their meanings:

Potentiation (Synergism). Sometimes a combination of two drugs can cause an effect which is **greater than** the **sum** of the individual effects of each drug alone. For example, penicillin and streptomycin, two antibiotic drugs, are given together in treatment for bacterial endocarditis because of their synergistic action.

Additive Action. In this drug action, the combination of two similar drugs is equal to the sum of the effects of each. For example, if drug A gives 10 per cent tumor kill as a cancer chemotherapeutic agent and drug B gives 20 per cent tumor kill, using A and B together would give 30 per cent tumor kill. If these drugs were synergistic in their action, a combination of drugs would give greater than 30 per cent tumor kill.

Cumulation. If a drug is given in short intervals and the body cannot dispose of it rapidly enough, the drug concentration will rise in the body tissues with each successive dose. This cumulation may cause toxic effects in the body. There are some instances, however, in which cumulation is desired for therapeutic purposes. The use of digitalis in management of cardiac insufficiency is an example of a therapeutic buildup of a drug to promote the efficient working of the heart.

Tolerance. In this drug action, the effects of a given dose diminish as treatment goes on, and larger doses must be given to maintain the desired effect. Tolerance is a feature of addiction to drugs such as morphine and meperidine (Demerol).

Idiosyncrasy. In some instances, a patient may display unexpected effects following the administration of a drug. Idiosyncratic reactions are produced in very few patients taking a drug, but may be life-threatening in those few instances. For example, in some individuals penicillin is known to cause an idiosyncratic reaction such as **anaphylaxis** (acute type of hypersensitivity, including asthma and shock).

VI. DRUG TOXICITY

Drug toxicity refers to the poisonous and potentially dangerous effects of some drugs. Idiosyncrasy is an example of an unpredictable type of drug toxicity.

Other types of drug toxicity are more predictable and based on the dosage of the drug given. If the dosage of certain drugs is increased, unfavorable effects may be produced. Physicians are trained to be aware of the potential toxic effects of all drugs they prescribe and must be cautious with their use. Disorders directly resulting from diagnostic or therapeutic efforts of a physician are known as **iatrogenic**, and are usually related to drug toxicity.

Side effects are toxic effects which routinely result from the use of a drug. They often occur with the usual therapeutic dosage of a drug and are usually tolerable. For example, nausea, vomiting, and alopecia are common side effects of the chemotherapeutic drugs used to treat cancer.

Contraindications are factors in a patient's condition which make the use of a drug dangerous and ill advised. For example, in the presence of renal failure, it is unwise to administer a drug which is normally eliminated by the kidneys.

Among the most dangerous toxic complications of drug usage are blood dyscrasias (blood diseases) such as aplastic anemia and leukopenia, cataract formation (eye disorder), cholestatic jaundice (biliary obstruction leading to yellow discoloration of skin), neuropathy, collagen disorders (connective tissue damage such as arthritis), and photosensitivity (abnormal sensitivity to light).

VII. COMBINING FORMS

Combining Form	Definition	Terminology	Meaning
pharmac/o	drug	pharmacology _____	
chem/o	drug	chemotherapy _____	

tox/o toxic/o	poison	toxemia _____
		toxic _____
		toxicology _____
lingu/o	tongue	sublingual _____
derm/o	skin	intradermal _____
		hypodermic _____
enter/o	intestine	parenteral _____
ven/o	vein	intravenous _____
thec/o	sheath *(covering of the spinal cord and brain)*	intrathecal _____
aer/o	air	aerosols _____
erg/o	work	synergism _____
idi/o	individual, distinct, own	idiosyncrasy _____
		idiopathic _____
iatr/o	physician	iatrogenic _____
cras/o	disease, mixture	dyscrasia _____
-phylaxis	protection	anaphylaxis _____
		Ana- means "excessive" in this word.
anti-	against	antipruritic _____
		antiseptic _____
		antipyretic _____
intra-	within	intramuscular _____
contra-	against	contraindication _____

VIII. EXERCISES

A. *Build medical words:*

1. Pertaining to against itching _____

2. The study of poisons _____

3. Treatment with chemicals _____

4. Pertaining to within a vein _____

5. Study of drugs _____

6. Pertaining to under the tongue _____

7. Pertaining to under the skin _____

8. Against infection _____

9. Produced by a physician _____

10. Pertaining to within a sheath _____

B. *Give the meaning of the following terms:*

1. parenteral _____

2. pharmacopeia _____

    _____

3. idiosyncrasy _____

4. synergism _____

5. contraindications _____

6. anaphylaxis _____

7. antidote _____

8. drug toxicity _____

9. aerosol _____

10. side effect _____

C. *Match the terms in Column I with associated terms in Column II:*

Column I

1. pharmacy _____
2. molecular pharmacology _____
3. brand name _____
4. generic name _____
5. chemical name _____
6. cumulation _____
7. additive action _____
8. potentiation _____
9. tolerance _____
10. absorption _____

Column II

a. Combination of two drugs together is equal to the sum of the effects of each.

b. Drug name which gives the chemical formula.

c. Combination of two drugs together gives an effect which is greater than sum of each drug alone.

d. Drugs passing into the bloodstream.

e. Building up of drug in the body due to inability to excrete it as fast as it is taken in.

f. Effects of a drug diminish as larger and larger doses are needed to produce desired effect.

g. Area to prepare, store, and dispense drugs.

h. Official name; legal and noncommercial name.

i. Trade name of drug privately owned by manufacturer.

j. Study of drug interaction with cells or subcellular entities.

D. *Give the meanings of the following abbreviations:*

1. PDR _____
2. FDA _____
3. I.V. _____
4. U.S.P. _____
5. I.M. _____
6. N.F. _____

E. *Match the routes of administration of drugs in Column I with the medications and procedures in Column II:*

Column I	Column II
1. intravenous _____	a. Lotions, creams, ointments
2. rectal _____	b. Tablets and capsules
3. oral _____	c. Used for allergy skin tests
4. topical _____	d. Lumbar puncture
5. inhalation _____	e. Deep injection, usually into buttocks
6. intrathecal _____	f. Suppositories
7. intramuscular _____	g. Used for blood transfusions
8. intradermal _____	h. Aerosols

ANSWERS

A.
1. antipruritic
2. toxicology
3. chemotherapy
4. intravenous
5. pharmacology
6. sublingual
7. subcutaneous, hypodermic
8. antiseptic
9. iatrogenic
10. intrathecal

B.
1. Pertaining to administration of drugs by injection in any region except the gastrointestinal tract.
2. Authoritative list of drugs, formulas, preparations, and information which sets a standard for drug manufacturing and dispensing.
3. Unpredictable, individual reaction to a drug.
4. Type of drug action in which the effect of two drugs given together is greater than the sum of each acting alone.
5. Conditions which forbid the use of a particular drug.
6. Hypersensitivity reaction to the presence of a foreign body or drug in the body.
7. Substance given to counteract a poison in the body.
8. Harmful effects and dangerous complications which may arise from use of a drug.
9. Drug suspended in air particles.
10. A toxic effect which results from the routine use of a drug.

C.
1. g
2. j
3. i
4. h
5. b
6. e
7. a
8. c
9. f
10. d

D.
1. Physicians' Desk Reference.
2. Food and Drug Administration.
3. Intravenous.
4. United States Pharmacopeia.
5. Intramuscular.
6. National Formulary.

E.
1. g
2. f
3. b
4. a
5. h
6. d
7. e
8. c

REVIEW SHEET 23

Combining Forms

aer/o	_____	lingu/o	_____
chem/o	_____	pharmac/o	_____
cras/o	_____	pyr/o	_____
cutane/o	_____	seps/o	_____
derm/o	_____	thec/o	_____
erg/o	_____	tox/o	_____
enter/o	_____	toxic/o	_____
iatr/o	_____	ven/o	_____
idi/o	_____		

Suffixes and Prefixes

anti-	_____	-phylaxis	_____
contra-	_____	-pruritic	_____
-genic	_____	syn-	_____
intra-	_____	-therapy	_____

Additional Terms

additive _____

anaphylaxis _____

antidote _____

antipruritic _____

brand name _____

chemical name

_____

chemotherapy

_____

contraindications

_____

cumulation

_____

drug toxcity

_____

Food and Drug Administration (FDA)

_____

generic name

_____

Hospital Formulary

_____

idiosyncrasy

_____

inhalation

_____

intracavitary injection

_____

interdermal injection

_____

intramuscular injection (I.M.)

_____

intrathecal injection

_____

intravenous injection (I.V.)

_____

molecular pharmacology

_____

National Formulary (N.F.)

_____

oral administration

_____

parenteral administration

_____

pharmacodynamics

_____

pharmacology

_____

Physician's Desk Reference (PDR)

_____

potentiation

_____

rectal administration

_____

side effects _____

subcutaneous injection _____

sublingual administration _____

suppositories _____

synergism _____

tolerance _____

topical application _____

toxicology _____

United States Pharmacopeia (U.S.P.) _____

CHAPTER 24

PHARMACOLOGY II

In this chapter you will:

Learn the names of the different classes of drugs and their use in patient care;

Become familiar with the names of some of the more common drugs in each class of drugs; and

Build medical terms using combining forms, prefixes, and suffixes which relate to drugs.

The chapter is divided into the following sections:

I. INTRODUCTION

This chapter concentrates on the major types of drugs and their effects on the body. Although most drug classes are presented, there are far too many drugs to include a description of all of them in a chapter of this length. Antineoplastic drugs are omitted in this chapter, but are discussed in Chapter 21.

If you are interested in learning more about drugs and their role in the physiology and pathology of the body, the following references should be helpful:

Garb, Solomon, Crim, Betty Jean, and Thomas, Garf: *Pharmacology and Patient Care.* 3rd edition. New York, Springer Publishing Company, 1970.

Goth, Andres: *Medical Pharmacology.* 8th edition. St. Louis, C. V. Mosby Company, 1976

Falconer, M. W., Patterson, H. R., and Gustafson, E. A.: *Current Drug Handbook 1976–78.* Philadelphia, W. B. Saunders Co., 1976.

In this chapter, the first letter of the brand names of drugs is capitalized to differentiate them from generic and chemical names, which are not capitalized.

II. VOCABULARY

acetylcholine	A chemical which is found in the body and acts as a transmitter of nerve impulses of the parasympathetic nervous system.
adrenergic agent	A drug which duplicates the effect of stimulating sympathetic nerve fibers. This agent is also called a sympathomimetic drug.
alcohol	Central nervous system depressant. Also used as a dilator of blood vessels and as an antiseptic.
amphetamine	Central nervous system stimulant.
anaphylactic shock	An acute allergic reaction to a drug, chemical, or foreign substance. Symptoms include asthma, fall in blood pressure, and swelling of the larynx (laryngeal edema).
anesthetics	Drugs which produce loss of sensation and block the awareness of painful stimuli. Examples of local anesthetics are procaine (Novocain), cocaine, and lidocaine (Xylocaine).
antacids	Drugs which neutralize acids in the stomach. Examples are magnesium trisilicate and magnesium hydroxide.
antiarrhythmic	Drug used to regulate heart rhythm.
antibiotic	Chemical substance, produced by a mold or bacteria, that inhibits the growth of other microorganisms. Examples of antibiotics are penicillin, erythromycin, and tetracyclines.
anticoagulants	Agents which prevent the clotting of blood. Examples are heparin and Coumadin.

anticonvulsants	Drugs which prevent and treat convulsions (involuntary contraction and spasm of muscles associated with loss of consciousness). They are used in the treatment of epilepsy. Examples are diphenylhydantoin (Dilantin) and phenobarbital.
antidiarrheals	Drugs which relieve loose bowel movements (diarrhea). An example is atropine.
antihistamines	Drugs which block the action of histamine in the body. Examples are diphenhydramine (Benadryl), meclizine (Bonine), and chlorpheniramine (Chlor-Trimeton).
antinauseants	Agents which relieve nausea and vomiting. Examples are dimenhydrinate (Dramamine) and meclizine (Bonine).
antineoplastic drugs	Drugs which are used to treat malignant tumors.
ascorbic acid	Vitamin C.
atropine	An agent used to decrease muscle contractions or spasms (antispasmodic) and block impulses of the parasympathetic nervous system.
barbiturates	Drugs which are used to induce sedation or sleep. Examples are phenobarbital and secobarbital.
belladonna	Drug containing atropine and used as an antispasmodic and sedative agent.
caffeine	Central nervous system stimulant.
cathartic	Agent which promotes defecation (bowel movement).
cholinergic agent	A drug which duplicates the effect of stimulating parasympathetic nerve fibers. An example is bethanechol.
depressants	Drugs which decrease the functioning of an organ or system.
digitalis glycosides	Drugs originating from or synthesized from an active ingredient of the foxglove, or digitalis, plant; useful in treating heart failure.

diuretics — Agents which promote urine production and reduce blood pressure. Examples are chlorothiazide and ethacrynic acid.

emetics — Drugs which induce vomiting. An example is syrup of ipecac.

gram-negative bacteria — A general class of bacteria which, when stained with the Gram stain and its "counter" stain, fails to retain the purple Gram stain, but takes on the red color of the "counter" stain. Examples are the bacteria which cause typhoid fever and urinary tract infections (*Escherichia coli*).

gram-positive bacteria — A general class of bacteria which, when stained with the Gram stain and its "counter" stain, retains the purple color of the Gram stain. Examples are staphylococci and streptococci.

histamine — A chemical found in all tissues of the body which when released in excess from cells causes allergic symptoms (rhinorrhea, edema, hives, itching, asthma).

hypnotics — Drugs which depress the central nervous system and produce sleep.

laxative — Mild purgative (promoting defecation).

narcotic — A depressant drug which produces stupor, sleep, or unconsciousness, and is habit-forming. Examples are opiates such as heroin and morphine, and synthetic drugs such as meperidine (Demerol).

neuropharmacologic drugs — Those drugs which affect the nervous system. They include autonomic and central nervous system drugs, e.g., cholinergic drugs (acting like parasympathetic nerves) and adrenergic drugs (acting like sympathetic nerves).

prophylaxis — Prevention of (protection against) disease.

purgatives — Drugs which promote defecation and relieve constipation.

pyridoxine — Vitamin B_6.

quinidine — Drug used to treat abnormalities in heart rhythm.

riboflavin	Vitamin B_2.
sedatives	Central nervous system depressants which relax and quiet a patient without producing sleep.
stimulants	Drugs which increase the functioning of an organ or system.
sulfonamides	"Sulfa drugs," used to inhibit the growth of bacteria. Gantrisin is an example of this type of drug.
thiamine	Vitamin B_1.
tranquilizers	Drugs which calm and quiet a patient, altering behavior without causing the drowsiness produced by sedatives.
vasoconstrictors	Drugs which cause constriction of the muscular wall of blood vessels and narrow their opening. An example of a vasoconstrictor is epinephrine. These agents are also called vasopressors.
vasodilators	Drugs which relax the muscular wall of blood vessels, causing the vessels to dilate. Examples are nitrites such as nitroglycerin.
vitamins	Substances found in foods and, in minute quantities, essential for good health, growth, and life itself.

III. DRUG CLASSES

1. Neuropharmacologic Drugs

These drugs act on the nervous system. There are two major types of neuropharmacologic drugs: autonomic drugs and central nervous system drugs.

Autonomic Drugs. These drugs influence the body in a manner similar to the action of the parasympathetic and sympathetic nerves of the autonomic nervous system.

The function of the sympathetic nerve network in the body is (1) to stimulate the flow of epinephrine from the adrenal gland, (2) to increase heart rate, (3) to constrict blood vessels, and (4) to dilate air passages.

Drugs which mimic the action of sympathetic nerves are called **sympathomimetic** or **adrenergic agents**. They stimulate the flow of epinephrine, increase heart rate, constrict blood vessels, and dilate air passages. Examples of sympathomimetic drugs are epinephrine (adrenaline) and norepinephrine (noradrenaline). These drugs are the same chemicals which are naturally released from the sympathetic nerve endings and adrenal glands during times of stress or emergency.

Drugs which mimic the action of parasympathetic nerves are called **parasympathomimetic** or **cholinergic agents**. These drugs oppose the actions of the sympathomimetic (adrenergic) drugs, which means that they slow down heart rate, constrict air passages, and stimulate involuntary muscles in the digestive tract and other organs. The parasympathetic agent which is produced normally at all times by parasympathetic nerve endings is called **acetylcholine**. Acetylcholine, unlike a drug such as epinephrine (adrenaline), cannot be administered to patients. This is because there are enzymes in the body called cholinesterases which inactivate acetylcholine almost as quickly as it is given. Other cholinergic drugs are, therefore, chosen as exogenous agents. One example of a cholinergic drug similar to acetylcholine in effect but longer lasting in the body is bethanechol. Bethanechol (Urecholine) is used in postoperative urinary retention to induce the constriction of the urinary bladder, aiding urination.

Other autonomic drugs are **parasympatholytic agents** which oppose the effect of parasympathetic nerve stimulation. Examples of these drugs are atropine and belladonna, which are also known as antispasmodic drugs because they act to relax the muscles in the gastrointestinal tract and decrease peristalsis.

Sympatholytic agents, which block the action of the sympathetic nervous system, include reserpine, guanethidine, and phentolamine. These drugs are used to decrease blood pressure and protect against the excess epinephrine secretion liberated by pheochromocytomas (tumors of the adrenal gland).

Figure 24–1 is a chart summarizing the various types of autonomic drugs.

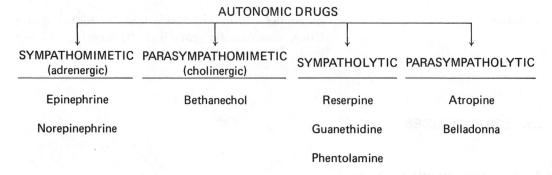

Figure 24–1

Central Nervous System Drugs. The drugs which affect the central nervous system are of two main types: those which stimulate the nerves in the brain and spinal cord, **stimulants**, and those which depress the nerves in the brain and spinal cord, **depressants**.

Stimulants. Central nervous system stimulants are used to speed up vital processes in cases of shock and collapse, and also to oppose the depressant effect of other drugs. Stimulants produce a temporary feeling of euphoria (well-being) and help to relieve lethargy. Examples of drug stimulants are **caffeine** and **amphetamine** (Benzedrine).

Side effects of caffeine, which is obtained from tea leaves and coffee beans, are tachycardia and irritability, as well as insomnia. Amphetamines are much more powerful than caffeine and can produce restlessness, insomnia, and nervousness, as well as hypertension (high blood pressure) and gastrointestinal disorders when given in high doses. Used in excessive doses, these drugs can produce convulsions.

Depressants. There are several types of central nervous system depressants, These include **analgesics, hypnotics, sedatives and barbiturates, tranquilizers, anticonvulsants, alcohol,** and **anesthetics.**

Analgesics are agents which act to relieve pain. Examples of analgesics are acetylsalicylic acid (aspirin), acetaminophen (Tylenol), and dextropropoxyphene (Darvon). Aspirin and Tylenol are **antipyretics** (agents against fever) as well as analgesics. Darvon is used to lessen any type of mild pain, especially in recurrent or chronic disease.

Acetylsalicylic acid, acetaminophen, and dextropropoxyphene are examples of non-narcotic analgesics. Examples of **narcotic** analgesics are opium, morphine, heroin, codeine, and meperidine (Demerol). Narcotics are drugs which, in moderate doses, can suppress the central nervous system and relieve pain, but in excessive doses produce unconsciousness, stupor, coma, and possibly death. Most of the narcotic analgesics are addictive and habit-forming.

Hypnotic drugs are those which depress the central nervous system and produce sleep. **Sedatives** are used to quiet and relax the patient without necessarily producing sleep. Some drugs act as sedatives in small doses and as hypnotics in larger doses. **Barbiturates**, such as phenobarbital, secobarbital, and pentobarbital, are the best known sedatives and hypnotics. Chloral hydrate is an example of another type of sedative. Depending on the dose and how it is administered, the response to a barbiturate may range from mild sedation to hypnosis and finally to general anesthesia.

Tranquilizers are drugs which alter behavior, allowing for control of nervous symptoms such as anxiety, depression, fear, or anger. Minor tranquilizers, such as chlordiazepoxide (Librium) and diazepam (Valium), are used primarily for control of less severe nervous states, while the major tranquilizers, such as phenothiazines (Thorazine, Stelazine), and tricyclic antidepressants, such as amitriptyline (Elavil), are used to control severe disturbances of behavior or psychoses (loss of contact with reality).

Anticonvulsant agents are used to treat epilepsy, a central nervous system disorder caused by abnormal electrical discharges within the brain which result in abnormal muscular movements, loss of consciousness, and other symptoms. Ideally, anticonvulsant drugs should depress the part of the brain which controls motor, or movement, activity and not the sensory and cognitive (thinking) parts of the brain. An example of an effective anticonvulsant drug is diphenylhydantoin (Dilantin). Barbiturates like phenobarbital are also used as anticonvulsant drugs.

Alcohol is another central nervous system depressant. It affects the cerebral cortex of the brain in several ways. One way is to block the processes which control or inhibit behavior. This effect accounts for the talkativeness and lack of inhibition which accompany consumption of even small amounts of alcohol in some people. Alcohol is also used as a dilator of blood vessels in vascular disease, as an antiseptic, and as a hypnotic.

Anesthetics are drugs which produce loss of sensation, and particularly loss of the appreciation of pain. General anesthetics produce loss of sensation throughout the entire body by depressing the central nervous system, producing sleep, unconscious-ness, and muscle relaxation. Examples of general anesthetics are diethyl ether, nitrous oxide, thiopental, and halothane. Local anesthetics relieve or prevent pain in a particular area of the body. The names of most of the local anesthetics have the suffix -caine. Examples are cocaine, procaine (Novocain), lidocaine (Xylocaine), and tetracaine (Pontocaine).

Figure 24–2 is a chart summarizing the different types of drugs affecting the central nervous system.

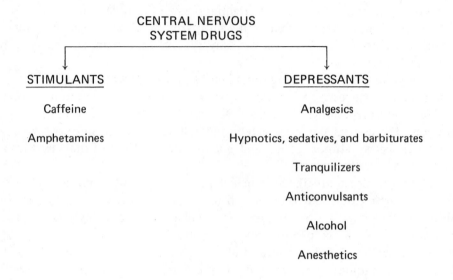

CENTRAL NERVOUS
SYSTEM DRUGS

STIMULANTS

Caffeine

Amphetamines

DEPRESSANTS

Analgesics

Hypnotics, sedatives, and barbiturates

Tranquilizers

Anticonvulsants

Alcohol

Anesthetics

Figure 24–2

2. Antihistamines

These are drugs which block the action of a chemical called **histamine** which is found in the body. Histamine is produced by most cells and especially by sensitive cells under the skin and in the respiratory system. When certain foreign antigens (protein substances which lead to the production of antibodies) enter the body, antibodies are made by cells. These antibodies attempt to inactivate, or neutralize, the offending antigens and, as a result, a chemical called histamine may be released by other cells. Histamine causes the characteristic allergic symptoms when it is liberated from cells: itching, hives, allergic rhinitis, bronchial asthma, hay fever, and, in some very serious cases, **anaphylactic shock**.

Antihistamines, by blocking the action of histamine in the body, can relieve the allergic symptoms which histamine produces. Antihistamines cannot cure the allergic reaction, but they can relieve its symptoms. Some potentially dangerous side effects of antihistamines are drowsiness, sedation, and blurred vision. Examples of antihistamines are diphenhydramine (Benadryl), meclizine (Bonamine), chlorpheniramine (Chlor-Trimeton) and tripelennamine (Pyribenzamine).

3. Cardiovascular Drugs

These drugs may be divided into three groups: drugs that **affect the heart**; drugs that **affect blood pressure**; and drugs that **prevent blood clotting**.

Drugs That Affect the Heart. Drugs may affect the heart in two major ways: changing the rate and forcefulness of the heartbeat and altering the rhythm of the heartbeat.

The most common drugs used to change the rate and forcefulness of the heartbeat are the **digitalis glycosides** (cardiac glycosides). These drugs are used to treat patients in heart failure (when the heart is not contracting with sufficient force). Most of the digitalis glycosides are obtained from the leaf of the digitalis (foxglove) plant, either as a crude mixture or as the purified glycoside from the leaf of the plant.

The important effects of the digitalis glycosides are the strengthening of the myocardium (heart muscle) and the slowing of the rate of contraction of the heart. Examples of digitalis glycosides are: digitalis, digoxin, and digitoxin.

Other drugs, which belong to the general class of sympathomimetics, are used to increase heart rate and the force of contraction. These include isoproterenol and epinephrine.

Drugs used to correct abnormal heart rhythm are called **antiarrhythmics**. Examples of these drugs are quinidine, procainamide, lidocaine (Xylocaine), and propranolol. These drugs help restore the heart rhythm to a regular cycle by depressing ectopic (outside, unwanted) myocardial impulses. Quinidine comes from the bark of the cinchona tree and is the primary drug used to treat arrhythmias. Quinidine decreases the number of times the heart muscle can contract in a given period of time. The cocaine derivatives procainamide and lidocaine (Xylocaine) are also useful in controlling abnormal cardiac rhythms.

Drugs That Affect Blood Pressure. **Vasodilators** are drugs which relax the muscles of vessel walls, thus increasing the size of blood vessels. These drugs are used in treating blood vessel diseases, heart conditions, and high blood pressure (hypertension). Blood flows more freely and blood pressure falls as blood vessels open and become dilated. Examples are sympatholytics (reserpine, guanethidine, and alpha-methyldopa) and other agents such as hydralazine.

Nitrites are drugs which are also used as vasodilators. Examples of nitrite drugs are glyceryl trinitrate (nitroglycerin) and amyl nitrite. Nitroglycerin dilates all smooth (involuntary) muscles in the body, but has a greater effect on the muscles of the coronary blood vessels. The relaxation of the muscle fibers around the blood vessels of the heart increases the width of these heart vessels and increases blood flow to the heart muscle. The pain (angina pectoris) caused by a lack of adequate blood flow to the heart is relieved by placing nitroglycerin under the tongue; from there the drug is quickly absorbed into the bloodstream. The other nitrite drugs work in a manner similar to that of nitroglycerin.

A third type of drug used to lower blood pressure is called a **diuretic**, an agent which promotes excretion of fluid and a shrinkage of the volume of blood within the vessels. An example of this type of drug is chlorothiazide (Diuril).

Vasoconstrictors are drugs which constrict muscle fibers around blood vessels and narrow the size of the vessel opening. They may act directly on the muscles of blood vessels or stimulate a region in the brain which relays the message to the vessels. Vasoconstrictors are needed to raise blood pressure, increase the force of heart action, and stop local bleeding. Examples of vasoconstrictor drugs are epinephrine (adrenaline), vasopressin, and Aramine (metaraminol).

Drugs That Prevent Blood Clotting. These drugs are called **anticoagulants**. They are used to prevent the formation of clots in veins and arteries. These clots may cause occlusion (thrombosis) of the blood supply to a vital organ, such as the brain, or may travel from their point of origin to a new site and produce a sudden occlusion of a distant organ (embolism). Anticoagulant drugs are also used to prevent coagulation in preserved blood stored for transfusions.

Heparin is an anticoagulant chemical substance found normally in human cells in the liver and lung. However, heparin can be made synthetically for commercial preparations by extracting it from the lungs of animals. When given intravenously or intramuscularly, heparin prevents the formation of clots within vessels.

Another anticoagulant is bishydroxycoumarin (Coumadin and Dicumarol). Coumadin is given orally and is effective in preventing the formation of new clots, as well as retarding the extension of those already formed.

Figure 24–3 is a chart reviewing the types of drugs used to treat cardiovascular disorders.

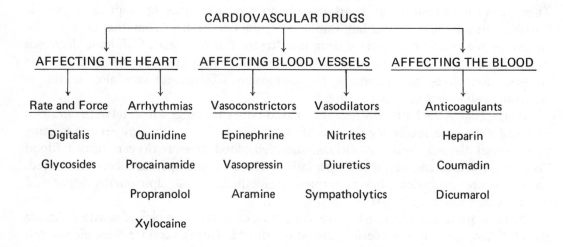

Figure 24–3

4. Gastrointestinal Drugs

There are a wide variety of gastrointestinal drugs. They each have different pharmacologic activities and are used mainly to relieve uncomfortable and potentially dangerous symptoms, rather than as cures for diseases. The following list gives the type of gastrointestinal drug, how it functions in the body, and examples of specific drugs of that type:

Type of Drug	Function	Example
Antacids	Neutralize (render inactive) acid in the stomach. Used for peptic ulcer symptoms, which are esophagitis (heartburn) and epigastric discomfort.	Magnesium trisilicate (given alone or combined with aluminum hydroxide in drug called Gelusil); magnesium hydroxide and aluminum hydroxide (Maalox); sodium bicarbonate (baking soda).
Emetics	Produce vomiting.	Solution of table salt; syrup of ipecac.
Purgatives: Laxatives (mild) Cathartics (strong)	Promote defecation and relieve constipation; there are four modes of action: (1) Irritants disturb the lining of the intestine and produce contractions. (2) Agents which swell in the presence of water and mechanically stimulate intestinal contractions. (3) Salt (saline) holds water in the intestine, promoting contraction of muscles. (4) Emollients soften the feces.	Bisacodyl (Dulcolax); castor oil. Agar (from seaweed). Milk of magnesia; magnesium sulfate (Epsom salts). Mineral oil.
Antinauseants	Relieve nausea and vomiting.	Dimenhydrinate (Dramamine); meclizine (Bonine); prochlorperazine (Compazine).
Antidiarrheals and antispasmodics	Treat diarrhea and decrease rapid movement of bowels (spasms).	Atropine; belladonna.

5. Antibiotics

An antibiotic is a chemical substance produced by a microorganism (bacterium or simple plant called a mold). The antibiotic can be **bacteriocidal** (able to kill microorganisms such as bacteria) or **bacteriostatic** (inhibit the growth of other microorganisms). Antibiotics have been synthesized in the laboratory and are used to treat serious bacterial infections.

The terms **gram-positive** and **gram-negative** are often used to describe types of bacteria which are destroyed or inhibited by antibiotics. Gram-positive bacteria are those which stain purple with the Gram stain. Gram-negative bacteria lose the Gram stain and take the red color of a "counter" stain. Examples of gram-positive bacteria are claustridia, staphylococci, and streptococci. Gram-negative bacteria are the bacteria causing meningitis, cholera, and typhoid fever.

The chart below gives the names of the major antibiotic groups, the bacterial organism affected, the disease prevented, and an example of a specific antibiotic drug of that group:

Drug Group	Bacteria	Disease	Example of Drug
Penicillin	cocci (berry-shaped)	pneumonia; streptococcal infection	
	bacilli (rod-shaped)	tetanus	ampicillin; penicillin G;
	treponema of syphilis	syphilis	penicillin V
	actinomyces	actinomycosis	
Erythromycin	some gram-positive cocci; some gram-negative cocci	streptococcal, staphylococcal and pneumococcal infections	erythromycin estolate
Streptomycin	tubercle bacilli; many gram-positive and gram-negative bacteria	tuberculosis; plague	streptomycin
Tetracyclines	streptococci; staphylococci; gram-negative bacteria; rickettsia (parasitic organisms)	bacterial infections; rickettsial infections	tetracycline; Aureomycin B; Terramycin
Antifungal agents	fungi (simple plants)	skin infections and fungal meningitis	nystatin; amphotericin B

The sulfonamides, or "sulfa drugs," are also used to inhibit the growth of bacteria. They are bacteriostatic, as opposed to bacteriocidal. These drugs are synthetic and made to resemble a substance bacteria need for making a necessary vitamin, folic acid. Sulfa drugs have been largely replaced by antibiotics which can act faster with fewer side effects. However, such sulfonamides as Gantrisin (sulfisoxazole) are effective in combating urinary tract infections.

6. Vitamins

Vitamins are necessary for normal body functioning, although none can be made by the body itself. They are found in plant and animal foods and are needed in only minute quantities for good health. Vitamins play important roles in the metabolic processes of the body, and can be synthesized in the laboratory.

The following list includes the major vitamins, the foods containing the vitamin, and diseases resulting from deficiency of the vitamin:

Vitamin	Other Names	Foods	Deficiency Disease
Vitamin A		carrots, egg yolks, green leafy vegetables	night blindness, dryness of eyes and skin
Vitamin B_1	thiamine	wheat germ, yeast, soybean	beriberi (neurological disorder)
Vitamin B_2	riboflavin	eggs, liver, poultry	pellagra (cutaneous, gastrointestinal, neurological, and mental disorder)
Vitamin B_6	pyridoxine	rice, yeast	dermatitis, neuritis, anorexia
Vitamin B_{12}	cyanocobalamin	liver, dairy products	pernicious anemia
Vitamin C	ascorbic acid	fresh vegetables, fruits (citrus), and juices	scurvy (abnormal bleeding, poor teeth and bone formation)
Vitamin D		milk, butter, egg yolks	rickets (poor bone formation and poor calcium absorption)
Vitamin E		lettuce and other green leafy vegetables	not well understood in humans
Folic acid		meats, yeast, green leafy vegetables	anemia
Vitamin K		most foods	hemorrhaging

IV. COMBINING FORMS

Combining Form	Definition	Terminology	Meaning
narc/o	numbness, stupor	narcotic _____	
		narcolepsy _____	
pyr/o	fever	antipyretic _____	
hypn/o	sleep	hypnosis _____	
		hypnogenic _____	
esthesi/o	feeling (nervous sensation)	anesthesia _____	
algesi/o	sensitivity to pain	analgesic _____	
hist/o	tissue	histamine _____	
		antihistamine _____	
vas/o	vessel	vasodilator _____	
		vasoconstrictor _____	
erg/o	work	adrenergic _____	
		cholinergic _____	
myc/o	mold (a type of fungus)	erythromycin _____ This antibiotic is produced by a red mold.	
		streptomycin _____	
vit/o vit/a	life	vitamin _____	
-cidal	pertaining to killing	bacteriocidal _____ Also spelled bactericidal.	
-static	pertaining to stopping, controlling	bacteriostatic _____	

-phoria	feeling *(mental state)*	eu<u>phoria</u> _____
-phylaxis	protection	ana<u>phylaxis</u> _____
-mimetic	to mimic, copy	sympatho<u>mimetic</u> _____
-lytic	destruction	sympatho<u>lytic</u> _____
		adreno<u>lytic</u> _____
anti-	against	<u>anti</u>biotic _____

V. EXERCISES

A. *Give the meaning of the following terms which relate to autonomic neuropharmacologic drugs:*

 1. sympathomimetic _____

 2. adrenergic agents _____

 3. parasympathomimetic _____

 4. cholinergic agents _____

 5. acetylcholine _____

 6. epinephrine _____

 7. parasympatholytic _____

 8. sympatholytic _____

B. *Match the neuropharmacologic drug in Column I with a term in Column II which describes its function:*

Column I		*Column II*
1. atropine _____		a. cholinergic (parasympathomimetic)
2. epinephrine _____		b. sympatholytic
3. reserpine _____		c. parasympatholytic

4. belladonna _____   d. sympathomimetic (adrenergic)

5. bethanechol _____

6. acetylcholine _____

C. *Give the meaning of the following terms which describe drugs affecting the central nervous system:*

1. depressants _____

2. stimulants _____

3. analgesics _____

4. anesthetics _____

5. anticonvulsants _____

6. hypnotics _____

7. antipyretics _____

8. narcotics _____

9. sedatives _____

10. barbiturates _____

11. tranquilizers _____

D. *Match the name of the drug in Column I with an appropriate drug term in Column II:*

Column I		*Column II*
1. chloral hydrate _____		a. anesthetic
2. morphine _____		b. tranquilizer
3. acetylsalicylic acid _____		c. sedative
4. caffeine _____		d. anticonvulsant
5. Dilantin _____		e. narcotic

6. amphetamine _____   f. stimulant

7. diethyl ether _____   g. analgesic

8. heroin _____

9. Thorazine _____

10. Novocain _____

E. *Give the meaning of the following terms:*

1. antihistamine _____

2. anaphylactic shock _____

3. Benadryl _____

4. Chlor-Trimeton _____

5. digitalis glycosides _____

6. antiarrhythmic _____

7. quinidine _____

8. vasodilators _____

9. nitroglycerin _____

10. diuretic _____

11. vasconstrictors _____

12. anticoagulant _____

F. *Match the name of the drug in Column I with the appropriate drug type in Column II:*

Column I   Column II

1. heparin _____   a. vasoconstrictor

2. Xylocaine _____   b. digitalis glycoside

3. reserpine _____   c. anticoagulant

4. Coumadin _____   d. vasodilator

5. epinephrine _____   e. sympathomimetic

6. nitroglycerin _____   f. sympatholytic

7. bethanechol _____   g. antiarrhythmic

8. digoxin _____   h. diuretic

9. amyl nitrite _____   i. cholinergic

10. Diuril _____

G. *Match the type of gastrointestinal drug in Column I with its function in Column II:*

Column I		*Column II*

1. laxative _____   a. produce vomiting

2. antidiarrheal _____   b. relieve nausea and vomiting

3. antacids _____   c. relieve diarrhea

4. antinauseant _____   d. promote defecation (mild drug)

5. cathartic _____   e. neutralize acid in the stomach

6. emetic _____   f. relieve spasms of the bowels

7. antispasmodic _____   g. promote defecation (strong purgative)

H. *In the following drugs, tell if each is an:*

(A) Emetic
(B) Purgative
(C) Antacid
(D) Antinauseant
(E) Antidiarrheal

1. Compazine _____   4. Gelusil _____

2. mineral oil _____   5. Dramamine _____

3. syrup of ipecac _____   6. Milk of magnesia _____

7. Maalox _____   9. Bonine _____

8. atropine _____   10. Dulcolax _____

I. *Give the meaning of the following terms:*

1. gram-positive bacteria _____

_____

2. gram-negative bacteria _____

_____

3. antibiotic _____

4. bacteriocidal _____

5. bacteriostatic _____

6. penicillin _____

7. erythromycin _____

8. streptomycin _____

_____

9. tetracycline _____

10. sulfonamides _____

J. *Match the name of the vitamin in Column I with its synonym in Column II:*

Column I   *Column II*

1. cyanocobalamin _____   a. vitamin B_6

2. riboflavin _____   b. vitamin B_1

3. thiamine _____   c. vitamin C

4. pyridoxine _____   d. vitamin B_{12}

5. ascorbic acid _____   e. vitamin B_2

K. *The following diseases are associated with what vitamin deficiency?*

1. beriberi _____

2. pernicious anemia _____

3. night blindness _____

4. scurvy _____

5. pellagra _____

6. rickets _____

ANSWERS

A.
1. Agents which produce effects similar to those caused by stimulating the sympathetic nervous system; increase heart rate, dilate air passages, constrict blood vessels, and stimulate the flow of epinephrine.
2. Those drugs which mimic the action of the sympathetic nerve fibers; sympathomimetics.
3. Agents which produce effects similar to those caused by stimulating the parasympathetic nervous system; slow down heart rate, constrict air passages, stimulate muscles in the digestive tract and other internal organs.
4. Drugs which mimic the action of the parasympathetic nervous system (whose nerve endings release acetylcholine); parasympathomimetics.
5. Chemical produced normally at all times by parasympathetic nerve endings.
6. Chemical normally released by the adrenal glands and endings of sympathetic nerves; increases heart rate, blood pressure, and dilates air passages.
7. Agents which produce effects resembling interruption of the parasympathetic nerve supply to a part of the body; atropine and belladonna are examples.
8. Agents which produce effects resembling interruption of the sympathetic nerve supply to a part of the body; reserpine and guanethidine are examples.

B.
1.	c	4.	c
2.	d	5.	a
3.	b	6.	a

C.
1. Agents which decrease the functioning of an organ or system.
2. Agents which increase the functioning of an organ or system.
3. Drugs which decrease sensitivity to pain; examples are aspirin and acetaminophen (Tylenol).
4. Drugs which produce a loss of nervous sensation and block the awareness of painful stimuli; examples are diethyl ether and lidocaine (Xylocaine).
5. Drugs which prevent convulsions; examples are Dilantin and phenobarbital.
6. Drugs which produce sleep.
7. Drugs which relieve fever.
8. Drugs which produce sleep and are habit-forming. Opiates, such as morphine and heroin, and synthetic drugs, such as meperidine (Demerol) are examples.
9. Drugs which depress the central nervous system; in small doses they cause relaxation and calm, and may produce sleep in large doses.
10. Drugs which have sedative and hypnotic action. Examples are phenobarbital and pentobarbital.
11. Drugs which alter behavior and control symptoms such as anxiety, depression, fears, and anger without a sedative effect of suppressing body reactions to stimuli.

D. 1. c   6. f
    2. e   7. a
    3. g   8. e
    4. f   9. b
    5. d   10. a

E. 1. Drug which blocks the action of histamine in the body.
    2. Acute allergic reaction to a drug, chemical, or foreign substance.
    3. Antihistamine drug which blocks the action of histamine in the body.
    4. Antihistamine drug.
    5. Drugs which increase the rate and force of the heartbeat when the heart is in failure. Synthesized or obtained from an active ingredient of the foxglove plant.
    6. Drug which is used to correct an abnormal heart rhythm.
    7. Antiarrhythmic drug; helps to restore the heart rhythm.
    8. Drugs which increase the size of blood vessels by relaxing the muscles in the vessel walls.
    9. Type of vasodilator with a great effect on the coronary arteries.
   10. Drug which increases the amount of urine (water) excreted, thereby reducing the volume of blood and lowering blood pressure.
   11. Drugs which constrict muscle fibers around blood vessels and narrow the size of the vessel opening.
   12. Drug which prevents blood clotting.

F. 1. c   6. d   *G.* 1. d   *H.* 1. D   6. B
    2. g   7. i   2. c   2. B   7. C
    3. d, f   8. b   3. e   3. A   8. E
    4. c   9. d   4. b   4. C   9. D
    5. a, e   10. h   5. g   5. D   10. B
                        6. a
                        7. f

I. 1. Bacteria which when stained with the purple Gram stain and its red counter stain take on the color of the red counter stain.
    2. Bacteria which when stained with the Gram stain and its counter still retain the purple color of the Gram stain.
    3. A substance, derived from a mold or bacteria, that inhibits the growth of other microorganisms.
    4. Causing the death of bacteria.
    5. Inhibiting or retarding the growth of bacteria.
    6. An antibiotic substance derived from a mold; it is bacteriostatic in its action but is also slightly bacteriocidal.
    7. An antibiotic substance derived from a red mold. It is generally more active against gram-positive bacteria than gram-negative.
    8. An antibiotic substance derived from a mold and active against the tubercle bacillus (bacterium causing tuberculosis) and a large number of gram-positive and gram-negative bacteria.
    9. Antibiotic substance derived from a mold. Tetracycline is effective against many types of bacteria.
   10. Sulfa drugs used to inhibit the growth of bacteria.

J. 1. d
    2. e
    3. b
    4. a
    5. c

K. 1. thiamine (vitamin B_1)
    2. cyanocobalamin (vitamin B_{12})
    3. vitamin A
    4. ascorbic acid (vitamin C)
    5. riboflavin (vitamin B_2)
    6. vitamin D

REVIEW SHEET 24

Combining Forms

adren/o _____   hypn/o _____

algesi/o _____   myc/o _____

bacteri/o _____   narc/o _____

erg/o _____   pyr/o _____

erythr/o _____   strept/o _____

esthesi/o _____   vas/o _____

hist/o _____   vit/o, vit/a _____

Suffixes and Prefixes

anti- _____   -mimetic _____

-cidal _____   -phoria _____

eu- _____   -phylaxis _____

-lepsy _____   -static _____

-lytic _____

Additional Terms

acetylcholine _____

adrenergic agent _____

alcohol _____

amphetamine _____

anaphylactic shock _____

anesthetics _____

antacids _____

antiarrhythmics _____

antibiotics _____

anticoagulants _____

anticonvulsants _____

antidiarrheals _____

antihistamines _____

antinauseants _____

antineoplastic drugs _____

ascorbic acid _____

atropine _____

bacteriocidal _____

bacteriostatic _____

barbiturates _____

belladonna _____

caffeine _____

cathartics _____

cholinergic agents _____

cyanocobalamin _____

depressants _____

digitalis glycosides _____

diuretics _____

emetics _____

erythromycin _____

gram-negative bacteria _____

gram-positive bacteria _____

heparin _____

histamine _____

hypnotics _____

laxatives _____

narcotics _____

neuropharmacologic drugs _____

parasympatholytic _____

parasympathomimetic _____

prophylaxis _____

purgatives _____

pyridoxine _____

riboflavin _____

sedatives _____

stimulants _____

streptomycin _____

sulfonamides _____

sympatholytic _____

sympathomimetic _____

tetracycline _____

thiamine _____

tranquilizers _____

vasoconstrictors _____

vasodilators _____

vitamins _____

GLOSSARY

PLURALS

The rules for commonly forming plurals of medical terms are as follows:

1. For words ending in **is**, drop the **is** and add **es**:

   Examples:

Singular	*Plural*
anastomosis	anastomoses
metastasis	metastases
epiphysis	epiphyses
prosthesis	prostheses

2. For words ending in **um**, drop the **um** and add **a**:

   Examples:

Singular	*Plural*
bacterium	bacteria
diverticulum	diverticula
ovum	ova

3. For words ending in **us**, drop the **us** and add **i**:

   Examples:

Singular	*Plural*
calculus	calculi
bronchus	bronchi
nucleus	nuclei

Some exceptions to this rule include viruses and sinuses.

4. For words ending in **a**, retain the **a** and add **e**:

   Examples:

Singular	Plural
vertebr<u>a</u>	vertebr<u>ae</u>
burs<u>a</u>	burs<u>ae</u>
bull<u>a</u>	bull<u>ae</u>

5. For words ending in **ix** and **ex**, drop the **ix** or **ex** and add **ices**:

   Examples:

Singular	Plural
ap<u>ex</u>	ap<u>ices</u>
var<u>ix</u>	var<u>ices</u>

6. For words ending in **on**, drop the **on** and add **a**:

   Examples:

Singular	Plural
gangli<u>on</u>	gangli<u>a</u>
spermatoz<u>oon</u>	spermatoz<u>oa</u>

ABBREVIATIONS

A.C.	Alternating current.
a.c.	Before meals (*ante cibum*).
ACTA	Automated computerized transverse axial scanner (machine for computerized axial tomography).
ACTH	Adrenocorticotropic hormone.
ADH	Antidiuretic hormone.
ad lib.	As desired.
AP view	Anteroposterior view (x-ray position).
aq.	Water (*aqua*).
Ara-C	Cytosine arabinoside (antineoplastic drug).
ASHD	Arteriosclerotic heart disease.
ATP	Adenosine triphosphate (energy storage substance in cell).
Au	Gold.
ausc.	Auscultation.
A-V	Arteriovenous, atrioventricular.
Ba	Barium.
B-cells	Lymphocytes produced in the bone marrow.
BCNU	Bischloroethylnitrosourea (antineoplastic drug).
BE	Barium enema.
b.i.d.	Twice a day (*bis in die*).
BMR	Basal metabolic rate.
BP	Blood pressure.
BPH	Benign prostatic hypertrophy.
BSP	Bromsulphalein (dye used in a liver function test; its retention is indicative of liver damage or disease).
BT	Bleeding time.
BUN	Blood, urea, nitrogen (test of kidney function).
C_1, C_2	First, second cervical vertebra.
C_{cr}	Creatinine clearance (test of kidney function).

Ca	Calcium.
CAT	Computerized axial tomography.
CBC, c.b.c.	Complete blood count.
cc.	Cubic centimeter (unit of mass; 1/1000 liter).
CCU	Coronary care unit.
CEA	Carcinoembryonic antigen.
CHF	Congestive heart failure.
Cl	Chlorine.
cm.	Centimeter (1/100 meter).
CNS	Central nervous system.
Co	Cobalt.
CO$_2$	Carbon dioxide.
COP	Cytoxin, Oncovin, prednisone (antineoplastic drugs given in combination chemotherapy).
COPD	Chronic obstructive pulmonary disease.
CPC	Clinicopathological conference.
CPK	Creatinine phosphokinase (enzyme released into blood following injury to heart or skeletal muscles).
Cr	Chromium.
Cs	Cesium.
CSF	Cerebrospinal fluid.
CVA	Cerebrovascular accident.
CVP	Cytoxin, vincristine, prednisone (antineoplastic drugs given in combination chemotherapy).
D$_1$, D$_2$	First, second dorsal (thoracic) vertebra.
D$_x$	Diagnosis.
D.C.	Direct current.
D & C	Dilation and curettage.
DES	Diethylstilbestrol.
diff.	Differential blood count (numbers of all types of blood cells).
DNA	Deoxyribonucleic acid.

DT's	Delirium tremens (mental confusion, hallucinations, incoherence of ideas—brought on by alcoholic withdrawal).
EBV	Epstein-Barr virus.
ECG	Electrocardiogram.
EEG	Electroencephalogram.
EKG	Electrocardiogram.
EM	Electron microscope.
Em	Emmetropia.
EMG	Electromyogram.
EMI scanner	Computerized axial tomography scanner developed by Electronic Music Instruments, Ltd.
FBS	Fasting blood sugar.
FDA	Food and Drug Administration.
Fe	Iron.
FFA	Free fatty acids (found in the blood).
FSH	Follicle-stimulating hormone.
5-FU	5-Fluorouracil (antineoplastic drug).
F.U.O.	Fever of undetermined origin.
Ga	Gallium.
GBS	Gallbladder series (x-rays).
GC	Gonorrhea.
GFR	Glomerular filtration rate (kidney function test).
GH	Growth hormone.
GI	Gastrointestinal.
Gm., gm.	Gram.
Grav. 1,2,3	First, second, third pregnancy.
GTT	Glucose tolerance test.
gtt.	Drops (*guttae*).
GU	Genitourinary.
H	Hydrogen.
Hb	Hemoglobin.

HCG	Human chorionic gonadotropin.	**LUQ**	Left upper quadrant.
HCl	Hydrochloric acid.	**LV**	Left ventricle.
HCT (Hct)	Hematocrit.	**mc**	Millicurie (dose of radiation).
He	Helium.	**MCH**	Mean corpuscular hemoglobin (amount of hemoglobin in each red blood cell).
H & E	Hematoxylin and eosin stains (for viewing tissues).		
Hg	Mercury.	**MCHC**	Mean corpuscular hemoglobin concentration (amount of hemoglobin per unit of blood).
HGB (Hgb)	Hemoglobin.		
H₂O	Water.	**MCV**	Mean corpuscular volume (measurement of size of individual red cell).
hpf	High power field (microscope).		
h.s.	At bedtime (*hora somni*).	**mEq.**	Milliequivalent (measurement of the concentration of a solution).
I	Iodine.		
¹³¹I	Radioactive isotope of iodine.	**mEq./L.**	Milliequivalent per liter.
IADH	Inappropriate antidiuretic hormone.	**mg.**	Milligram (1/1000 gram).
		MI	Myocardial infarction (heart attack).
ICU	Intensive care unit.		
I.M.	Intramuscular (injection).	**ml.**	Milliliter (1/1000 liter).
IPPB	Intermittent positive-pressure breathing (asthma and emphysema therapy).	**mm.**	Millimeter (1/1000 meter; 0.039 inch).
		mm. Hg	Millimeters of mercury.
IUD	Intrauterine device.	**mμ**	Millimicron (1/1000 micron; a micron is 10^{-3} mm.).
I.V.	Intravenous (injection).		
IVP	Intravenous pyelogram.	**μg.**	Microgram (one-millionth of a gram).
K	Potassium.	**MOPP**	Nitrogen mustard, Oncovin, prednisone, procarbazine (antineoplastic combination chemotherapy drugs).
kg.	Kilogram (1000 grams).		
KUB	Kidney, ureter, and bladder (abdominal x-ray).		
		6-MP	6-Mercaptopurine (antineoplastic drug).
L.	Liter.		
L₁, L₂	First, second lumbar vertebra.	**mRNA**	Messenger RNA.
LB	Large bowel.	**MTX**	Methotrexate.
LDH	Lactic dehydrogenase (an enzyme whose concentration is a measure of liver function).	**N**	Nitrogen.
		Na	Sodium.
		NB	Newborn.
L.E.	Lupus erythematosus.	**N.F.**	National Formulary.
LH	Luteinizing hormone.	**NPO**	Nothing by mouth (*nulli per os*).
LLQ	Left lower quadrant.		
LMP	Last menstrual period.	**O₂**	Oxygen.
LP	Lumbar puncture.	**OB**	Obstetrics.

O.D.	Right eye (*oculus dexter*).
O.S.	Left eye (*oculus sinister*).
OT	Old tuberculin (test for tuberculosis).
P	Phosphorus.
PAC	Premature atrial contractions.
Para 1,2,3	Unipara, bipara, tripara (number of viable births).
PAT	Paroxysmal atrial tachycardia.
PA view	Posteroanterior view (x-ray position).
PBI	Protein-bound iodine (test of thyroid function).
p.c.	After meals (*post cibum*).
PDA	Patent ductus arteriosus.
PDR	Physicians' Desk Reference.
PEG	Pneumoencephalography.
pH	Hydrogen ion concentration (alkalinity and acidity measurement).
P.I.D.	Pelvic inflammatory disease (gonorrhea).
PKU	Phenylketonuria.
PMN	Polymorphonuclear leukocytes.
PNH	Paroxysmal nocturnal hemoglobinuria.
p.o.	Orally (*per os*).
polys	Polymorphonuclear leukocytes.
POMP	Prednisone, Oncovin, methotrexate, 6-mercaptopurine (antineoplastic combination chemotherapy drugs).
PPD	Purified protein derivative (test for tuberculosis).
p.r.n.	As required (*pro re nata*).
Pro. time	Prothrombin time (test of blood clotting).
P.S.P.	Phenylsulfonphthalein (dye test for kidney impairment).
PTH	Parathyroid hormone.
PVC	Premature ventricular contraction.

q.d.	Every day (*quaque die*).
q.h.	Every hour (*quaque hora*).
q.i.d.	Four times daily (*quarter in die*).
q.n.s.	Quantity not sufficient.
R$_x$	Take (prescription).
Ra	Radium.
rad	Radiation absorbed dose (unit of measurement for ionizing radiation).
RAI	Radioactive iodine.
RBC	Red blood count or red blood cell (corpuscle).
Rh	Rh factor (antigen in blood of some individuals).
RLQ	Right lower quadrant.
RNA	Ribonucleic acid.
RP	Retrograde pyelogram.
RUQ	Right upper quadrant.
S$_1$, S$_2$	First, second sacral vertebra.
S-A	Sinoatrial.
Sed. rate	Sedimentation rate (rate of blood sedimentation).
SGOT	Serum glutamic-oxaloacetic transaminase (enzyme test for myocardial infarction and liver disease).
SGPT	Serum glutamic-pyruvic transaminase (enzyme measured as a test of liver function; elevated in acute and toxic hepatitis and hepatocellular damage).
SH	Serum hepatitis (virus infection of liver transmitted by unsterilized needles and syringes or administration of infected blood).
S.O.B.	Shortness of breath.
Sr	Strontium.
Staph.	Staphylococcus.
stat.	Immediately (*statim*).
STH	Somatotropin (growth hormone).

Strep.	Streptococcus.
S.T.S.	Serological test for syphilis (measurement of antibodies in serum).
SV-40	Simian vacuolating virus.
T₁, T₂	First, second thoracic vertebra.
TB	Tuberculosis.
TBI	Total body irradiation.
Tc	Technetium.
TCA	Tetrachloracetic acid (used to precipitate proteins out of solution).
T-cells	Lymphocytes produced in the thymus gland.
t.i.d.	Three times daily (*ter in die*).
TNI	Total nodal irradiation.
TP	Testosterone propionate (male hormone).
TPI	Treponema pallidum immobilization (test for syphilis).
TPR	Temperature, pulse, and respiration.
tRNA	Transfer RNA.
TSH	Thyroid-stimulating hormone.
TUR	Transurethral resection (for prostatectomy).
URI	Upper respiratory infection.
U.S.P.	United States Pharmacopeia.
VD	Venereal disease.
VDRL	Venereal Disease Research Laboratory (an antibody test for syphilis).
VMA	Vanillylmandelic acid (test for pheochromocytoma).
WBC	White blood count; white blood cell.

MEDICAL TERMS → ENGLISH

Combining Form, Suffix, or Prefix	Pronunciation	Meaning	Page
a-	ā	no; not; without	8, 77
ab-	ăb	away from	77
abdomin/o	ăb-dom′ĭ-nō	abdomen	21, 45, 58
-ac	ăk	pertaining to	7, 63
acanth/o	ă-kăn′thō	thorny; spiny	363
acetabul/o	ăs-ĕ-tăb′ū-lō	acetabulum (hip socket)	329
acou/o	ă-koo′ō	hearing	395
acr/o	ăk′rō	extremities	58
acu/o	ăk′ū-ō	sharp	58
ad-	ăd	toward	78
aden/o	ăd′ĕ-nō	gland	5, 21, 451
adenoid/o	ăd′ĕ-noyd-ō	adenoids	255
adip/o	ăd′ĭ-pō	fat	45, 363
adren/o	ă-drē′nō	adrenal glands	425
adrenal/o	ă-drē′năl-ō	adrenal glands	427
aer/o	ā′ĕr-ō	air	551
agglutin/o	ă-gloo′tĭn-ō	clumping; sticking together	287

-al	ăl	pertaining to	7, 63
alb/o	ăl′bō	white	362
albumin/o	ăl-bū′mĭn-ō	protein	141
algesi/o	ăl-jē′zē-ō	pain, excessive sensitivity to	205, 572
-algia	ăl′jē-ăh	pain	7, 60
alveol/o	ăl-vē′ō-lō	alveolus	257, 452
		air sac	257
		small sac	257, 452
ambly/o	ăm′blē-ō	dull; dim	386
amni/o	ăm′nē-ō	amnion (sac in which embryo develops)	75, 166
amphi-	ăm′fĭ	on both sides	334
amyl/o	ăm′ĭ-lō	starch	103, 107
an-	ăn	no; not; without	8, 77
an/o	ā′nō	anus	106
ana-	ăn′ăh	up; again; backward	8, 37, 48, 78, 452
andr/o	ăn′drō	male	183, 427
aneurysm/o	ăn-ū-rĭz′mō	aneurysm	234
angi/o	ăn′jē-ō	vessel	21, 233
ankyl/o	ăn′kĭ-lō	crooked; bent; stiff	334
ante-	ăn′tē	before; forward	78
anter/o	ăn′tĕr-ō	front	46
anteri/o	ăn-tĕr′ĭ-ō		
anthrac/o	ăn′thră-kō	coal dust	257
anti-	ăn′tĭ	against	78, 551, 573
aort/o	ā-ōr′tō	aorta	233
aponeur/o	ăp-ō-nū′rō	aponeurosis (type of tendon)	337
append/o	ă-pĕn′dō	appendix	106
appendic/o	ă-pĕn′dĭ-kō		
aque/o	ăk′wē-ō	water	386
-ar	ēr	pertaining to	63
-arche	ăr′kē	beginning	167
arteri/o	ăr-tē′rē-ō	artery	58, 233
arteriol/o	ăr-tē-rē-ōl′ō	arteriole; small artery	233
arthr/o	ăr′thrō	joint	5, 58, 333
articul/o	ăr-tĭk′ū-lō	joint	333
-ary	ĕr′ē	pertaining to	63
-ase	āz	enzyme	103, 107
-asthenia	ăs-thē′nē-ăh	lack of strength	206
atel/o	ăt′ĕ-lō	incomplete	205
ather/o	ăth′ĕr-ō	yellowish plaque; fatty substance; paste, porridge	234
atri/o	ā′trē-ō	atrium	234

audi/o	ăw'dē-ō	hearing	395
aur/i	ăw'rĭ	ear	395
aur/o	ăw'rō		
auto-	ăw'tō	self	8, 78
axill/o	ăk'sĭ-lō	armpit	21
azot/o	ăz'ō-tō	urea; nitrogen	140
bacteri/o	băk-tē'rē-ō	bacteria	141
balan/o	băl'ă-nō	glans penis	182
bartholin/o	băr'tō-lĭn-ō	Bartholin's glands	165
bas/o	bā'sō	base	286
bene-	běn'ě	good	20
bi-	bī	two	22, 78
bi/o	bī'ō	life	5, 58
bil/i	bĭl'ĭ	gall; bile	106
bilirubin/o	bĭl-ĭ-roo'bĭn-ō	bilirubin	106
-blast	blăst	embryonic; immature	77, 287, 327
blephar/o	blěf'ăr-ō	eyelid	206, 386
bol/o	bŏl'ō	cast; throw	37, 46, 75, 471
brachi/o	brā'kē-ō	arm	205
brady-	brăd'ē, brād'ē	slow	78
bronch/o	brŏng'kō	bronchial tube	256
bronchi/o	brŏng'kē-ō		
bronchiol/o	brŏng-kē'ōl-ō	bronchiole; small bronchus	257
bucc/o	bŭk'ō	cheek	105, 119
burs/o	bŭr'sō	bursa (sac of fluid near joints)	333
calc/o	kăl'kō	calcium	425
calcane/o	kăl-kā'nē-ō	calcaneus (heel bone)	330
calci/o	kăl'sē-ō	calcium	326
cali/o	kăl'ĭ-ō	calyx	139
-capnia	kăp'nē-ăh	carbon dioxide	258
carcin/o	kăr'sĭn-ō	cancer	6, 58, 451, 496
cardi/o	kăr'dē-ō	heart	6, 233
carp/o	kăr'pō	carpus (wrist)	329
cata-	kăt'ăh	down	37, 48, 78
caud/o	kăw'dō	tail; lower part of body	46
caus/o	kăw'sō	burn	363
cauter/o	kăw'těr-ō	heat; burn	498
cec/o	sē'kō	cecum (first part of large intestine)	106, 119
-cele	sēl	hernia	60

celi/o	sē′lē-ō	belly; abdomen	105, 119
-centesis	sĕn-tē′sĭs	surgical puncture to remove fluid	60
cephal/o	sĕf′ă-lō	head	6, 58
cerebell/o	sĕr-ĕ-bĕl′ō	cerebellum	205
cerebr/o	sĕr′ĕ-brō	brain; cerebrum	6, 204
cerumin/o	sĕ-roo′mĕn-ō	cerumen (wax in inner ear)	395
cervic/o	sĕr′vĭ-kō	neck	21, 46, 327
		neck of uterus; cervix	165
cheil/o	kī′lō	lip	105, 119
chem/o	kē′mō	drug; chemical	497, 550
chir/o	kī′rō	hand	58
chol/e	kō′lē	gall; bile	106, 119
cholecyst/o	kō-lē-sĭst′ō	gallbladder	106, 119
choledoch/o	kō′lē-dŏk-ō	common bile duct	106, 119
chondr/o	kŏn′drō	cartilage	46, 58, 333
chori/o	kō′rē-ō	chorion; extra-embryonic membrane	166
chrom/o	krō′mō	color	46, 285, 472
chron/o	krŏn′ō	time	58
cib/o	sĭ-bō	meals	76
-cidal	sīd′ăl	killing	498, 572
cine/o	sĭn′ē-ō	movement	531
cis/o	sī′zō	cut	6, 76
-clast	klăst	break	327
clavicul/o	klă-vĭk′ū-lō	clavicle (collar bone)	328
-clysis	klī′sĭs	irrigation; washing	118
-coccus	kŏk′ŭs	berry-shaped	60
(-cocci, pl.)	kŏk′sī		
coccyg/o	kŏk′sĭ-gō	tailbone; coccyx	47, 206
col/o	kō′lō	colon; large intestine	58, 106, 119
colp/o	kŏl′pō	vagina	165
con-	kŏn	with; together	78
coni/o	kō′nē-ō	dust	257, 260
conjunctiv/o	kŏn-jŭnk′tĭ-vō	conjunctiva	386
contra-	kŏn′trăh	against; opposite	78, 551
cor/o	kō′rō	pupil	384
core/o	kōr′ē-ō	pupil	384
corne/o	kōr′nē-ō	cornea	384
coron/o	kōr′ŏ-nō	heart	233
cortic/o	kōr′tĭ-kō	cortex	137, 427
cost/o	kŏs′tō	ribs	76, 328
crani/o	krā′nē-ō	skull	47, 328

cras/o	krā′zō	disease; mixture	551
crin/o	krĭn′ō	secrete	6
-crine	krĭn	secrete; separate	77
-crit	krĭt	separate	22
cry/o	krī′ō	cold	183, 498
crypt/o	krĭp′tō	hidden	183
culd/o	kŭl′dō	cul-de-sac	165
-cusis	kū′sĭs	hearing	396
cutane/o	kū-tā′nē-ō	skin	21, 362
cyan/o	sī′ăn-ō	blue	238, 257
cycl/o	sī′klō	ciliary body of eye	384
-cyesis	sī-ē′sĭs	pregnancy	77, 166
cyst/o	sĭs′tō	urinary bladder	140
		cyst; sac of fluid	452
cyt/o	sī′tō	cell	6
-cyte	sīt	cell	7, 60
-cytosis	sī-tō′sĭs	cells, condition of	287
dacry/o	dăk′rē-ō	tear	385
dacryoaden/o	dăk′rē-ō-ăd′ē-nō	tear gland	385
dacryocyst/o	dăk′rē-ō-sĭs′tō	tear sac; lacrimal sac	385
dactyl/o	dăk′tĭl-ō	fingers or toes	58
de-	dē	lack of	208, 234
dent/i	dĕn′tĭ	tooth	105, 119
derm/o	dĕr′mō	skin	6, 362, 551
dermat/o	dĕr-măh′tō	skin	6, 362
-desis	dē′sĭs	binding	327
di	dī	complete	334
dia-	dī′ăh	complete; through	8, 78, 334
diaphor/o	dī′ă-fō-rō	sweat	363
dips/o	dĭp′sō	thirst	140, 427
dist/o	dĭs′tō	far	47
dors/o	dōr′sō	back (of body)	47
-drome	drōm	run	77
duct/o	dŭk′tō	carry; to lead	76
duoden/o	dŭ-ō-dē′nō	duodenum (first part of small intestine)	106, 119
dur/o	dūr′ō	dura mater (outer layer of meninges)	205
dys-	dĭs	bad; painful; difficult	79
ec-	ĕk	out; outside	79
ech/o	ĕk′ō	sound	530

-ectasia	ĕk-tā′zē-ăh	stretching; dilation	118
-ectasis	ĕk′tă-sĭs	stretching; dilation	118
ecto-	ĕk′tō	out; outside	79
-ectomy	ĕk′tō-mē	removal; excision; resection	7, 60
electr/o	ē-lĕk′trō	electricity	6
em-	ĕm	in	258
-emesis	ĕm′ĕ-sĭs	vomiting	118
-emia	ē′mē-ăh	blood condition	7, 60, 67, 287
emmetr/o	ĕm′ĕ-trō	in due measure	386
-emphraxis	ĕm-frăk′sĭs	obstruction; blockage	396
en-	ĕn	in; within	79
encephal/o	ĕn-sĕf′ă-lō	brain	6, 58, 204
endo-	ĕn′dō	within	8, 22, 79
enter/o	ĕn′tĕr-ō	small intestine	6, 106, 119, 551
eosin/o	ē-ō-sĭn′ō	rosy; dawn-colored	58, 285
epi-	ĕp′ĭ	above; upon	8, 48, 79, 452
epididym/o	ĕp-ĭ-dĭd′ĭ-mō	epididymis	182
epiglott/o	ĕp-ĭ-glŏt′ō	epiglottis	255
episi/o	ē-pĭz′ē-ō	vulva	166
-er	ĕr	one who	63
erg/o	ĕr′gō	work	551, 572
erythem/o	ĕr-ĭ-thē′mō	flushed; redness	362
erythr/o	ĕ-rĭth′rō	red	6, 285
eso-	ĕs′ō	inward	22
esophag/o	ĕ-sŏf′ă-gō	esophagus	105, 119
esthesi/o	ĕs-thē′zē-ō	feeling (nervous sensation)	206, 572
estr/o	ĕs′trō	female	427
ethm/o	ĕth′mō	sieve	319
eti/o	ē′tē-ō	cause	108
eu-	ū	good	79
ex-	ĕks	out	8, 79
exo-	ĕk′sō	outside	8
fasci/o	făsh′ē-ō	fascia	337
femor/o	fĕm′ō-rō	femur (thigh bone)	329
fibr/o	fī′brō	fibers; fibrous tissue	337
fibrin/o	fī′brĭn-ō	fibrin; threads of a clot	286
fibros/o	fī-brō′sō	fibrous tissue	333
fibul/o	fīb′ū-lō	fibula (smaller of two leg bones)	329
fluor/o	floo′ōr-ō	luminous	531
follicul/o	fō-lĭk′ū-lō	follicle; small sac	452
furc/o	fŭr′kō	forking; branching	76
-fusion	fū′zhŭn	pour	77

gangli/o	găng′glē-ō	ganglion	204
gastr/o	găs′trō	stomach	6, 105, 119
gen/o	jĕn′ō	producing; beginning	6
-genesis	jĕn′ĕ-sĭs	producing, condition of; forming, condition of	60
germ/o	jĕr′mō	sprout; seed	496
gingiv/o	jĭn′jĭ-vō	gums	105, 119
glauc/o	glăw′kō	gray	386
gli/o	glī′ō	glue; neuroglial tissue	206
-globin	glō′bĭn	protein	64, 287
-globulin	glŏb′ū-lĭn	protein	287
glomerul/o	glō-mĕr′ū-lō	glomerulus	137
gloss/o	glŏs′ō	tongue	76, 105, 119
gluc/o	gloo′kō	sugar	107, 427
glyc/o	glī′kō	sugar	76, 107, 119, 427
glycogen/o	glī′kō-jĕn′ō	glycogen	107
gnos/o	nō′sō	knowledge	6, 76
gon/o	gŏn′ō	seed	58, 64
gonad/o	gō′năd-ō	sex glands	427
-grade	grād	go	77
-gram	grăm	record	7, 22, 61, 531
granul/o	grăn′ū-lō	granules	58, 286
-graph	grăf	instrument for recording	61, 531
-graphy	grăf′ē	recording, process of	61, 531
gravid/o	grăv′ĭ-dō	pregnancy	166
gynec/o	gī′nĕ-kō jin′ĕ-kō	woman; female	6
hem/o	hē′mō	blood	6, 285
hemat/o	hĕm′ăh-tō	blood	6, 285
hemi-	hĕm′ē	half	79
hepat/o	hĕp′ăh-tō	liver	21, 58, 106, 119
herni/o	hĕr′nē-ō	hernia	107, 119
hidr/o	hĭd′rō	sweat	363
hist/o	hĭs′tō	tissue	47, 572
histi/o	hĭs′tē-ō	tissue	363
home/o	hō′mē-ō	sameness; unchanging; constant	425
humer/o	hū′mĕr-ō	humerus (upper arm bone)	328
hydr/o	hī′drō	water	58
hyper-	hī′pĕr	above; excessive	8, 79
hypn/o	hĭp′nō	sleep	572
hypo-	hī′pō	deficient; below	8, 79
hyster/o	hĭs′tĕr-ō	uterus; womb	165

-ia	ē'ăh	condition; process	7, 62
-iasis	i'ăh-sĭs	condition	107
iatr/o	i-ăt'rō	physician	551
-ic	ĭk	pertaining to	8, 63
idi/o	ĭd'ē-ō	individual; own; self	221, 551
ile/o	ĭl'ē-ō	ileum (third part of small intestine)	106, 120
ili/o	ĭl'ē-ō	ilium	47, 329
immun/o	ĭm'ū-nō	safe; protection	279, 287
in-	ĭn	not	79
		in	79
infra-	ĭn'frăh	below; inferior	79
inguin/o	ĭng'gwĭ-nō	groin	21, 47
inter-	ĭn'tĕr	between	22, 48, 79, 531
intra-	ĭn'trăh	within	22, 80, 531, 551
ion/o	i'ŏn-ō	ions; charged particles	497
		wander; going	530
ir/o	ĭr'-ō	iris (colored portion of eye)	384
irid/o	ĭr'ĭd-ō		
is/o	i'sō	same; equal	285, 386, 530
isch/o	ĭs'kō	hold back	58
ischi/o	ĭs'kē-ō	ischium (part of hip bone)	329
-ist	ĭst	specialist	8, 63
-itis	i'tĭs	inflammation	8, 61
jejun/o	jē-joo'nō	jejunum (second part of small intestine)	106, 120
kal/i	kā'lē	potassium	427
kary/o	kăr'ē-ō	nucleus	36, 47, 287, 471
kerat/o	kĕr'ăh-tō	horny; hard; cornea	362, 384
kinesi/o	kĭ-nē'sē-ō	movement	206
kyph/o	ki'fō	humpback	327
labi/o	lā'bē-ō	lips	105, 120
lacrim/o	lăk'rĭ-mō	tear; tear duct	319, 385
lact/o	lăk'tō	milk	166, 427
lamin/o	lăm'ĭ-nō	lamina (part of vertebral arch)	327
lapar/o	lăp'ăh-rō	abdominal wall; abdomen	21, 58
laryng/o	lăh-rĭng'ō	larynx; voice box	58, 255
later/o	lăt'ĕr-ō	side	21, 47
leiomy/o	li-ō-mi'ō	smooth (visceral) muscle	337, 452
leuk/o	lū'kō	white	6, 285, 362

ligament/o	lĭg-ăh-mĕn'tō	ligament	333
lingu/o	lĭng'gwō	tongue	105, 120, 551
lip/o	lĭp'ō	fat	103, 107, 120, 363, 452
lith/o	lĭth'ō	stone; calculus	59, 67, 107, 120
lob/o	lō'bō	lobe	257
-logy	lō'jē	study	8
lord/o	lōr'dō	swayback; curve	327
luc/o	lū'sō lū'kō	light; transparent	530
lumb/o	lŭm'bō	lower back; loins	47, 327
lymph/o	lĭm'fō	lymph	19, 21, 295
lymphaden/o	lĭm-făd'ĕ-nō	lymph gland	295
lymphangi/o	lĭm-făn'jē-ō	lymph vessels	295
-lysis	li'sĭs	break down; separate; destruction	22, 61, 77, 118
-lytic	lĭt'ĭk	destruction	573
macro-	măk'rō	large	80
mal-	măl	bad	20, 80
-malacia	măh-lā'shē-ăh	softening	61, 327
mamm/o	măm'ō	breast	166
mandibul/o	măn-dĭb'ū-lō	lower jaw bone	328
mast/o	măs'tō	breast	166
mastoid/o	măs-toi'dō	mastoid process	396
maxill/o	măk'sĭl-ō	upper jaw; upper jaw bone	59, 328
medi/o	mē'dē-ō	middle	47
medull/o	mĕ-dŭl'ō	medulla (inner section of an organ)	137
		middle; soft	452
-megaly	mĕg'ăh-lē	enlargement	22, 61
melan/o	mĕl'ăh-nō	black	362
men/o	mĕn'ō	menses; menstruation	166
mening/o	mĕ-nĭng'gō	meninges (membranes around brain and spinal cord)	205
meningi/o	mĕ-nĭn'jē-ō	meninges, membranes	205
meso-	mĕz'ō	middle	80
meta-	mĕt'ăh	beyond; change; near	20, 22, 48, 80, 453
metacarp/o	mĕt-ăh-kăr'pō	metacarpals (hand bones)	329
-meter	mē'tĕr	measure	77
metr/o	mē'trō	uterus	165
metri/o	mē'trē-ō	uterus	165
mi/o	mi'ō	small; less than	386
micro-	mi'krō	small	80

-mimetic	mĭ-mĕt′ĭk	mimic; copy	573
mit/o	mĭ′tō	thread	472, 498
mon/o	mŏn′ō	one; single	286
morph/o	mōr′fō	shape; form	59, 66, 76, 287
mort/o	mōr′tō	death	76
muc/o	mū′kō	mucus	59
mut/a	mū′tăh	mutation; genetic change	471, 496
my/o	mĭ′ō	muscle	47, 165, 206, 337
myc/o	mĭ′kō	fungus; mold	363, 386, 572
myel/o	mĭ′ĕ-lō	spinal cord	59, 205, 327
		bone marrow	59, 286, 327
myocardi/o	mĭ-ō-kăr′dē-ō	heart muscle	337
myos/o	mĭ′ō-sō	muscle	337
myring/o	mĭ-rĭng′gō	eardrum	395
myx/o	mĭk′sō	mucus	429
narc/o	năr′kō	numbness; stupor	572
nas/o	nā′zō	nose	254, 319
nat/i	nā′tē	birth	76
natr/o	nā′trō	sodium	427
necr/o	nĕ′krō	death	59
nect/o	nĕk′tō	bind; tie; connect	76
neo-	nē′ō	new	19, 22
nephr/o	nĕf′rō	kidney	6, 137
neur/o	nū′rō	nerve	6, 204
neutr/o	nū′trō	neither; neutral	286
noct/i	nŏk′tē	night	141
norm/o	nōr′mō	rule; order; normal	76, 287
nucle/o	nū′klē-ō	nucleus	287, 471
ocul/o	ŏk′ū-lō	eye	384
odont/o	ō′dŏn′tō	tooth	105, 120
-odynia	ō-dĭn′ē-ăh	pain	61
-oid	ŏyd	resembling	63, 452
-ole	ōl	little; small	62
olecran/o	ō-lĕk′răn-ō	elbow	328
olig/o	ŏl′ĭ-gō	scanty	141
-ology	ŏl′ō-jē	study of	61
-oma	ō′măh	tumor	8, 19, 61, 449, 452
onc/o	ŏng′kō	mass; tumor	6, 451, 496
onych/o	ŏn′ĭ-kō	nail	363
oo/o	ō′ō-ō	egg	163

oophor/o	ō-ŏf'ō-rō ō'ō-fōr-ō	ovary	163
opac/o opaq/o	ō-păs'ō ō-pāk'ō	dark; impervious to light rays	530
ophthalm/o	ŏf-thăl'mō	eye	6, 59, 384
-opia	ō'pē-ăh	vision	387
opsy	ŏp'sē	view	8, 61
-or	ōr	one who	62
or/o	ō'rō	mouth	105, 120
orch/o orchi/o orchid/o	ōr'kō ōr'kē-ō ōr'kĭd-ō	testis	182
-orrhagia	ōr-rā'jē-ăh	bursting forth of blood	118
-orrhaphy	ōr'ă-fē	suture	118
-orrhea	ō-rē'ăh	flow; discharge	77, 118
-orrhexis	ō-rĕk'sĭs	rupture	118
orth/o	ōr'thō	straight	258
-osis	ō'sĭs	condition, abnormal	8, 22, 61, 67
-osmia	ŏz'mē-ăh	smell	258
oste/o	ŏs'tē-ō	bone	6, 59, 326, 452
-ostomy	ŏs'tō-mē	make a new opening	61
ot/o	ō'tō	ear	59, 395
-otomy	ŏt'ō-mē	incision; cut into	61
-ous	ŭs	pertaining to	22, 63
ov/o	ō'vō	egg	163
ovari/o	ō-vā'rē-ō	ovary	163
ox/o	ŏk'sō	oxygen	76, 234, 257
pachy/o	păk'ē-ō	thick; heavy	362
palat/o	păl'ăh-tō	palate	105
pan-	păn	all	22, 80
pancreat/o	păn'krē-ăh-tō	pancreas	106, 120, 427
papill/o	pă-pĭl'ō păp'ĭ-lō	nipple-like; finger-like	452
para-	păr'ăh	near; beside; abnormal	80
-para	păh'răh	births (viable offspring)	166
parathyroid/o	păr-ăh-thī'rŏyd-ō	parathyroid glands	425
-paresis	păh-rē'sĭs	slight paralysis	207
-partum	păr'tŭm	birth; labor	77
patell/o	păh-tĕl'ō	patella	329
path/o	păth'ō	disease	7
-pathy	păth'ē	disease process	22, 61
pector/o	pĕk'tōr-ō	chest	257

pelv/i	pĕl′vē	pelvic bone; hip	47, 329
pelv/o	pĕl′vō		
-penia	pē′nē-ăh	decreased number	22, 61
-pepsia	pĕp′sē-ăh	digestion	118
per-	pŭr	through	23, 80
peri-	pĕr′ē	surrounding	9, 80
perine/o	pĕr-ĭ-nē′ō	perineum	166
peritone/o	pĕr-ĭ-tō-nē′ō	peritoneum	21, 59, 106
perone/o	pĕr-ō-nē′ō	fibula	330
-pexy	pĕk′sē	fixation	62
phag/o	făg′ō	eat; swallow	21, 59, 286
-phagia	fā′jē-ăh	eating; swallowing	118
phalang/o	făh-lăn′gō	phalanges (finger and toe bones)	329
pharmac/o	făr′mă-kō	drug; chemical	495, 550
pharyng/o	făh-rĭng′gō	throat; pharynx	105, 255
phas/o	fā′zō	speech	206
phe/o	fē′ō	dusky	430
-pheresis	fĕr-ē′sĭs	removal	288
phil/o	fĭl′ō	like; love; attraction to	59
-philia	fĭl′ē-ăh	attraction for (increase in numbers)	287
phleb/o	flĕb′ō	vein	233
phob/o	fō′bō	fear	59
-phobia	fō′bē-ăh	fear	62
-phonia	fō′nē-ăh	voice	258
		sound	396
-phoresis	fō-rē′sĭs	carrying; transmission	288
-phoria	fōr′ē-ăh	feeling (mental state)	573
phot/o	fō′tō	light	386
phren/o	frĕn′ō	diaphragm	257
		mind	257
-phylaxis	fī-lăk′sĭs	protection	551, 573
physi/o	fĭz′ē-ō	nature	7
-physis	fī′sĭs	grow; growth	77, 326, 428
plas/o	plăz′ō	development; formation	59
-plasia	plā′zē-ăh	formation; development; growth	22, 62, 77, 452
-plasm	plăzm	growth; formation	19, 22, 452
-plasty	plăs′tē	surgical repair	62, 118
ple/o	plē′ō	more	452
-plegia	plē′jē-ăh	paralysis; palsy	207
pleur/o	ploor′ō	pleura	257
plex/o	plĕk′sō	plexus; nerve network	204
pne/o	nē′ō	breathing; breath	76

-pnea	nē′ăh	breathing	258
pneum/o	nū′mō	lung	59, 64, 257
pneumon/o	nū-mō′nō	lung	257
-poiesis	poy-ē′sĭs	formation	62, 288
poikil/o	pyo′kĭl-ō	varied; irregular	285
polio-	pō′lē-ō	gray matter of brain and spinal cord	80, 206
poly-	pŏl′ē	many	66, 80
polyp/o	pŏl′ĭ-pō	polyp; growths	452, 498
pont/o	pŏn′tō	pons	205
-porosis	pō-rō′sĭs	passage	328
post-	pōst	after; behind	23, 80
poster/o	pŏs′tĕr-ō	back (of body)	47
-prandial	prăn′dē-ăl	meal	107
pre-	prē	before; in front of	80
presby/o	prĕs′bē-ō	old age	386
pro-	prō	before	9, 80
proct/o	prŏk′tō	anus and rectum	106, 120
prostat/o	prŏs′tăh-tō	prostate gland	182
prot/o	prō′tō	first	47
prote/o	prō′tē-ō	first; protein	472
proxim/o	prŏk′sĭ-mō	near	47
pseud/o	sū′dō	false	80
psych/o	sī′kō	mind	7
-ptosis	tō′sĭs	drooping; sagging; prolapse	62
-ptysis	tĭ′sĭs	spitting	118, 258
pub/o	pū′bō	pubis (part of hip bone)	329
pulmon/o	pŭl′mō-nō	lung	257
pupill/o	pū′pĭl-ō	pupil	384
py/o	pī′ō	pus	141
pyel/o	pī′ĕ-lō	renal pelvis	21, 139
pylor/o	pī-lōr′ō	pylorus	120
pyr/o	pī′rō	fever	572
rachi/o	rā′kē-ō	spinal column; vertebrae	327
radi/o	rā′dē-ō	radius (lateral lower arm bone)	329
		rays (x-rays)	7, 59, 498, 530
re-	rē	back	8, 23
rect/o	rĕk′tō	rectum	59, 106, 120
ren/o	rē′nō	kidney	21, 139
reticul/o	rĕ-tĭk′ū-lō	network	287

retin/o	rĕt'ĭ-nō	retina	384, 496
retro-	rĕt'rō	behind	9, 23, 81
rhabdomy/o	răb-dō-mĭ'ō	striated (skeletal) muscle	337, 452
rhin/o	rī'nō	nose	7, 254
rib/o	rī'bō	sugar	471
roentgen/o	rĕnt'gĕn-ō	x-rays	530

sacr/o	sā'krō	sacrum	47
salping/o	săl-pĭng'gō	fallopian tubes; oviducts	163, 395
		eustachian tube	395
-salpinx	săl'pĭnks	fallopian tubes	165
sarc/o	săr'kō	flesh (connective tissue)	20, 21, 337, 449, 451
scapul/o	skăp'ū-lō	scapula; shoulder blade	328
scint/i	sĭn'tĭ	spark	526, 531
scirrh/o	skĭr'ō	hard	452
scler/o	sklē'rō	sclera (white of eye)	384
-sclerosis	sklē-rō'sĭs	hardening	62
scoli/o	skō'lē-ō	crooked; bent	327
scop/o	skō'pō	examination (usually visual)	7
-scope	skōp	instrument for visual examination	8, 62
scot/o	skō'tō	darkness	390
seb/o	sē'bō	sebum	363
secti/o	sĕk'shē-ō	cut	7, 76
semi-	sĕm'ē	half	81
seps/o	sĕp'sō	infection	76
sial/o	sī'ăh-lō	saliva	105, 120
sialaden/o	sī-ăl-ăh'dĕn-ō	salivary glands	105
sider/o	sĭd'ĕr-ō	iron	287
sigmoid/o	sĭg-moy'dō	sigmoid colon	106
sinus/o	sī'nŭs-ō	sinus; cavity	257
som/o	sō'mō	body	471
somat/o	sō-măh'tō	body	427
somn/o	sŏm'nō	sleep	76
son/o	sō-nō	sound	76, 530
-spasm	spăzm	contraction of muscles (sudden) twitching	118
sperm/o	spĕr'mō	spermatozoa	182
spermat/o	spĕr'măh-tō		
sphen/o	sfē'nō	wedge, sphenoid bone	318
spher/o	sfē'rō	globe-shaped; round	285
sphygm/o	sfĭg'mō	pulse	234

spin/o	spī'nō	spine (backbone)	47
spir/o	spī'rō	breathing	257
splen/o	splē'nō	spleen	107, 120, 295
spondyl/o	spŏn'dĭ-lō	vertebrae (backbones)	47, 326
squam/o	skwā'mō	scale	363
-stalsis	stăl'sĭs	constriction	118
staped/o	stăh'pē-dō	stapes (middle ear bone)	395
staphyl/o	stăf'ĭl-ō	clusters; grapes	59
-stasis	stā'sĭs	control; stop	20, 22, 62, 77, 118, 288
-static	stăt'ĭk	stopping; controlling	572
steat/o	stē'ăh-tō	fat	107, 120
-stenosis	stĕn-ō'sĭs	tightening, stricture	118
ster/o	stĕr'ō	solid structure	425
stere/o	stĕr'ē-ō	solid; three-dimensional	531
stern/o	stĕr'nō	sternum; breastbone	328
steth/o	stĕth'ō	chest	234
-sthenia	stē'nē-ăh	strength	337
stomat/o	stō'măh-tō	mouth	105, 120
strept/o	strĕp'tō	twisted chains	59
sub-	sŭb	under, below	81
submaxill/o	sŭb-măk'sĭl-ō	lower jaw bone	328
supra-	soo'prăh	above	81
sym-	sĭm	together; with	81
syn-	sĭn	together; with	81, 334
syndesm/o	sĭn'dĕs-mō	ligament	334
synovi/o	sĭ-nō'vē-ō	synovia (joint fluid)	333
syring/o	sĭ-rĭng'gō	tube	549
tachy-	tăk'ē	fast	81
tax/o	tăk'sō	order; coordination	206
tele/o	tĕl'ē-ō	distant; far	528, 530
ten/o	tĕn'ō	tendon	333
tend/o	tĕn'dō		
tendin/o	tĕn'dĭn-ō		
terat/o	tĕr'ăh-tō	monster	184, 452
test/o	tĕs'tō	testis; testicle	182, 427
thalam/o	thăl'ăh-mō	thalamus	205
thalass/o	thăh-lăs'ō	sea	289
the/o	thē'ō	put; place	76
thec/o	thē'kō	sheath; meningeal covering	551
thel/o	thē'lō	nipple	47, 76
-therapy	thĕr'ăh-pē	treatment	62

therm/o	thĕr′mō	heat	530
thorac/o	thō′răh-kō	chest	48, 59, 327
-thorax	thō′răks	pleural cavity	258
thromb/o	thrŏm′bō	clot	7, 21, 59, 286
thym/o	thī′mō	thymus gland	295, 427
thyr/o	thī′rō	shield; thyroid gland	76, 425
thyroid/o	thī′royd-ō		
tibi/o	tĭb′ē-ō	tibia; shin bone	329
-tic	tĭk	pertaining to	63
-tocia	tō′sē-ăh	labor; birth	166
-tocin	tō′sĭn	labor; delivery	428
tom/o	tō′mō	cut	7, 21, 531
-tome	tōm	instrument to cut	8, 62
-tomy	tō′mē	cutting, process of; incision; section; cut into	8, 22
tonsill/o	tŏn′sĭl-ō	tonsils	59, 105, 255
top/o	tŏp′ō	place; position; location	76
tox/o	tŏk′sō	poison	76, 497, 551
toxic/o	tŏk′sĭ-kō	poison	425, 498, 551
trache/o	trā′kē-ō	trachea; windpipe	59, 255
trans-	trăns	across	9, 81
-tresia	trē′zē-ăh	opening	118
trich/o	trĭk′ō	hair	363
-trophy	trō′fē	nourishment; development	62, 77, 337
-tropia	trō′pē-ăh	turn	387
-tropin	trō′pĭn	nourish; develop; stimulate	427
tympan/o	tĭm′păh-nō	eardrum; middle ear	395
-ule	ūl	little; small	62
uln/o	ŭl′nō	ulna (medial lower arm bone)	328
ultra-	ŭl′trăh	beyond; excess	81
ungu/o	ŭng′gwō	nail	363
ur/o	ū′rō	urine; urinary tract	7, 139, 425
ureter/o	ū-rē′tĕr-ō	ureter	22, 140
urethr/o	ū-rē′thrō	urethra	140
-uria	ū′rē-ăh	urination; urine	140
uter/o	ū′tĕr-ō	uterus	165
uve/o	ū′vē-ō	vascular layer of eye	385
vagin/o	văj′ĭ-nō	vagina	165
valv/o	văl′vō	valve	234
vas/o	văs′ō	vessel; duct; vas deferens	182, 233, 572

ven/o	vē′nō	vein	22, 59, 77, 233, 551
ventr/o	vĕn′trō	belly side of body	48
ventricul/o	vĕn-trĭk′ū-lō	ventricle (of brain)	205
		(of heart)	234
venul/o	vĕn′ūl-ō	venule; small vein	234
vertebr/o	vĕr′tĕ-brō	vertebrae (backbones)	48, 326
vesic/o	vĕs′ĭkō	urinary bladder	140
vesicul/o	vĕ-sĭk′ū-lō	seminal vessels	182
vir/o	vī′rō	virus; poison	497
viscer/o	vĭs′ĕr-ō	internal organs	48
vit/a	vī′tăh	life	572
vit/o	vī′tō		
vitre/o	vĭt′rē-ō	glassy	386
vulv/o	vŭl′vō	vulva	166
xanth/o	zăn′thō	yellow	362
xer/o	zē′rō	dry	362, 386, 498, 530
-y	ē	condition; process	8, 62
zo/o	zō′ō	animal life	183
zym/o	zī′mō	leavening agent; catalyst	472

ENGLISH → MEDICAL TERMS

Meaning	Combining Form, Prefix, or Suffix	Page
abdomen	abdomin/o	21, 45, 58
	celi/o	105, 119
abdominal wall	lapar/o	21, 58
abnormal	para-	80
above	epi-	8, 48, 79
	hyper-	8, 79
	supra-	81
acetabulum	acetabul/o	329
across	trans-	9, 81
adenoids	adenoid/o	255
adrenal glands	adren/o	425
	adrenal/o	427
after	post-	23, 80
again	ana-	8, 452

against	anti-	78, 551, 573
	contra-	78, 551
air	aer/o	551
	pneumon/o	257
	pneum/o	257
air sac	alveol/o	257
all	pan-	22, 80
alveolus	alveol/o	257, 452
amnion	amni/o	75, 166
aneurysm	aneurysm/o	234
animal life	zo/o	183
anus	an/o	106
anus and rectum	proct/o	106, 120
aorta	aort/o	233
aponeurosis	aponeur/o	337
appendix	append/o	106
	appendic/o	106
arm	brachi/o	205
arm bone, lower (lateral)	radi/o	329
arm bone, lower (medial)	uln/o	328
arm bone, upper	humer/o	328
armpit	axill/o	21
arteriole	arteriol/o	233
artery	arteri/o	58, 233
artery, small	arteriol/o	233
atrium	atri/o	234
attraction for	-philia	287
attraction to	phil/o	59
away from	ab-	77
	ex-	8, 79
back	dors/o	47
	poster/o	47
	re-	8, 23
	retro-	81
back, lower	lumb/o	47, 327
backbone	spin/o	47
backward	ana-	8, 452
bacteria	bacteri/o	141
bad	dys-	79
	mal-	20, 80
Bartholin's glands	bartholin/o	165
base	bas/o	286
before	ante-	78

	pre-	80
	pro-	9, 80
beginning	-arche	167
	gen/o	6
behind	post-	80
	retro-	9, 23, 81
belly	celi/o	105, 119
belly side	ventr/o	48
below	hypo-	8, 79
	infra-	79
	sub-	81
bent	ankyl/o	334
	scoli/o	327
berry-shaped	-coccus	60
beside	para-	80
between	inter-	22, 48, 79, 531
	meta-	80
beyond	hyper-	79
	meta-	20, 22, 48, 80, 453
	ultra-	81
bile	bil/i	106
	chol/e	106, 119
bile duct, common	choledoch/o	106, 119
bilirubin	bilirubin/o	106
bind	nect/o	76
binding	-desis	327
birth	nat/i	76
	-para	166
	-partum	77
	-tocia	166
black	melan/o	362
bladder (urinary)	cyst/o	140
	vesic/o	140
blockage	-emphraxis	396
blood	hem/o	6, 285
	hemat/o	6, 285
blood condition	-emia	7, 60, 67, 287
blue	cyan/o	238, 257
body	som/o	471
	somat/o	427
bone	oste/o	6, 59, 326, 452
bone marrow	myel/o	59, 286, 327
both sides	amphi-	334
brain	cerebr/o	6, 204
	encephal/o	6, 58, 204
branching	furc/o	76

chest	pector/o	257
	steth/o	234
	thorac/o	48, 59, 327
	-thorax	258
chorion	chori/o	166
ciliary body	cycl/o	384
clavicle	clavicul/o	328
clot	thromb/o	7, 21, 59, 286
clumping	agglutin/o	287
clusters	staphyl/o	59
coal dust	anthrac/o	257
coccyx	coccyg/o	47, 206
cold	cry/o	183, 498
collar bone	clavicul/o	328
colon	col/o	58, 106, 119
color	chrom/o	46, 285, 472
common bile duct	choledoch/o	106, 119
complete	di-	78, 334
	dia-	8
condition	-ia	7, 62
	-iasis	107
	-y	8, 62
condition, usually abnormal	-osis	8, 22, 61, 67
conjunctiva	conjunctiv/o	386
connect	nect/o	76
constant	home/o	425
constriction	-stalsis	118
contraction of muscles (sudden)	-spasm	118
control	-stasis	20, 22, 62, 77, 118, 288
controlling	-static	572
coordination	tax/o	206
copy, to	-mimetic	573
cornea	corne/o	384
	kerat/o	362, 384
cortex	cortic/o	137, 427
crooked	ankyl/o	334
	scoli/o	327
cul-de-sac	culd/o	165
curve	lord/o	327
cut	cis/o	6, 76
	secti/o	7, 76
	tom/o	7, 21, 531
cut into	-otomy	61
	-tomy	8, 22
cyst	cyst/o	452

eat	phag/o	21, 59, 286
	-phagia	118
egg cell	oo/o	163
	ov/o	163
elbow	olecran/o	328
electricity	electr/o	6
embryonic	-blast	77, 287, 327
enlargement	-megaly	22, 61
enzyme	-ase	103, 107
epididymis	epididym/o	182
epiglottis	epiglott/o	255
equal	is/o	285, 386, 530
esophagus	esophag/o	105, 119
eustachian tube	salping/o	395
examination (visual)	scop/o	7
excess	ultra-	81
excessive	hyper-	8, 79
excision	-ectomy	7, 60
extremities	acr/o	58
eye	ocul/o	384
	ophthalm/o	6, 59, 384
eyelid	blephar/o	206, 386
fallopian tubes	salping/o	163, 395
	-salpinx	165
false	pseudo-	80
far	dist/o	47
	tele/o	530
fascia	fasci/o	337
fast	tachy-	81
fat	adip/o	45, 363
	lip/o	103, 107, 120, 363, 452
	steat/o	107, 120
fatty substance	ather/o	234
fear	phob/o	59
	-phobia	62
feeling	-esthesi/o	206, 572
	-phoria	573
female	estr/o	427
	gynec/o	6
femur	femor/o	329
fever	pyr/o	572
fibers	fibr/o	337
fibrin	fibrin/o	286

fibrous tissue	fibr/o	337
	fibros/o	333
fibula	fibul/o	329
	perone/o	330
finger	dactyl/o	58
finger bones	phalang/o	329
finger-like	papill/o	452
first	prot/o	47
	prote/o	472
fixation	-pexy	62
flesh	sarc/o	20, 21, 337, 449, 451
flow	-orrhea	77, 118
flushed	erythem/o	362
follicle	follicul/o	452
forking	furc/o	76
form	morph/o	59, 66, 76, 287
formation	plas/o	59
	-plasia	22, 62, 77, 452
	-plasm	19, 22, 452
	-poiesis	62, 288
forming, condition of	-genesis	60
forward	ante-	78
front	anter/o	46
fungus	myc/o	363, 386, 572
gall	bil/i	106
	chol/e	106, 119
gallbladder	cholecyst/o	106, 119
ganglion	gangli/o	204
	ganglion/o	204
genetic change	mut/a	471, 496
gland	aden/o	5, 21, 451
glans penis	balan/o	182
glassy	vitre/o	386
globe-shaped	spher/o	285
glomerulus	glomerul/o	137
glue	gli/o	206
glycogen	glycogen/o	107
go	-grade	77
going	ion/o	530
good	bene-	20
	eu-	79
grapes	staphyl/o	59
gray	glauc/o	386

gray matter	polio-	80, 206
granules	granul/o	58, 286
groin	inguin/o	21, 47
grow	-physis	77, 326, 428
growth, condition expressing	-plasia	22, 62, 452
	plasm	19, 22, 452
gum	gingiv/o	105, 119
hair	trich/o	363
half	hemi-	79
	semi-	81
hand	chir/o	58
hand bones	metacarp/o	329
hard	kerat/o	362
	scirrh/o	452
hardening	-sclerosis	62
head	cephal/o	6, 58
hearing	acou/o	395
	audi/o	395
	-cusis	396
heart	cardi/o	6, 233
	coron/o	233
heart muscle	myocardi/o	337
heat	cauter/o	498
	therm/o	530
heavy	pachy/o	362
heel bone	calcane/o	330
hernia	-cele	60
	herni/o	107, 119
hidden	crypt/o	183
hip	pelv/i	47
	pelv/o	47
hip socket	acetabul/o	329
hold back	isch/o	58
horny	kerat/o	362, 384
humerus	humer/o	328
humpback	kyph/o	327
ileum	ile/o	106, 120
ilium	ili/o	47, 329
immature	-blast	77, 287, 327
in	em-	258
	en-	79
	in-	79

in due measure	emmetr/o	386
incision	-otomy	61
	-tomy	8, 22
incomplete	atel/o	205
individual	idi/o	551
infection	seps/o	76
inferior	infra-	79
inflammation	-itis	8, 61
instrument to cut	-tome	8, 62
instrument to record	-graph	61, 531
instrument for visual examination	-scope	8, 62
internal organs	viscer/o	48
intestine, large	col/o	58, 106, 119
intestine, small	enter/o	6, 106, 119, 551
inward	eso-	22
ion	ion/o	497
iris	ir/o	384
	irid/o	384
iron	sider/o	287
irregular	poikil/o	285
irrigating	-clysis	118
ischium	ischi/o	329
jaw bone, lower	mandibul/o	328
	submaxill/o	328
jaw bone, upper	maxill/o	59, 328
jejunum	jejun/o	106, 120
joint	arthr/o	5, 58, 333
	articul/o	333
joint fluid	synovi/o	333
kidney	nephr/o	6, 137
	ren/o	21, 139
killing	-cidal	498, 572
kneecap	patell/o	329
knowledge	gnos/o	6, 76
labor	-partum	77
	-tocia	166
	-tocin	428
lack of	de-	234
lacrimal duct	lacrim/o	385
lacrimal sac	dacryocyst/o	385
lamina	lamin/o	327

large	macro-	80
large intestine	col/o	58, 106, 119
larynx	laryng/o	58, 255
lead, to	duct/o	76
leavening agent	zym/o	472
life	bi/o	5, 58
	vit/a	572
	vit/o	572
ligament	ligament/o	333
	syndesm/o	334
light	phot/o	386
	luc/o	530
like, to	phil/o	59
lip	cheil/o	105, 119
	labi/o	105, 120
little	-ole	62
	-ule	62
liver	hepat/o	21, 58, 106, 119
lobe	lob/o	257
location	top/o	76
loins	lumb/o	327
love	phil/o	59
luminous	fluor/o	531
lung	pneum/o	59, 64, 257
	pneumon/o	257
	pulmon/o	257
lymph	lymph/o	19, 21, 295
lymph gland	lymphaden/o	295
lymph vessels	lymphangi/o	295
male	andr/o	183, 427
many	poly-	66, 80
mass	onc/o	6, 496
mastoid process	mastoid/o	396
meal	-prandial	107
	cib/o	76
measure	-meter	77
medulla	medull/o	137
membranes	mening/o	205
	meningi/o	205
meninges	mening/o	205
	meningi/o	205
menses	men/o	166
menstruation	men/o	166

normal	norm/o	287
nose	nas/o	254, 319
	rhin/o	7, 254
not	a-, an-	8, 77
	in-	79
nourishment	-trophy	62, 77, 337
	-tropin	425
nucleus	kary/o	36, 47, 287, 471
	nucle/o	287, 471
numbness	narc/o	572
obstruction	-emphraxis	396
old age	presby/o	386
on	epi-	79
one	mon/o	286
one who	-er	63
	-or	62
one's own	idi/o	221, 551
opening	-tresia	118
opening, new	-ostomy	61
opposite	contra-	78
order	norm/o	76
	tax/o	206
out	ec-	79
	ecto-	79
	ex-	8, 79
outside	ec-	79
	ecto-	79
	exo-	8
ovary	oophor/o	163
	ovari/o	163
oviducts	salping/o	163, 395
oxygen	ox/o	76, 234, 257
pain	-algia	7, 60
	-odynia	61
pain, excessive sensitivity to	algesi/o	205, 572
painful	dys-	79
palate	palat/o	105
palsy	-plegia	207
pancreas	pancreat/o	106, 120, 427
paralysis	-plegia	207
paralysis, slight	-paresis	207
parathyroid glands	parathyroid/o	425
passage	-porosis	328

paste	ather/o	234
patella	patell/o	329
pelvic bone and cavity	pelv/o	47, 329
perineum	perine/o	166
peritoneum	peritone/o	21, 59, 106
pertaining to	-ac	7, 63
	-al	7, 63
	-ar	63
	-ary	63
	-ic	8, 63
	-ous	22, 63
	-tic	63
phalanges	phalang/o	329
pharynx	pharyng/o	105, 255
physician	iatr/o	551
place	top/o	76
place, to	the/o	76
pleura	pleur/o	257
pleural cavity	-thorax	258
plexus	plex/o	204
poison	tox/o	76, 497, 551
	toxic/o	425, 498, 551
	vir/o	497
polyp	polyp/o	452, 498
pons	pont/o	205
porridge	ather/o	234
position	top/o	76
potassium	kal/i	427
pour, to	-fusion	77
pregnancy	-cyesis	77, 166
	gravid/o	166
process	-ia	7
	-y	8, 62
producing	gen/o	6
	-genesis	60
prolapse	-ptosis	62
prostate gland	prostat/o	182
protection	immun/o	279, 287
	-phylaxis	551, 573
protein	albumin/o	140
	-globin	64, 287
	-globulin	287
	prote/o	472
pubis	pub/o	329
pulse	sphygm/o	234
puncture (surgical) to remove fluid	-centesis	60

pupil	cor/o	384
	core/o	384
	pupill/o	384
pus	py/o	141
put	the/o	76
pylorus	pylor/o	120
radioactivity	radi/o	530
radius	radi/o	329
rays	radi/o	7, 59, 329, 497, 530
record	-gram	7, 22, 61, 531
recording, process of	-graphy	61, 531
rectum	rect/o	59, 106, 120
red	eosin/o	285
	erythr/o	6, 285
redness	erythem/o	362
removal	-ectomy	7, 60
	-pheresis	288
renal pelvis	pyel/o	21, 139
resection	-ectomy	7
resembling	-oid	63, 452
retina	retin/o	384, 496
ribs	cost/o	76, 328
rosy	eosin/o	58, 285
round	spher/o	285
rule	norm/o	76, 287
run	-drome	77
rupture	-orrhexis	118
sac, small	alveol/o	257, 452
	follicul/o	452
sac of fluid	cyst/o	452
sacrum	sacr/o	47
safe	immun/o	279, 287
sagging	-ptosis	62
saliva	sial/o	105, 120
salivary glands	sialaden/o	105
same	is/o	285, 530
sameness	home/o	425
scale	squam/o	363
scanty	olig/o	141
scapula	scapul/o	328
sclera	scler/o	384

sea	thalass/o	289
sebum	seb/o	363
secrete	-crine	77
	crin/o	6
section	-tomy	8
seed	germ/o	496
	gon/o	58, 64
self	auto-	8, 78
	idi/o	221
seminal vessels	vesicul/o	182
sensation	esthesi/o	206, 572
separate	-crine	77
	-crit	22
	-lysis	22, 77
sex glands	gonad/o	427
shape	morph/o	59, 66, 76, 287
sharp	acu/o	58
sheath	thec/o	551
shield	thyr/o	76
shin bone	tibi/o	329
shoulder blade	scapul/o	328
side	later/o	21, 47
sieve	ethm/o	319
sigmoid colon	sigmoid/o	106
single	mon/o	286
sinus	sinus/o	257
skeletal muscle	rhabdomy/o	337, 452
skin	cutane/o	21, 362
	derm/o	6, 362, 551
	dermat/o	6, 362
skull	crani/o	47, 328
sleep	hypn/o	572
	somn/o	76
slow	brady-	78
small	micro-	80
	mi/o	386
	-ole	62
	-ule	62
small intestine	enter/o	6, 106, 119, 551
smell	-osmia	258
sodium	natr/o	427
soft	medull/o	452
softening	-malacia	61, 327
solid	stere/o	531
solid structure	ster/o	425

sound	ech/o	530
	-phonia	396
	son/o	76, 530
spark	scint/i	526, 531
specialist	-ist	8, 63
speech	phas/o	206
spermatozoa	sperm/o	182
	spermat/o	182
sphenoid bone	sphen/o	318
spinal column	rachi/o	327
spinal cord	myel/o	59, 205, 327
spine	spin/o	47
spiny	acanth/o	363
spitting	-ptysis	118, 258
spleen	splen/o	107, 120, 295
sprout	germ/o	496
stapes	staped/o	395
starch	amyl/o	103, 107
sternum	stern/o	328
sticking together	agglutin/o	287
stiff	ankyl/o	334
stomach	gastr/o	6, 105, 119
stone	lith/o	59, 67, 107, 120
stop	-stasis	20, 22, 62, 77, 118, 288
stopping	-static	572
straight	orth/o	258
strength	-sthenia	337
strength, lack of	-asthenia	206
stretching	-ectasia	118
	-ectasis	118
stricture	-stenosis	118
study of	-logy	8
	-ology	61
stupor	narc/o	572
sugar	gluc/o	107, 427
	glyc/o	76, 107, 119, 427
	rib/o	471
surgical repair	-plasty	62, 118
surrounding	peri-	9, 80
suture	-orrhaphy	118
swallow	phag/o	21, 59, 286
swallowing	-phagia	118
swayback	lord/o	327

sweat	diaphor/o	363
	hidr/o	363
synovia	synovi/o	333
tail	caud/o	46
tailbone	coccyg/o	47, 206
tear	dacry/o	385
	lacrim/o	319, 385
tear duct	lacrim/o	385
tear gland	dacryoaden/o	385
tear sac	dacryocyst/o	385
tendon	ten/o	333
	tend/o	333
	tendin/o	333
testis (testicle)	orch/o	182
	orchi/o	182
	orchid/o	182
	test/o	182, 427
thalamus	thalam/o	205
thick	pachy/o	362
thigh bone	femor/o	329
thirst	dips/o	140, 427
thorny	acanth/o	363
thread	mit/o	472, 498
threads of a clot	fibrin/o	286
three-dimensional	stere/o	531
throat	pharyng/o	105, 255
through	dia-	8, 78
	per-	23, 80
throw	bol/o	37, 46, 75, 471
thymus gland	thym/o	295, 427
thyroid gland	thyr/o	425
	thyroid/o	425
tibia	tibi/o	329
tie	nect/o	76
tightening	-stenosis	118
time	chron/o	58
tissue	hist/o	47, 572
	histi/o	363
toe	dactyl/o	58
toe bones	phalang/o	329
together	con-	78
	sym-	81
	syn-	81, 334

vein	phleb/o	233
	ven/o	22, 59, 77, 233, 551
vein, small	venul/o	234
ventricle	ventricul/o	205, 234
venule	venul/o	234
vertebrae	rachi/o	327
	spondyl/o	47, 326
	vertebr/o	48, 326
vessel	angi/o	21, 233
	vas/o	182, 233, 572
view, to	-opsy	8, 61
virus	vir/o	496
visceral muscle	leiomy/o	337, 452
vision	-opia	387
voice	-phonia	258
voice box	laryng/o	58, 255
vomiting	-emesis	118
vulva	episi/o	166
	vulv/o	166
wander	ion/o	530
washing	-clysis	118
water	aque/o	386
	hydr/o	58
wax (ear)	cerumin/o	395
wedge	sphen/o	318
white	alb/o	362
	leuk/o	6, 285, 362
white of eye	scler/o	385
windpipe	trache/o	59, 255
with	con-	78
	sym-	81
	syn-	81
within	en-	79
	endo-	8, 22, 79
	intra-	22, 80, 531, 551
without	a-, an-	8, 77
woman	gynec/o	6
work	erg/o	551, 572
wrist bones	carp/o	329
yellow	xanth/o	362
yellowish plaque	ather/o	234
x-rays	radi/o	7, 497, 530
	roentgen/o	530

INDEX

Page numbers in *italics* refer to illustrations.

Pre-Dead Nov⁸, 79